MANAGING WITHOUT BLOOD

THE MEDICAL, LEGAL AND ETHICAL CHALLENGES

Second Edition 2016

Richard Daniel

Barrister

Published by Daniel Medico-Legal

danielmedleg@aol.co.uk

www.danielmedicolegal.co.uk

British Library Cataloguing-in-Publication data

A catalogue record for this book is available from the British Library

ISBN: 978-0-9573803-0-2

First Published 2012

Second Edition 2016

DISCLAIMER

Whilst the author and publisher have taken all reasonable care and believe that the material set out in this book is accurate and reliable, the reader must take his or her own professional advice from a registered medical practitioner on any proposed medical treatment, advice on drug and other product usage, surgical techniques and clinical processes and decide whether or not to act upon it. No liability is accepted for any injury, loss or damage due to reliance upon the published material and/or implementation of any ideas or use of any product described herein.

Printed and bound in Great Britain by:

CPI London
38 Ballards Lane
Finchley Central
London
N3 2BJ

Contents

Dedication

This work is respectfully dedicated:

- to the many patients and parents who have taken a courageous stand for what they believe is right;
- to the clinicians who have been skilful and bold enough to push back the boundaries of conventional medical and surgical practice and to respect and follow their patients' choice of non-blood treatment; and
- to the lawyers who have staked their professional reputations and courted grave unpopularity in upholding the patient's legal right to do so.

Acknowledgments

A work like this does not just come together from a single author. It represents the culmination of some 30 years professional experience in medical law cases that has been a sharp learning curve to which a number of people have contributed.

I gratefully acknowledge firstly the input from medical professionals who have helped a layman to start to come to terms with some highly complex technical issues in blood transfusion and non-blood management. Notable amongst these were:

- the late Mr Raphael Marcus MD Ch M FRCS;
- the late Dr Jim Watt MD (Hons) Aberdeen, FRCPath, former Reader in Pathology at Liverpool University Medical School;
- the late Nigel Vukovich SRN RMN;
- Dr Mervyn Thomas MRCOG formerly of Guy's Hospital and later in practice in Nanaimo BC. Canada;
- Professor Michael Tynan MD FRCP formerly Joseph Levy Professor of Paediatric Cardiology at Guy's Hospital;
- Dr Rosemary Radley Smith MRCP FRCP formerly Consultant Paediatric Cardiologist at Harefield Hospital;
- Mr Michael Gough FRCS formerly Consultant Paediatric Urological Surgeon at Manchester Children's Hospital;
- Professor Len Doyal formerly Professor of Medical Ethics at St Bartholomew's and the Royal London Hospitals;
- Professor Vitaliy Slepushkin Consultant Anaesthetist at the Caucasus Medical Centre Beslan Hospital, Vladikavkaz, North Ossetia; and
- many others, including surgeons, anaesthetists, haematologists, ITU specialists and nurses, some recounted in Case Histories in this book, whose input into the miscellaneous treatments was magnificent.

A feature in each case was not merely their exceptional level of professional skill but their kindness and gentle consideration shown to the parents and child involved, often in very emotional circumstances of life and death.

Secondly an acknowledgement of the lawyers from whom I have learnt so much. Outstanding amongst these was the late Glen How QC, an exceptional lawyer and advocate at the Canadian Bar. He was deservedly the recipient of the Courageous Advocate of the Year Award from the American Bar Association, the only Canadian to be so honoured. After winning many cases in the Canadian Supreme Court that helped to lay the foundation for the Charter of Rights, Glen continued to fight for the right to choose non-blood management. This culminated in the decision in *Malette v Shulman* that has become the leading case on Advance Medical Directives in Common Law jurisdictions throughout the world, and *re LDK* that stands as a landmark decision for children. I was privileged to have had the benefit of his wisdom, experience and guidance.

I also take this opportunity to acknowledge the magnificent support of John Reeves F. Inst. L Ex., together with Robin Williams, and their respective valuable contributions to the preparation and conduct of many of the earlier English High Court cases recounted.

Another to whom I owe a great debt is my friend and colleague Tony Brace whose brilliant thesis for his Master's Degree in Medical Law deserves publication in its own right. His tact and diplomacy have curbed some of my wilder moments and I value his input.

There are many source materials cited—indeed one of the main purposes of the work has been precisely to bring together into one volume such widely scattered and diverse material. I readily acknowledge the collective professional experience and wisdom that they represent.

Finally, but by no means least, to my dear wife Jan who has loyally supported me through these past 30 years. In those early days before computers and electronically-stored precedents, Jan typed and re-typed pleadings, affidavits and skeleton arguments well into the night and, in many urgent cases, often through the weekend. She has helped with proof reading and formatting the multiple drafts of this book (always willingly) and without her huge and unstinting efforts this work would never have seen the light of day.

Others have kindly reviewed the manuscript and made welcome suggestions for improvements, but the ultimate responsibility for the work and any errors rests with me. Hopefully it will fill a niche in the better understanding between those who choose non-blood management and the clinicians, lawyers and judges who even now are still adjusting to that choice.

Richard Daniel
London
2016

Preface

More than 5 years have passed since the research and writing of this work was started and more than 3 years since it was first published. Much has happened, been judicially decided and been published in the medico-legal world during that time. The following is a brief summary of some of the additional material that has been incorporated into this second edition

Consent

Since the first edition, the major case of *Montgomery* on appeal from Scotland to the Supreme Court has changed the legal landscape almost beyond recognition.

The concept used to exist in the UK that, for members of the medical profession in general and the treating clinician in particular, the fact of informing the patient of the existence of a less invasive or non-invasive alternative was optional 'best practice' and in the discretion of that treating clinician. The decision in *Birch v UCH* in 2008 became, in law, part of main-stream practice along with the confirmed legal duty to advise on the non-blood alternatives and the risk/benefit.

But the law on Consent has further crystallised in *Montgomery* which is dealt with in some detail in the text, mainly in chapter 9 from §9.27 onwards. After a lengthy development of the law on the duty and extent of disclosure starting with *Sidaway,* 'medical paternalism' as a legal concept has finally been laid to rest by this judgment.

It has been replaced by the patient's legal right to bodily integrity, to choose treatment options and, for that choice to be properly informed, to be told in clear and understandable terms of the risks and benefits of alternatives, especially non-invasive or less invasive, before choosing which, if any, treatment option to accept.

Whilst fully accepted and acted upon by (*inter alia*) the better informed clinicians and clinical negligence/medical lawyers, there are demonstrably residual pockets of misunderstanding, downright ignorance and even resistance amongst many medical practitioners and some lawyers advising them.

The ever increasing practice of team working, involving often not merely specialists but sub-specialists, brings an increasing risk of the lines of responsibility for the obtaining of consent becoming blurred, whereas it always remains the ultimate responsibility of the treating clinician in charge. But Informed Consent is now the law in the UK.

Confidentiality

The Hippocratic principle remains unchanged but the extensive practice of 'information sharing' between professionals and often between different professions has resulted in the need for more formalised structures and guidelines. These were the subject of extensive review by the distinguished Professor Caldicott resulting in the publication of her further Report and the clarification of the Principles. These are addressed in this second edition at chapter 11.

The creation of the relationship of doctor and patient

The rapid advance of Bioethics, Genetic and DNA testing, has resulted in some interesting consequences. The case of *ABC v St George's Healthcare NHS Trust* held on the facts that there was no relationship in law of doctor and patient and the duty of confidentiality owed to the primary patient, the father, had to be respected.

The Court of Appeal has given leave and the case may well go to the Supreme Court and possibly even onwards to Strasbourg.

A change in the law may yet have to be addressed by Parliament especially with regard to the interests of unborn children to whom a known hereditary condition may be, or may have been, transmitted because of a simple failure to disclose highly relevant information.

Advance Directives/Decisions

The law relating to the right of competent adult patients to choose their treatment options and the lawfulness and applicability of Advance Directives/Decisions has come under close scrutiny both in the UK and in the comparable common law jurisdiction of the Namibia Supreme Court.

In the former, the starting point is the common law. Following the leading Canadian case of *Malette v Shulman*, in the case of *AK (Adult patient) (Medical Consent)* [2001] 1 FLR 129 Hughes J. (as he then was) reviewed the authorities and his succinct conclusions are set out.

The very tight statutory provisions under ss.24–6 of the Mental Capacity Act 2005 are considered. Notably the draftsman of the statute changed the wording from 'Advance ***Directives***' to 'Advance ***Decisions***'. There seems to have been a subtle shift in emphasis in the statute from the absolute right of the competent patient to *direct* that which he did and did not want by way of medical treatment once he had lapsed into lack of capacity. That appears to have changed to a mere expression of his *decision* that the court is empowered to review and, if it thought fit, to interfere. Whether that was a necessary or correct shift of emphasis is discussed.

Further under the statute the age at which a binding decision can be expressed in writing is stated to be 18 years whereas at common law the test of validity is competence and not age. Whether that statutory age is Convention compliant remains to be determined.

In Namibia, the decision in the case of *ES v AC* has overwhelmingly upheld the common law principles of *Malette v Shulman.* It is a decision that is likely to impact upon South Africa as one of the judges was seconded from their Constitutional Court and carries the authority of that position. This too is covered in more detail in this second edition in chapter 21.

The specific provisions of the Assisted Decision Making (Capacity) Act 2015 in Ireland that only passed into law on 30 December 2015 are discussed in greater detail in chapter 17. No commencement date has yet been set while the extensive drafting of the Regulations and Code of Practice is undertaken. The best guess is some time in 2017.

Pre-operative work up

At last some serious professional attention is being given to this and to treating anaemia pre-operatively thereby avoiding unnecessary transfusion. The arithmetic is simple. Accepting the recommended threshold for transfusion as Hb 7gd/l, (although there are compelling arguments for a lower threshold) the higher the level of Hb at the commencement of surgery, the greater the margin for blood loss and the avoidance of allogeneic blood. That is demonstrable fact. On 6 September 2015 the British Committee for Standards in Haematology (BCSH) published guidelines based on the combined research and experience of a team of highly qualified experts that was then peer-reviewed before publication. They not only rely on their extensive combined professional experience but cite over 70 medical articles by leading experts in their respective fields in support of the various conclusions that they reach and the recommendations that they make.

Better outcomes for patients, costs savings for the NHS and less reliance on the ever diminishing blood donor pool are all explicitly demonstrated. So hopefully pre-operative work-up and especially the crucial level of Hb will now receive greater attention than it has traditionally had in the past.

Obstetrics

There remain concerns in Obstetric practice about the implementation of choice of non-blood management by many mothers. Monitoring of Hb at an early stage of pregnancy; through to delivery; and then on to the post-natal stage is not consistent throughout the NHS and frequently opportunities are missed for good pre-delivery management to ensure the mother goes down to the delivery room with as high a margin of safety as is practicable. In many NHS units the take-up and training in the use of alternatives to allogeneic blood, for instance cell salvage, vary from excellent to patchy despite the accumulated evidence of the benefit to delivering mothers, of whatever religious persuasion or none. And too often there is a rush to transfuse neonates (especially premature) with insufficient consideration given to alternatives. These issues are discussed.

Mature Minors

There is growing concern about the state of the common law relating to mature minors and their right to choose treatment options which of necessity includes refusal of at least one option. The UK courts have acknowledged at common law a right to consent but not to refuse. The consequence has been highlighted by what many regard as the truly dreadful court decision in Sydney, Australia in 2013 to compel treatment on a mature minor (found by the court to be such and having capacity) just 3 months short of his 18th birthday upon which he attained his majority. That flawed decision was compounded by the use of 3 apparently medically untrained and unqualified hospital security guards to overpower the resisting patient by brute force to facilitate the sedation and thus compulsory transfusion to which he so profoundly objected. The ethical implications are discussed in chapter 11 in the hope of ensuring that such an incident is unlikely either to occur in an NHS hospital or be approved on an application to the courts in the UK.

Ethics

Several further issues have arisen since writing the first edition including the publication of further UK guidelines on physical restraint and on the proper approach to the consent of the under-age patient to his or her choice of non-blood management.

The judicial role

A review of the law reports shows that cases involving the decisions and treatment of patients, whether adults, mature minors, infants or expectant mothers, are coming before the courts with increasing frequency. The role of the judge is crucial and the authoritative writings of two eminent US judges are considered.

Relative costs of blood v non-blood

Ever increasing budgetary pressure on the NHS in the UK and elsewhere in the world, combined with the known risks of the contamination of blood by HIV and the vCJD prion (for which there is currently neither a satisfactory blood test nor the means of elimination even if identified), have resulted in closer examination of the relative costs of allogeneic blood against non-blood alternatives. The estimated cost of addressing the mere prion problem given in a Parliamentary Answer was a formidable £200 million.

The financial implications of harvesting, processing and distributing blood from providers whether paid or unpaid for their contributions, have escalated. The impact has been especially dramatic in the commercial world of blood in the US where diminishing demand has led not only to significant financial losses among blood harvesters, processors, brokers and sellers but also to the reduction of the workforce engaged in the activity. These issues are considered in a new chapter 12.

The imported plasma scandal

The importation of plasma harvested from paid providers, as well as the highly controversial sale to a US investment company of the major shareholding in the UK's principal plasma processing facility at Elstree, Herts are each discussed and the implications examined. There is an important and indeed forthright contribution from Lord Owen, who speaks with the wide ranging triple authority of a distinguished Member of the House of Lords; a qualified doctor and a former Minister of Health. Additionally, two articles are cited, one by Dr Lucy Reynolds of the prestigious London School of Hygiene and Tropical Medicine. The second is by a US journalist who, short of his rent money, succumbed to the blandishments of a commercial harvester of plasma. He relates his somewhat disconcerting experience of the health risk of twice-weekly harvesting against the world-wide standard (as set by WHO) of once every two weeks. It seems that the commercial imperative or pressure may be winning against patient safety.

AAGBI Consolidated Guidelines 2016

There has been an important development in the Guidelines issued by AAGBI, the professional association of anaesthetists for the UK and Ireland. As recently as July 2016 the new Guidelines entitled 'The use of blood components and their alternatives 2016' were published. Its 14 distinguished contributors bring together in one updated document previous guidelines of 2005, 2008 and 2010. These are discussed in an amended chapter 6.

'The Children Act' by Ian McEwan

The publication of the novel *The Children Act* by the well-respected author Ian McEwan cannot pass without mention. His is of course just a work of fiction, embellished by artistic/fictional licence and informed by a reading of an early draft of this book. He rightly acknowledges his story to be based on facts analogous to *re E* recounted in chapter 15.6 (chapter 12 of the first edition). The decision of Ward J. as he then was in that case has been the subject of much discussion and writing.

Finally, the author continues to have no conflicts of medical or financial interests to declare.

Richard Daniel
November 2016

Preface to First Edition

'In England we have come to rely on a comfortable time-lag of fifty years or a century intervening between the perception that something ought to be done and a serious attempt to do it.' — H.G. Wells

Sixty years ago the relationship between doctor and patient was largely one of benevolent paternalism. There was an aura, almost a mystique, surrounding the medical profession and patients were for the most part uninformed and compliant, content to say 'Yes, doctor—you know best. Do whatever you think.' Discussion of medical matters was primarily confined to the professional journals with occasional articles by medical correspondents in some of the heavier broadsheets. The very idea of suing a doctor was anathema save in the most egregious and blatant cases of negligence such as amputating the wrong limb, removing the sound instead of the diseased organ, or sewing up and leaving some swabs or metal clamps inside the patient. These indefensible cases were usually settled by the medical defence insurers discreetly with a denial of liability and a confidentiality clause as a condition of the payment so that even they rarely made the headlines. The courts broadly supported the medical profession in trying to curtail accountability for mistakes or even sub-optimal treatment.

> 'It is easy to be wise after the event and to condemn as negligence that which was only a misadventure. We ought always to be on our guard against it, especially in cases against hospitals and doctors. Medical science has conferred great benefits on mankind, but these benefits are attended by considerable risks. Every surgical operation is attended by risks. We cannot take the benefits without taking the risks. Every advance in technique is also attended by risks. Doctors, like the rest of us, have to learn by experience and experience often teaches in a hard way. Something goes wrong and shows up a weakness, and then it is put right…
>
> We should be doing a disservice to the community at large if we were to impose liability on hospitals and doctors for everything that happens to go wrong. Doctors would be led to think more of their own safety than of the good of the patients. Initiative would be stifled and confidence shaken. A proper sense of proportion requires us to have regard to the conditions in which hospitals and doctors have to work'. (*Roe v Minister of Health* [1954] 2 QB 66 at 83 *per* Denning LJ.)

The overwhelming culture in the National Health Service (NHS) when something did go wrong was for years 'Never apologise; never explain'. It took the Access to Health Records Act 1990 as subsumed in the Data Protection Act 1998 to give to the patient, or authorised relative, a legal right to access clinical notes outside the formalities of actual litigation. Even since then it has taken a marked shift in attitude to begin to change the culture that sadly still persists in some hospitals. Whilst loyalty to professional colleagues is an admirable quality, the indefensible is still defended with disconcerting frequency and 'written back' clinical notes still turn up too often for comfort.

Due largely to the extended coverage by the media, today's generation of patients are not merely better informed but are much more likely to want to be involved in their treatment plan and to know what is contemplated and why before giving consent. And the law on consent to treatment has been more explicitly developed and spelt out in a progression of cases through the courts.

Over that same period, one medical procedure, the transfusion of donor blood or blood products, has moved from being the perceived 'gold standard' of inexpensive and life-saving treatment to an expensive and comparatively scarce resource for which conservative strategies are now firmly recommended and the clinical risk/benefit of which is now being seriously questioned.

Many patients have read about the blood scandals that have rocked the medical world and are much more aware that there are risks attached, to the point that a sizable number will choose not to have blood simply on medical grounds and perceived risk. Indeed one eminent Professor of Surgery is on record as saying 'No doctor would have blood.'

Throughout that time one group of patients has stood firm and has not bent to the changing wind of medical and public opinion. With a belief firmly based in their understanding of Scripture but to a large extent now reinforced by conventional medical material, Jehovah's Witnesses have attracted serious unpopularity over their stand for non-blood management, especially when it comes to the emotive issue of children.

The author has some 30 years' experience of representing them when court proceedings have been instituted to overrule their choice of management options. In the course of many cases he has had to research and attempt to master not only the law but also the complex medical arguments for and against transfusion.

Much of this material is widely scattered in medical and legal literature; clinical notes and case law and many unreported children's case decisions buried in the archives of the Family Division of the High Court. In one of those quirks of the English system, there are no central records or database kept by hospitals, NHS Trust lawyers or the court; many of the judges previously involved have retired and are no longer on the Bench; and consequently a significant proportion of this material is not known to clinicians, lawyers or the present generation of judges. There is no formal follow up to those cases in which a permissive order has been made in the High Court, at great expense to public funds, but no blood has in fact ever been given. The author's personal records suggest a hit rate of blood actually transfused of a mere 36% overall, mainly in the blood disorders such as Haemophilia, Thalassaemia, Sickle Cell anaemia or Rhesus conflict and also anaemia of prematurity. However the rate is zero in surgical cases, including complex cardiac and neurosurgery, which seems a questionable use in litigation of scarce NHS funds that could more usefully have been applied to patient care.

The purpose of this book is to draw together that diversely scattered material into one reference source so that both the patients (or parents) directly affected and those who have to deal with these often difficult cases can make an informed judgment on the risk/benefit evaluation and whether or not the clinical facts and the relevant law properly support efforts to override the choice of non-blood treatment.

When no less an authority than the Royal College of Surgeons describes these beliefs as a 'deeply held core value', then there is a compelling argument that the medico-legal apparatus should be slow to interfere.

Additionally, but looming ever larger in an NHS desperate to cut costs, there is the issue of cost/benefit. The complexities of blood harvesting, processing and attempting to ensure a safe product involving now the known risks of the vCJD prion and other risks yet to be identified are inevitably increasing year on year. The costs rise inexorably in line with those complexities and a key factor in overall cost is unnecessarily prolonged hospital bed stay. In parallel with that rise there is, despite the recent relaxation of the ban on homosexual donors in certain circumstances, a constantly diminishing pool of eligible blood donors.

The prospects of some form of rationing or at the least prioritisation are now very real. And so the comparative costs of donor blood and blood products are being closely examined in comparison with the range of non-blood alternatives as reduction in hospital bed stay features ever more prominently, primarily in the interests of the patient but additionally in NHS Trust budgets.

These are important issues that the author addresses and with which the reader is encouraged to come to terms.

Table of Cases

Chapter One

Outline history of blood transfusion and the risk/benefit of donor blood

'…a Hospital…should do the sick no harm'
Florence Nightingale—*Notes on Hospitals*

1.1 The practice of blood transfusion did not get off to a very auspicious start. The first recorded case[1] was in 1492 involving Pope Innocent VIII who had sustained an apoplectic stroke. Three 10-year-old boys were ex-sanguinated and their blood transfused into the ailing 80-year-old Pope in a doomed and hopeless experiment to try and rejuvenate him. The idea that 3 non-consenting minors should give their lives for a geriatric with a hopeless prognosis is not one likely to commend itself to a modern Ethics Committee. Thereafter, there were some slightly more scientific experiments and in 1666 Richard Lower was the first to infuse animals with allogeneic blood. A year later half a pint of lamb's blood was administered by Jean Baptiste Denis into a 15-year-old boy who, remarkably, survived. Thereafter there were various experiments, usually with cadaverous blood, and in 1828 James Blundell progressed to transfusion from one live donor to the patient.

1.2 The concept was simplicity itself. P the patient needs blood; D the donor is able to provide it. So transfer blood from D to P. Unfortunately there was little or no scientific understanding of what was being done. Indeed Karl Landsteiner, the well-known Austrian scientist, only discovered blood grouping in 1900. Then with the advent of the 1914–18 War, grotesquely injured victims who had sustained major blood loss were given blood and the first Blood Bank was established in 1916. The world's first civilian blood transfusion service was established by the British Red Cross in 1926. However the practice and techniques of transfer developed faster than the scientific and clinical knowledge of the implications of what the practitioners were doing. There was then a lull through the 1930's until the outbreak of the Spanish Civil War, with the consequent civilian and combatant casualties, when the practice resumed.

1.3 It was not until 1940 that Landsteiner made the discovery of the Rhesus factor that now plays so crucial a part in blood grouping. So no one will ever know

[1] Diario Della Citta di Roma di Stefano Infessura 275,276 (O. Tommasini ed 1890)

how many patients, transfused before that finding, died not from their injuries and blood loss but from seriously incompatible blood.

1.4 During the 1939–45 war the practice and techniques were developed on a pragmatic basis but still without any proper clinical controlled evaluation of the benefits against the hazards and side effects. However, the process of consent lagged far behind. Those of us who did National Service in the armed forces, which continued right through the 1950's, recall only too well that the concept of consent to any medical treatment was a joke, let alone informed consent. The first weekend of our induction the entire platoon formed up, as ordered, in the Medical Room in a line, stark naked, and a Lance Corporal in the RAMC, (of dubious qualifications but bearing the intimidating stripe) administered a jab that was a multi-cocktail containing whatever the army thought was good for us. To this day we have no idea what was in it apart from anti-tetanus. In those days before disposables, we were lucky if we had a clean needle if not a sharp one. That was merely symptomatic of medical treatment in the services for us conscripts. Upon presenting oneself to a doctor whose word as a Commissioned Officer was final, he simply went ahead and did what he thought was the right thing. It was the ultimate benevolent paternalism to which a whole generation of national servicemen submitted without question.

1.5 It is scarcely surprising that this ethos was carried over into the early days of the National Health Service founded in 1948. Examination of the early records of the appointees shows that many of the consultants first appointed to the NHS had formerly held senior rank in the armed forces, often Lt. Colonel or equivalent. They had been accustomed to submissive and compliant service patients and expected the same of their civilians. Thus the usual response was: 'Yes, doctor, you know best—go ahead and do what you think!' Informed consent was a long way in the future and any who questioned the advice and proposed treatment were regarded as, at best, difficult. Blood transfusion was then such a standard practice that it was administered almost routinely to any patient whom the treating team thought, rightly or wrongly, might possibly benefit. Those who, whether for religious or other reasons, chose not to have donor blood were regarded as religious fanatics or mildly potty.

1.6 There was comparatively little regulation or control of donor blood until, after the Thalidomide disaster, the Sainsbury Committee[2] was established to consider the relationship between the NHS and the pharmaceutical industry. It reported that about two-thirds of all drugs on the market were therapeutically effective while the other third were described as 'undesirable'. It is the view of many that a proportion as high as one-third was and is truly unacceptable. Ensuing legislation, the Medicines Act 1968, created the Committee on Safety of Medicines. For the first time there were realistically imposed strict procedures from laboratory experiments, through controlled trials on animals; then progressively on human volunteers with extremely careful monitoring of adverse incidents. Only after such close scrutiny and scientific evaluation by independent experts was the tested product finally awarded a Product Licence that then enabled it to be marketed. The criteria were 'safety, efficiency and quality'.[3]

1.7 However, the immensely powerful pharmaceutical industry successfully lobbied for a Product Licence of Right intended to be given to those existing products that had stood the test of time and were, so far as could be established, risk-free or the side effects of which were well known. It was on the back of this that donor blood slipped through without the scientific testing put in place for new products and was given a Product Licence of Right. Under the Medicines Act it was awarded the automatic status of a medicine that could accordingly only be administered on the authority of a registered medical practitioner. That was the deemed safeguard. Hindsight is a wonderful attribute but, in the light of what was to come, a major opportunity for a full scientific evaluation of the risks and benefits of donor blood was thereby missed.

Hazards of Donor (Allogeneic) Blood—The risk/benefit equation

> 'What's out there, in terms of transfusion safety, undoubtedly includes a mixture of the known and the unknown, and there is always the danger of watching closely the unknown and failing to appreciate the changing threat of the already known'.
>
> Alan Kitchen PhD. Head, National Transfusion Microbiology Reference Laboratory, London.

1.8 The fundamental claim is made that blood donated within the UK is intrinsically safe because it depends entirely on voluntary rather than paid

---

[2] Lord Sainsbury—Report of Committee of Enquiry into the relationship of the Pharmaceutical Industry with the NHS (HMSO London Cmd 3410, 1967)

[3] Medicines Act 1968 s.19

donations. Volunteer donors are treated as altruistic and responsible people who can be trusted fully to disclose high risk factors when asked. It is a process known as voluntary de-selection or self-deferral.

1.9 Whilst the theory is fine, in practice there are self-evident flaws. Basically it depends on the assumption that the donor is either celibate or in a stable and exclusive sexual relationship with a similar partner and is not engaging in unprotected sexual activity with any other person, whether same or other sex. Further, that the donor is not, and has never been, a user of non-prescribed drugs especially by injection, nor the sexual partner of such a user. Finally, that the donor has never been the recipient of a transfusion of allogeneic blood or blood products. In our modern society this is a high standard to achieve and, some would argue, unrealistic.

1.10 Early warnings of the dangers of donor blood were given but largely ignored. As far back as 1956, Dr Zeitlin, the then Director of the South London Blood Transfusion Centre, gave a very clear warning. An editorial in the (then) *Manchester Guardian*[4] entitled 'Warning on over-free use of blood transfusions' stated:

> 'The transfusion of blood has now become so commonplace and simple that nowadays in some hospitals pints of blood are dispensed more liberally than beer. As a result, blood transfusion, which is by no means as straightforward as it might seem, is causing a substantial number of deaths among hospital patients in this country every year. A warning by an expert on the extent of the risks involved which is published in "The Medical World Today" should have a welcome effect on the ardour of the over enthusiastic transfusionist'.

The article quoted Dr Zeitlin as saying:

> 'The ease with which blood is obtained encourages what have been called "cosmetic transfusions" which are performed more for the benefit of the relatives and the peace of mind of the doctor than for the well-being of the patient. Every year about two hundred deaths result from transfusions in Britain...the drama and glamour of a transfusion will often influence the resident doctor to give an unnecessary transfusion in borderline cases of haemorrhage. If blood transfusions were as safe as is commonly supposed it would still be difficult to justify them in cases such as these'.

---

4 Manchester Guardian, April 25 1956

1.11 His warning was followed soon after by Dr J.H. Dible, Professor of Pathology, who wrote:[5]

> 'Medical progress is a study of trial and error, of false paths, of whole generations under the sway of wrong ideas leading to wrong treatment and God knows what in the way of casualties—and the old tale goes on. A friend of mine said to me the other day "In the 18th century hundreds of people lost their lives through blood being taken out of them needlessly; today people are being killed through blood being put into them needlessly." And I, who only that morning had seen the body of a young man, dead as the result of an incompatible blood transfusion given after an operation of convenience, could only sadly agree with him'.

1.12 By 1960 the issue of actions for professional negligence, and its concomitant response of the medical profession in 'Defensive Medicine', was discussed in a pithy article by a Canadian doctor entitled 'Why do people sue their doctors?' [6] He wrote:

> 'First and foremost is the very nature of medical practice itself. In a field of rapid discovery, the accepted treatment of today was risky yesterday and will be obsolete tomorrow. During the period of yesterday, the treatment was new and hazardous, perhaps experimental in the eyes of the court and few doctors would come to its defence. During the period of tomorrow it is obsolete, antiquated, proven to be wrong, condemned in the witness box and accepted as negligent by the court. It is only during the period of today that the treatment is right and proper and this period is made ever shorter by the rate of discovery'.

1.13 The references above to the peace of mind of the doctor and a placebo for anxious relatives are perhaps early examples of defensive medicine. The practice of medicine in the UK has for years been conducted very largely on the basis of standard practice. The *Bolam*[7] test for negligence was the yardstick by which the actions of any doctor were measured:

> 'The true test for establishing negligence in diagnosis or treatment is whether he had been proved to be guilty of such failures that no doctor of ordinary skill would be guilty if acting with ordinary care. A doctor is not negligent if he was acting in accordance with a practice accepted as proper by a responsible body of men skilled in that art, merely because there is a body which takes a contrary view'.

---

5 Article 'Chance, Design and Discovery in Medicine', Postgraduate Journal Vol 29 p. 59

6 (1960) 3 Canadian Bar Journal, 222

7 *Bolam v Friern Barnet Hospital Management Committee* [1957] 1 WLR 582

Although in a case in 1998[8] a gloss was put on this formulation if the court was not convinced that the body of opinion is reasonable or responsible, the underlying test remained much the same.

1.14 Hence for many years judicial approval was given to the standard practice. If a doctor, from consultant to junior house officer, adhered to the generally recognised standard practice he was likely to remain immune from criticism from his peers, his employers, coroners and High Court judges and to be unquestioningly supported by his Professional Indemnity Insurers in negligence actions. The defence 'We did what we could—we even gave blood transfusion' was accepted without any real question.

1.15 The so-called Rule of Ten referred to elsewhere, whereby the transfusion trigger or threshold was established in 1942 as a haemoglobin level of 10 grammes per decilitre (g/dl), never did have any real proven scientific basis. As one doctor, quoted in the authoritative *Krever Interim Report* (1995) into the Canadian blood fiasco, so graphically expressed it:

> 'For almost half a century, clinicians believed that a hemoglobin level of 10g/dl was necessary before subjecting a patient to anesthesia and surgery. The aetiology of this requirement is cloaked in tradition, shrouded in obscurity, and unsubstantiated by clinical or experimental evidence'.

It was accepted as the standard practice to transfuse at that figure, again as a form of defensive medicine. Hence grew the practice of transfusing by numbers rather than by clinical signs and indications.

1.16 This question of transfusion practice and the threshold was considered in an editorial in the professional journal of anaesthetists[9] and several significant extracts are set out:

> 'Do we always honestly ask ourselves whether a blood transfusion is absolutely necessary or do we sometimes use this precious fluid just for the pleasure of seeing a ruddy glow come to our patient's cheeks? If we are convinced that a transfusion is really required, do we see that every drop is given to the greatest advantage of the patient, with the least morbidity using the most modern techniques and are we sure that blood is the great panacea that some would have us believe?

---

8 *Bolitho v City of Hackney Health Authority* [1998] AC 232 at 243C

9 Anaesthesia 1975 Vol 30 pp. 149-151

> Man is fortunately endowed with at least 25% more haemoglobin than is actually necessary. It can be shown that the ideal balance between oxygen carrying capacity and lowered viscosity promoting flow through the capillaries is achieved at a haematocrit of 30% rather than the normal 40% (Gruber U.F. (1970) British Journal of Hospital Medicine, 4, 631) and much lower levels can be tolerated without cellular damage provided that adequate inhaled oxygen is administered. Such knowledge is certainly reassuring wherever blood replacement is necessary and blood is not immediately available, but it may be life-saving in extreme stagnant hypoxaemic shock for, in such a condition, the administration of viscous blood as the initial transfusion may well tip the patient over into a condition of irreversible disseminated intravascular coagulation (DIC)...The best policy is often to avoid whole blood transfusion—hypovolaemia being a far more potent killer than anemia'.

Further down the article goes on to state:

> 'It is worth remembering also that the haemoglobin of stored, citrated red cells is not fully available for the transfer of oxygen to the tissues for some 24 hours after transfusion (Valtis and Kennedy (1954) Lancet 1, 119); rapid blood transfusion must therefore be regarded primarily as a mere volume expander in the initial stages. There is therefore much to be said for using other plasma expanders for blood replacement during elective operations to replace brisk moderate loss and to reserve whole blood for more leisurely administration in the post-operative period should this be necessary...
>
> Blood should be warmed and handled with care and generally treated with the respect accorded to a rare red wine for, as with wine, abuse and excessive consumption can lead to tragedy'.

How many surgeons and/or anaesthetists and/or risk managers (for whom this entire article should have been required reading) have actually read and applied this wise advice?

1.17 Other infections

Hepatitis C became a very serious issue in Ireland in 1994 and this is discussed in further detail in chapter 17. It remains even today a problem in the UK. The reality is that there has been no automatic reporting mechanism from hospitals back to GP's when blood has been transfused. So those recipients, some of whom may have been uncomprehending children at the time, may well be unaware that they could be within the current group who carry the virus.

Over the years, the hazards of transmission of, for example, syphilis and cytomegalovirus were addressed and the tests for hepatitis, although far from certain, were much improved. But then came the HIV epidemic.

1.18 In 1988 it was recognised retrospectively that 1977 had been a crucial cut-off year. The criteria for de-selection of donors at risk were simply stated in the publicity material of the blood donor service and reported in an article by the then Health Correspondent in the Sunday Times of October 9 as follows:

> 'But the AIDS epidemic has led to several groups being barred from giving blood including:
>
> - any men who have had sex with another man on any occasion since 1977;
> - anybody who has injected drugs since that year;
> - anyone who has visited or lived in Africa (south of the Sahara) since 1977 and had sex with men or women living there; and
> - the sexual contacts of those in the above groups'.

1.19 This policy remained in force for nearly 23 years but the rule on self-deferral was modified following a review by the Advisory Committee on the Safety of Blood, Tissues and Organs (SABTO) in 2011. From November of that year new guidelines provided that homosexual men are eligible to give blood but only if they have not had sex with another man in the past year. Despite protests of discrimination, SABTO said that the precaution was still necessary because of the much higher prevalence of HIV and Hepatitis B in the homosexual population. A shorter deferral period was considered but ruled out because Hepatitis B has an average incubation period of 67 days, during which the virus remains undetectable. The new guidelines bring the criteria for homosexual men in line with other high risk groups including women who have slept with a man who has had sex with another man; people who have slept with prostitutes and those who have had sex with an intravenous drug user. The guidelines say that people can never give blood if they have had syphilis, human T-lymphotropic virus (HTLV) or Hepatitis B or C and a lifetime ban remains in place for both men and women who have ever been a commercial sex worker or injected non-prescription drugs.

1.20 The questions inevitably arise as to how realistic is the standard set and how reliable can this self-policing policy ever be? In the age in which we live, the single or unattached donor may have casual sexual relationships with many different partners. Even the most conscientious, wanting to keep scrupulously to the de-selection criteria, may simply not have the information that he no longer meets the criteria. How can he or she be expected to ask their casual sexual partner(s) whether they have ever lived south of the Sahara; or ever had sex with one of the high risk groups, or an earlier partner of such, or been a drug abuser? This is simply not going to happen in the real world. So, however well-intentioned the self-de-selection process and criteria may be, the harsh reality is that there is a substantial risk that many high-risk donors have donated and are still donating. This is not mere speculation and two examples from the US demonstrate the problem.

a) **The Texas donor**

In one of the many transatlantic enquiries into the contaminated blood scandals there, details emerged of a high-risk homosexual donor from Texas who was promiscuous to the point of being predatory. He was initially asymptomatic with HIV but made paid donations of blood on 48 occasions between 1982 and 1983, when he died of AIDS. He simply lied about being in a high-risk group. Plasma from his donated blood infected 65,000 doses of blood-clotting agents that were commercially distributed to 14 countries worldwide including Canada, France, Jordan and Israel. The chain went on so far that it will never be possible to establish just how many recipients were infected or where.

b) **The Arkansas Prison Blood Scandal**

From 1964 and for over 20 years a squalid little scheme was in train to make money out of blood harvested from prisoners at the Cummins Unit of the Arkansas Department of Correction in the US, where the local State law forbids paying prisoners for their labour. A corporation, Health Management Associates Inc., was set up with political connivance and protection specifically as a commercial way of channelling money at significant profit from plasma. Prisoners were paid $US7 per unit in scrip and HMA sold it on for $US50 per unit. Not surprisingly, a venture that had as its harvesting source captive donors in its most literal sense and a profit mark-up of $US43 per unit (86% of receipts) was well protected.

One report[10] describes it thus:

10 'Arkansas Prison Blood Scandal'—Guy Lancaster: *Encyclopedia of Arkansas History and Culture*

> 'The problems with the prison plasma program were legion. Prisoners were not adequately screened for disease and state investigators later confirmed allegations that some prisoners were not paid in cash but in drugs. Other misdeeds included an inmate clerk in the prison's plasma center selling the 'right to bleed' to fellow inmates who had been excluded because they likely were infected with hepatitis B (a possible indicator of HIV infection)'.

Corruption among the administrators of the prison blood program and poor supervision resulted in disease-tainted blood being knowingly shipped to blood brokers. HMA sold plasma to Canada's largest blood broker, that sold on the plasma to companies in Europe and Japan and to a Toronto based company that sold blood products needed by haemophiliacs throughout Canada.

When the scandal broke and the tainted blood that had gone to Canada came under the close scrutiny of the Krever Commission, they reported that amongst the many misdeeds revealed, the shipping papers accompanying the plasma by using the acronym 'ADC' had not revealed that the plasma centre from which the product emanated was located in a prison. Other investigations discovered instances in which the cover corporation HMA had violated its state contract in 40 areas, including poor health assessment and record keeping and the hiring of unlicensed, uncertified and unqualified staff.

1.21 The proponents of blood will point to the increasingly sophisticated testing and treatment of donated blood (especially leucodepletion) as an additional scientific safeguard designed precisely to catch and eliminate the infected donation before it enters the chain for distribution. But again, history demonstrates, and the current state of scientific knowledge and testing procedures suggests, that there can be no guarantee of safety.

Still the question remains—who is to take the final decision of whether to accept transfusion based on a realistic risk assessment?

1.22 There was a perceived smugness in the 'Little Englander' approach that we are an island protected from the unsafe practices and risks inherent in paid donors from abroad. It is as though the Atlantic Ocean and the English Channel afforded protection from these risks and that the scientific *Drakes* responsible for the distribution of blood in the UK had dealt comprehensively with the invasion Armada of contaminated blood. When the facts of what happened in the US and Canada, then in France, and later in Ireland are examined, they suggest a very different conclusion.

1.23 In the wake of the major contaminated blood scandals of the 1980's, America and Canada had been much more open in their Public Inquiries, notably the Krever Commission Inquiry[11] the published Report of which was professional, thorough and impartial. A great deal of information has been gathered and published. To any patients who have received blood these reports are likely to make troubling reading.

1.24 First came the warnings that went unheeded. As early as 1982, the possibility of HIV transmission through blood transfusion was being reported. In 1983, high-risk groups of paid donors were supposedly identified and de-selected from donating. By 1984, a formal study reported 28 cases of HIV where the sole identified risk factor was blood transfusion. Recognising the proven risks of contamination in blood from commercial donors in the US, the Council of Ministers of the Council of Europe recommended that such imports should be discontinued and any stocks held destroyed. Despite this authoritative warning, it went unheeded in the UK as well as Germany and France (in the EU) and Canada and Japan further afield. All these countries continued to rely substantially on what proved to be heavily contaminated supplies from paid donors in the US.

1.25 The highest risk group of recipients were self-evidently the unfortunate haemophiliacs. At the annual meeting of the World Haemophilia Federation in June 1983 a courageously outspoken Dutchman Cees Smit, Coordinator of the Netherland Haemophilia Society, tried in vain to convince the Federation to warn haemophiliacs of the impending danger. There seems to have been a general paralysis of those at the top who perhaps could not face up to the enormity of the crisis that was about to engulf them, especially as at that time there were very few alternatives to allogeneic blood products that they could offer to their patients.

1.26 That is the generous interpretation. However, the public inquiries that were later to follow turned up some unsavoury details about the commercial factors also involved. In Canada all blood was collected and distributed by the Canadian Red Cross. There came a time when there was incontrovertible evidence that large quantities of Factor VIII, the clotting factor so desperately needed by haemophiliacs, was contaminated with HIV. Techniques of heat-

---

11 The Commission of Inquiry on the Blood System in Canada—Mr Justice H Krever, 1993-97. Final Report 21 November 1997

treating were simultaneously being developed so that safer batches of concentrates were gradually becoming available. With a cynical disregard for the interests of patients and with a much greater regard for the Balance Sheet, a deliberate decision was taken, on purely commercial grounds, to distribute the potentially lethal stocks rather than stand the commercial loss of destroying them.

1.27 As new batches of treated concentrates became available, they were still only distributed to certain selected groups who were put on what later became tragically (and ironically) known among the haemophiliac community as ‘Schindler’s List’. In 1984 the Canadian Red Cross were on notice that a particular batch of concentrates contained pooled plasma from three donors provenly diagnosed HIV positive and yet made no attempts whatsoever to trace, recall and destroy this potentially lethal product.

1.28 Worse was to come. Untreated products that were rejected in one city were returned to the central Red Cross warehouse in Ottawa and then redistributed to another area in an attempt to use up stocks and avoid the commercial loss of destroying them. By their actions, those responsible purportedly saved $CAN2 million. But the consequence was that more than 1,200 patients were infected with HIV directly through these contaminated batches. When the truth finally came out, the Canadian government picked up a bill for more than $CAN1 *billion* in compensation. So much for cost effective management of contaminated supplies!

For those who want to understand in greater detail how such a situation could have arisen on a major public health issue that caused the death of an estimated 2,000 Canadians, the reader is encouraged to read the leading account[12] by André Picard. One review describes it as ‘a shocking, deeply moving, often frightening analysis of the greatest preventable medical scandal in our history.’

1.29 Although it was little satisfaction to those infected, the closing chapter of this sorry saga was that criminal charges were finally brought (successfully) against the Red Cross as a corporate body and against five doctors employed in senior positions of responsibility in various organisations alleging ‘criminal negligence and common nuisance by endangering the public’.

---

[12] *The Gift of death—confronting Canada’s tainted blood tragedy,* André Picard—ISBN 9780002554152

The unanswered question is: How many of these contaminated products were imported to the UK and how many patients now donating here, albeit unpaid and probably unaware, have in fact been exposed to them?

1.30 It is easy to forget that France is a mere 22 miles across the Channel. A combination of efficient ferry services (and later the Tunnel) with the EU/Schengen concept of freedom of movement means that there is currently for all practical purposes an unimpeded interchange of people, goods and services. A cash-strapped NHS, unable to meet waiting time targets set by the government, has even sent patients to France for earlier surgery. Thus, what goes on in France should be of considerable concern to those in the UK.

1.31 The experience was remarkably similar to that of Canada. France originally paid its donors and also imported supplies from Canada and the US. But the driving force in the scandal of contaminated blood that was to break was commercial greed. Dr Michel Garetta was former head of the French National Blood Transfusion Centre. With a conflict of interest that we in the UK would find quite astounding, he was also a major shareholder in one of the main commercial suppliers of concentrate and was later proved to have channelled more than €1 million to companies that he controlled. When the scandal finally broke and criminal charges followed, Dr Garetta was ultimately sentenced to 4 years imprisonment; fined the equivalent of €100,000 and ordered to pay compensation of €3 million to 70 victims. Two associates were sentenced to 4 years imprisonment (2 suspended) and 4 years suspended respectively.

1.32 One source of paid donors was French prisons. Most other countries, with the notable exception of the State of Arkansas as recounted, had long abandoned the harvesting of blood from the prison population because of the known high risk of hepatitis but France continued the practice until 1985. That proved to be a key year. By that time the French government was aware that blood supplies were probably contaminated with HIV and it was known that the US had developed a screening test. However for purely political and commercial reasons, the French authorities declined to authorise the use of the US test, so as to give a domestic French company time to develop their own. During the 6 months delay patients were infected.

1.33 Later that same year, the French government banned the use of untreated blood concentrates. However, for the same commercial reasons as had prevailed in Canada, a substantial quantity, 3.2 million units, was not destroyed or written off as a commercial loss. On the contrary, this material was illegally exported to at least 5 countries in the European Union, namely West Germany, Italy, Spain, Portugal and Greece. Additional recipients of this lethal batch outside the EU were Argentina, Egypt, Iraq, Libya, Saudi Arabia and Tunisia. Thus there is a strong case for enlarging the de-selection criteria for donors in the UK to include any from these named countries along with their sexual partners.

1.34 But, as in Canada, the story gets worse. The French government banned imports of concentrates from the US but that did not stop the importing. To fill the gap, there grew up what have become known in the industry as 'vampire shops', usually Third World countries where the hard-pressed poor can make some much needed money by selling their blood. The later Inquiry revealed that France was secretly importing blood from these frequently untested sources. Again, the motive was commercial. The failure to destroy contaminated stocks and the delay in implementing a domestic HIV testing procedure saved a comparatively modest €4 million. But the ultimate cost in lives and the huge compensation schemes that became necessary dwarf that sum.

The real risk is the widespread, apparently uncontrolled, and largely unrecorded, distribution of these contaminated products throughout many EU countries, some of which are highly likely to have filtered back to the UK. Indeed, the risk to haemophiliacs is demonstrated by the statistic that up to 1988 70% of Factor VIII was imported and sourced predominantly from paid providers.

1.35 To the objective bystander, it would have made a great deal of sense and logic to apply a simple formula:

- blood is known to become infected;
- the infection is known to be transmitted by blood transfusion;
- *ergo* no one who has ever received a blood transfusion should be permitted to be a blood donor.

Unfortunately the opposite was the case. There was an unscientific but emotional element in the appeal to donate along the lines: 'Someone saved your life by donating their blood so you can repay the debt and do the same for someone else.' It has taken the vCJD scare finally to make the UK government face up to the reality that no recipient of blood should thereafter be a donor and in late 2004 this belatedly became official policy.

1.36 But again the problem arises of how a prospective donor is to know that he has received blood and should accordingly de-select himself. For decades its use has been so routine that, although categorised by many professionals as equivalent to a tissue transplant, there has been limited record keeping or information passed on. For instance it was unusual for a hospital, when reporting to a GP in a discharge letter, to refer to the fact that a blood transfusion was given. Thus, the only record is likely to be in the hospital notes and nothing may appear on the GP's notes. The chances of a check, perhaps many years later when the hospital notes have long been archived, will be remote. Even allowing for the modern computerisation of the NHS it is far from certain.

1.37 The reference in an Australian article in 1957 to 'recent graduates' finds an echo in the foreword to an official *BMJ* publication[13] in 1990 entitled *ABC of Transfusion,* edited by Dr Marcela Contreras, the then Director of the North London Blood Transfusion centre. Her introduction included this frank but also somewhat disturbing comment:

> 'The essentials of blood transfusion are still not adequately covered in the curriculum of most medical schools. Not infrequently a houseman will be called on to administer a blood component without knowing how to do it'.

The patient not unreasonably is entitled to ask whether, if the junior doctor does not know **how** to do it, does he really appreciate **what** he is doing and the undoubted risks associated with it? The second edition of the publication in 1992 contained the same sentence so, despite the very frank admission of a major defect in the training of young doctors, nothing had changed.

Although much attention has been given over the past ten years to mandatory training in transfusion practice, it appears to have had only partial success. As the annual report of the committee for Serious Hazards of Transfusion (SHOT) 2011[14] states:

> 'To limit avoidable patient morbidity and mortality arising from blood transfusion, including in relation to inappropriate and unnecessary transfusions, it

13 ABC of Transfusion—*British Medical Journal* 1990

14 Serious Hazards of Transfusion—2011 Annual SHOT Report of Steering Group

> remains essential that knowledge of transfusion medicine must be part of the core curriculum for all clinicians, as was recommended for doctors in training last year'.

1.38 Since 1942 the so-called *Rule of Ten* had prevailed, largely to provide a legal comfort zone of defensive medicine for practitioners against complaints by professional peers, coroners or judges. The issue was revisited at a Consensus Conference of the Royal College of Physicians in Edinburgh in 1994 under the headline 'How did we get a "Magic Number" for pre-operative haematocrit/haemoglobin level?' A report in *The Lancet*[15] stated:

> 'Despite more than five decades of established practice, doctors still do not agree about precisely when and why they should transfuse red cells and how efficacy can be assessed...One message was clear, the traditional transfusion trigger—i.e. the critical haemoglobin value justifying transfusion intervention—needs to be considerably revised...And despite the diversity of views, there was little dissension from the idea that a therapy that costs so much...deserved to be put on an altogether more substantial scientific basis'.

It is this lack of any proper scientific basis or evaluation that causes such disquiet.

1.39 Whilst much of the emphasis has inevitably been placed on the HIV problems, these are far from being the only concerns. Studies[16] have shown that 'blood transfusion is associated with a 35% greater risk of bacterial infection and a 52% greater risk of pneumonia.' Also that blood transfusions[17] 'have a negative long-term impact...including increased risk of infections, complicated wound healing and acceleration of local growth and/or dissemination of tumours... and should be viewed as the transplantation of cellular and soluble elements and that they cause substantial alterations in the immune responsiveness of recipients'.

The true scale of those infectious agents that are transmissible by transfusion of allogeneic blood[18] is demonstrated by the following partial table grouped under

---

15 Napier, Towards more rational use of red cells, *The Lancet* May 21 1994 at p. 1280

16 Carson et al, Risk of bacterial infection associated with allogeneic blood transfusion among patients undergoing hip fracture repair, *Transfusion* 1999 Jul; 39(7): 694-70

17 Grzelak, Zaleska & Olszewski, Blood transfusions downregulate hematopoiesis and subsequently downregulate the immune response. *Transfusion* 1998 Nov-Dec; 38 (11-12) 1104-14

18 Kitchen AD, Barbara JA., Current information on the infectious risks of allogeneic blood transfusion. *Transfusion Alternatives Transfus Med* 2008; 10 (3): 102-111

4 main headings:

Viruses

Hepatitis virus with variants A, B, C, D (which requires co-infection with B) and E

Retroviruses Human immunodeficiency virus I and II (with other sub-types)
Human T-cell leukaemia virus I and II
Herpes (including virus 8)
Cytomegalovirus
Epstein-Barr virus
Parovirus (including B19)
GBV-C (previously designated Hepatitis G)
Transfusion Transmitted virus (TTV)
West Nile virus

Bacteria

Endogoneous

Treponema pallidum (syphilis)
Borrelia burgdorferi (Lyme disease)
Brucella melitensis (brucellosis)
Yersinia enterocolitica
Salmonella spp

Exogenous (environmental species and skin commensals)

Staphylococcal spp
Pseudonomas
Serratia spp
Rickettsia riketsii (Rocky Mountain spotted fever)
Coxiella burnettii (Q fever)

Protozoa

Plasmodium spp (malaria)
Trypanosoma cruzi (Chagas disease)
Toxoplasma gondii (toxoplasmosis)
Babesia microti/divergens (babesiosis)
Leishmania spp (leishmaniasis)

Prions

Variant Creutzfeldt-Jakob disease

1.40 Those concerned with ensuring safe blood will doubtless contend that the risks of many of these are so statistically remote as to be completely discounted. But the undeniable major risk currently being addressed is the vCJD prion. The formidable cost of £200 million **per annum** for research, to try and find both a fail-safe test to identify the prion in donated blood and then a mechanism or procedure to eliminate it, is a serious indicator of just how seriously the problem is being taken.

Serious Hazards of Transfusion

1.41 Due to an increasing awareness of problems relating to the transfusion of allogeneic blood, discussions began in 1994 about setting up a confidential reporting system. The very sensible response was to form a Steering Group (affiliated to the Royal College of Pathologists) which now includes members from 20 organisations including the Royal Colleges and others associated with and concerned with blood transfusion. As a result of this, SHOT began reporting in 1996.

The acronym SHOT tells its own story. It is, in effect, a belated attempt to put in place a proper scientifically based system of monitoring the adverse effects of donor blood and blood products. It produces an annual report which commands respect. It is well constructed and addresses the issues particularly under the headings 'Analysis; Commentary; Learning point and Recommendations'.

1.42 The 2011 report, published in July 2012, runs to some 183 pages, includes 101 references and, perhaps as an indication of the complexities of the medical world, a glossary of over 200 acronyms. It picks up and addresses a number of major concerns, some of which seem to have their origin in the quality and content of the training of young doctors. The Foreword at page 5 includes the following:

> 'About half the reported events are due to mistakes. Analysis of the 'near miss' data for the past two years indicates that for every 'wrong blood in tube' error that results in a wrong blood incident, there are about 100 'near miss' sample mistakes…
>
> The need for education and training about blood transfusion has been a recurring theme in SHOT reports and competency assessment was first recommended in the 2001-2 report. Although progress is being made with this, it is clear that it is still not sufficiently effective, and that it needs to be underpinned by better knowledge and understanding of transfusion serology in the laboratory and of transfusion medicine in the clinical area. Work is therefore in progress…to assess knowledge

> and to develop better competency assessments. To limit avoidable patient morbidity and mortality arising from blood transfusion, including in relation to inappropriate and unnecessary transfusions, it remains essential that knowledge of transfusion medicine must be part of the core curriculum for all clinicians, as was recommended for doctors in training last year. Knowledge of prescribing or authorising of blood components should also be recognised as a core clinical requirement'.

The report then goes on to identify a number of specific areas to which attention needs to be directed.

Lack of Reporting

1.43 At page 10, the report draws attention to the failure of a number of organisations to comply with reporting. This prompted new guidance from the GMC entitled 'Good Medical Practice 2012' which includes a specific section on a doctor's duty to report poor practice.

Consent

1.44 At page 13 the report deals with consent for transfusion and the recommendations published by SaBTO in October 2011. It also contains the statement:

> 'Valid consent should be obtained for blood transfusion and documented in the patient's case notes according to General Medical Council (GMC) standards. This does not require a signed form'.

Transfusion of blood is, by any definition, an invasive procedure for which in law the consent of the patient is required. The review determined that this needed to be put on a more formal basis but not to the point of making the signature of the patient a requirement.

There is also an interesting comment relating to undergraduate training on this specific issue of consent which the report recommends should be included in undergraduate curricula.

Key Messages

1.45 Page 21 of the report is significant where it reports the number of deaths in which transfusion or lack of it played a role and the instances of major morbidity albeit in the context of the total number of units issued.

What is troubling is the continued level of errors resulting in wrong transfusions, inappropriate, unnecessary and under/delayed transfusions, poor handling of components and the high proportion of 'near miss' reporting. Comparisons are drawn with similar problems with drug prescribing. The level of errors in prescription of medications has been reported by the General Medical Council[19] with the highest error rate in foundation year 1 (8.4%) and year 2 (10.3%). The report states:

> 'The authors note "that a 'safety culture' was conspicuous by its absence" in the reports and discussions... As a result of this research the authors identified a need to target undergraduate and foundation year education programs at the very least'.

Inappropriate, Unnecessary or Under/Delayed Transfusion (I&U)

1.46 Two definitions are given at chapter 9 of the report:

- 'Transfusions given on the basis of erroneous, spurious or incorrectly documented laboratory testing results for haemoglobin, platelets and coagulation tests.
- Transfusions given as a result of poor understanding and knowledge of transfusion medicine, such as the decision to transfuse either puts the patient at significant risk or was actually harmful'.

1.47 At page 71 the report identifies two case histories that highlight the problem. In Case 13, an 85-year-old woman with iron deficiency received an unnecessary blood transfusion. She was prescribed 3 units of red blood cells by her GP; however, she only received one of the units after the GP was contacted and the request challenged. Oral iron was started. The note concludes that this transfusion was particularly inappropriate since a patient of this age is at risk of transfusion associated circulatory overload. Oral or IV iron are preferred treatment.

In Case 14 a 27-year-old pregnant patient at 39 weeks gestation had an Hb of 8.1g/dl. A junior doctor agreed with a consultant haematologist that the patient should have a transfusion of 2 units of red cells but this was outside the obstetric guideline threshold of 7g/dl. The learning point notes that blood transfusion is not an appropriate treatment for iron deficiency.

[19] Dornan, T, Ashcroft D, Heathfield H. et al. An in depth investigation into causes of prescribing errors by foundation trainees in relation to their medical education

Near Misses

1.48 It has for many years been standard procedure in the aviation industry that flight crew and ground controllers are expected to report near misses for the obvious reason that there are lessons likely to be learned to avoid such events in the future. At page 165 in the context of medical treatment the report quotes The Medicines and Healthcare products Regulatory Agency (MHRA) definition of a Serious Adverse Event as:

> 'Any untoward occurrence associated with the collection, testing, processing, storage and distribution, of blood or blood components that might lead to death or life-threatening, disabling or incapacitating conditions for patients or which results in, or prolongs, hospitalisation or morbidity'.

The Report sets out the total of near miss events which are then analysed and the appropriate table sets out the categories. By far the greatest numbers are 'simple errors'. In descending order the next category is 'laboratory, procedural or testing errors'. The third highest incidence is the category 'laboratory, component selection errors'.

A 2014 Report

1.49 The Annual Report for 2014 shows continuing progress but there is clearly still a long way to go. Figure 2 in the Annual Report Summary sets out some illuminating figures on 15 different aspects. Principally there were 359 anti D immunoglobulin events; 343 acute transfusion reactions; 278 cases of incorrect component transfused; 188 handling and storage errors; 185 cases of avoidable, delayed or under transfusion and 151 cases of alloimmmunisation.

The 2015 'PREVENTT' Study

1.50 A more recent study was published online 4 June 2015 and was due to conclude in August 2016. The study protocol was published in September 2015; the authors include some distinguished practitioners in their respective fields and the paper cites 32 references.

The discussion in the published paper includes the following:

> 'The problem of anaemia in patients undergoing major surgery is being increasingly recognised.[20] No major clinical trial has been conducted to address

---

[20] Musallam et al. Preoperative anaemia and postoperative outcomes in non-cardiac surgery; a retrospective cohort study. *Lancet* 2011; 378; 1396-407

the correction of iron deficiency and anaemia by the use of parenteral iron in patients undergoing major surgery. The NHS Enhanced Recovery Partnership Program (ERP)[21] has highlighted the need to address anaemia in surgical patients as a correctable condition, but no specific recommendations or guidelines for the evaluation or treatment of anaemia in these patients have been proposed'.

1.51 The PREVENTT trial is designed 'as a randomised, double-blind, parallel group, placebo-controlled, multicentre study'. Its purpose is to investigate the efficacy and safety of IV iron compared to that of placebo in a patient population with anaemia undergoing major surgery.

There is an interesting comparison with the case history of Natalie M recounted in chapter 15 which goes back some 12 years. That case demonstrated quite clearly that preoperative haemoglobin could safely be raised at the rate of 1 gramme per week by the combined use of erythropoietin and *Venofer*®, albeit off-licence. Things have moved on and the current trial is based on *Ferinject*®,[22] a later generation successor to *Venofer*® but using ferric carboxymaltose (FCM).

1.52 The PREVENTT paper in the discussion continues at page 4:

> 'The paradigm of patient blood management is becoming increasingly accepted in order to reduce unnecessary blood transfusions and to improve outcomes after surgery. It is defined as the timely application of evidence-based medical and surgical concepts designed to maintain haemoglobin concentration, optimise haemostasis and minimise blood loss in an effort to improve patient outcome'.

Although as mentioned 12 years have elapsed since it was demonstrated in the case of Natalie M that this combination worked effectively, it seems that the requirements of product licensing and official authorisation are still demanding evidence-based trials of this kind. But it does represent a major step in the right direction.

Summary

1.53 Drawing all this together, on the one hand it is encouraging to see that such a multidisciplinary group of highly qualified professionals are getting to grips with this range of problems. On the other hand, it is disquieting to learn

---

[21] Department of Health (UK) Delivering enhanced recovery-helping patients to get better sooner after surgery: best practice guidance, 2010

[22] Vifor Pharma UK, Bagshot UK

about such continuing deficiencies in the undergraduate and foundation training of doctors.

However late, the extent of the problem on the wards has been acknowledged with every acute hospital now obliged to have a specially trained Transfusion Practitioner whose principal assignment is haemovigilance and blood conservation. The costs of such training and staffing levels are a significant additional charge on individual NHS Trusts and perhaps reflect the gravity of the risk.

Chapter Two

The Development of Bloodless Surgery in the UK

2.1 Dr Jim Watt qualified as a doctor in time to volunteer and serve for 3 years as a Surgeon Lieutenant in the Fleet Air Arm during the Second World War in which he saw some serious action. A quiet and modest man, he was like many who had seen at the sharp end the true horrors of death and mutilation, reluctant to talk about his war experiences but they had undoubtedly left a deep mark. Although raised a Scottish Catholic, his strong Christian faith and abhorrence of the violence that he had seen at first hand, much of it religiously motivated, led him to seek out a religion that was committed to non-violence. He abandoned his previous church, studied the Bible with Jehovah's Witnesses and was baptised into that faith.

2.2 Recognising the force of the Scriptural precept to 'keep abstaining from blood',[23] he realised that he could not in all conscience practice clinical medicine in the NHS where the transfusion of blood was at that time still regarded as the standard practice which his contractual terms of service would require him to follow, as would his professional indemnity insurers. He devoted himself to pathology and teaching, and became a well-respected Reader in Pathology at Liverpool University.

2.3 As one of the few (if not the only) Registered Medical Practitioners among the small community of Jehovah's Witnesses in the UK in those early years of the NHS, Jim Watt was often asked for assistance by fellow members of his faith who were seeking treatment and surgery without the use of blood. He struck up a close professional relationship and personal friendship with Mr Raphael Marcus a remarkable surgeon whose life story featured in an impressive obituary[24] in both the *BMJ* and in the *Journal of the Burma Star Association*. The only child of Eastern European immigrants, Mr Marcus grew up in Liverpool and retained an abiding affection for his roots in that city. He had just gained his primary FRCS at the outbreak of war and immediately volunteered for service in the Royal Army Medical Corps. He served with

---

23 Acts Chapter 15: 28, 29

24 Raphael Marcus FRCS Obituary *BMJ* 2002; 324: 1587 (29 June) 2000

distinction in Burma where, cut off with the long range Chindits in the notorious Imphal Box, he and a colleague, Eric Parry, 'provided a surgical emergency service in the jungle where, under extreme battle conditions, they developed the art of triage, resuscitation and fluid balance. This was at a time before antibiotics and when anaesthesia was only rudimentary'. Triage is described as a system whereby a group of casualties is sorted according to their injuries so that treatment priorities can be allocated between them. In emergency situations with multiple casualties it is designed to maximise the number of survivors and is a crucial skill in Accident and Emergency departments. As an example of the extreme battle conditions they often used a highly polished jerry can to provide extra reflected lighting for surgical operations.

2.4 In his experiences in battle conditions in Burma and having to try and save lives and improvise with only the most rudimentary facilities, Raphael Marcus was following in a long and honourable tradition. History relates how the outstanding French surgeon Ambroise Paré as far back as 1537 was acting as a medical officer with the French army at the siege of Turin.[25] His primary task was treating gunshot wounds which at that time involved amputating limbs and then cauterizing the stumps with heated oil. According to the accepted practice of the time cauterization was necessary because of the toxic effects of gunpowder. As any battlefield surgeon knows, re-supply is often interrupted and in Paré's case he simply ran out of oil. In desperation he had to make do with what was available and so he treated patients with a home brewed mixture of egg yolk, oil of roses and turpentine. He had little hope of these patients surviving overnight but in the morning he found that those treated with his mixture had rested and healed well but those whose wounds had been cauterized in accordance with the accepted practice had swollen and painful wounds. Upon such circumstances do medical advances often turn!

2.5 When Raphael Marcus was demobilised in 1945 (in the rank of Lt. Colonel, which itself speaks volumes for the man) he returned to complete his studies at Liverpool University, finally qualifying MD. Ch M. FRCS, and there met up with Jim Watt. They collaborated in original research, not only in diverticular disease but also for inflammatory bowel disease. Their model is still being used worldwide for research into ulcerative colitis.

---

[25] Nuland SB—*Doctors: the biography of medicine*. New York 1988 Knopf pp. 97-100

2.6 In 1953 Mr Marcus was appointed Consultant General Surgeon at the Clatterbridge Hospital, Bebington, Merseyside, where his reputation soon became legendary both throughout Merseyside and North Wales. He was of the Jewish faith and recognised the strength of the Scriptural arguments against the use of blood but more especially the undoubted right of the competent patient to choose non-blood management. At that time, conventional surgeons and anaesthetists would have regarded the avoidance of blood as such an extreme departure from standard practice as to be on the verge of professional misconduct. It might also have brought him into potential conflict with the defence organisations that provided professional indemnity insurance cover, a legal requirement for practice in the NHS. The *Bolam* test of standard practice approved by a body of professional men was very much to the forefront of medico-legal considerations of professional standards and it was most unlikely that, back in the 1960's, he could have found a responsible body of professional men willing to support him. But very quietly and discreetly Mr Marcus, relying in part on his skills and experience of surgery in most basic conditions in the Burma jungle and also on the skills of his anaesthetic colleagues, pioneered techniques of non-blood surgery that were way ahead of their time. Thus his Obituary was headed:

> 'One of the few surgeons in the world prepared to operate on patients who refused blood transfusions'.

2.7 An outstanding example of their joint work was the bloodless surgery performed as early as December 1964 on a 10-year-old girl with renal carcinoma, normally regarded as highly malignant. The successful outcome in that case led them to publish a joint article entitled 'Renal Carcinoma in Children' which appeared in the British Journal of Surgery.[26] What is not mentioned in that article is that the patient was a member of a family of Jehovah's Witnesses and being brought up in that faith.[27] Mr Marcus carried out the surgery as the only surgeon known in the UK at that time willing to undertake such procedures without the routine use of blood and, with the usual full co-operation of his anaesthetist colleague, he completed the procedure without recourse to blood transfusion. Unusually for a teacher and non-practitioner Jim Watt was present in theatre throughout the procedure. There

---

[26] *British Journal of Surgery* 1966 Vol 53, No 4, April pp. 352-353
[27] Personal communication to the author

was no question of having to inform the child care authorities of the time, let alone seeking a court order, and the surgery was carried out solely on the consent of the parents. The child made a full and uneventful recovery.

2.8 It is perhaps an interesting reflection on the mutual trust and professional respect that existed between Jim and Raphael that when Jim himself needed major surgery it was to Raphael that he turned. Jim went down to theatre for a major procedure with a pre-operative Hb of a mere 6.5g/dl, which would raise eyebrows even today amongst some surgeons and anaesthetists experienced in non-blood management, but this procedure was carried out without blood and Jim made a full and uneventful recovery.

2.9 Whilst Raphael Marcus and Jim Watt were advancing bloodless surgery, Nigel Vukovich was quietly helping many patients to avoid or to prepare for surgery by enhancing their level of Hb with natural iron and vitamins, a simple forerunner of what has now come to be known and encouraged as pre-operative work up. His work was largely unreported but several thousand patients have good reason to be grateful for his care. He was one of the most skilful practitioners in finding the right mix of sound nutrition with mineral and vitamin supplements.

Nigel Vukovich came to the UK from wartime occupied Yugoslavia and from a background that accounted in part for his unbounded enthusiasm for the topic. Having trained as a surgeon, he was serving as a medic with the partisans in the mountains fighting the Nazi occupation when the Gestapo caught him. Before he escaped (itself a remarkable event) he was subjected to unspeakable brutalities and faced near fatal starvation. It was that first-hand experience that strengthened his belief in the body's natural needs for good nutrition and also its capacity to survive, to fight off infection and to recover even from serious illness. Like Dr Jim Watt, after the war he too sought a non-violent faith based on the Bible and became one of Jehovah's Witnesses.

2.10 On arrival in the UK, family commitments prevented him from fulfilling his ambition of going back to medical school to obtain the necessary UK qualifications that would enable him to practise as a doctor. Instead he qualified as both State Registered Nurse and Registered Mental Nurse and later within the NHS manned a specialist wound healing clinic where he achieved results that amazed even vastly experienced conventional practitioners. Although an exceptionally modest man, to friends he would occasionally open up and share some of his experiences. He was particularly pleased with his achievement in helping an elderly female patient with chronic diabetic leg ulcers. The treating team had tried everything available to them in the way of conventional pharmaceutical treatments but they were driven back to advising the patient that the ulcers were incurable and progressive and that there really was no alternative to amputation. In despair, the patient asked if there was not anything else to be tried and received the response: 'Well as a last resort you could try Nigel Vukovich but don't be too optimistic.' Nigel treated her without any pharmaceutical products and had the ulcers completely cleared up in a matter of weeks.[28]

2.11 Later he set up his own Clinic in private practice, first in North London and later in St Albans, and literally thousands of grateful patients came to him from all over the UK and even further afield. He continued devoting himself energetically to those patients until his death in his mid-eighties. Throughout those many years he was an ardent supporter of non-blood management and indeed, by good nutrition and sensible supplements with iron and other vitamins, helped many patients to achieve haemoglobin levels that avoided the need for blood transfusion.

2.12 Nigel Vukovich was especially passionate about the health of expectant mothers and their special needs for optimum nourishment of both the mother and the foetus. Indeed it was his nutritional regimen that helped the mother in Estonia (recounted elsewhere in this work) who had major Rhesus complications to pull through a difficult pregnancy, carry her baby to near term, and avoid the transfusion of the neonate. He promised 'This baby will have beautiful skin' and so it turned out, as remarked spontaneously by several observers and even recorded in the medical notes. This book has its genesis in a proposal he made late in life that we might collaborate in writing a work on this very topic. He would write the medical side and the author would deal with the law. Sadly his health deteriorated with his final years and we were never able to achieve that joint goal. But unreserved admiration is expressed for an exceptional man to whom many owe an enormous debt.

2.13 Whilst this quiet progress was being made with non-blood clinical management techniques, the on-going hostile attitude of some practitioners towards patients choosing not to have blood transfusion was demonstrated in

[28] Personal communication to the author

the early 1980's at a Seminar held by the Society of Anaesthetists at the prestigious National Heart Hospital in London at which the author was present. Dr Watt was one of the invited speakers but was preceded by a senior official of a well-respected national medical organisation. Although the Seminar was not conducted under 'Chatham House' rules, the author feels that more than 30 years later it is inappropriate to identify either the speaker or the organisation. However, it is what was said that demonstrates the deeply ingrained opposition to bloodless clinical management.

> 'We all know of Jehovah's Witnesses who had signed consent forms excluding blood who were given blood during surgery and then left theatre with a "clean" giving set'.

That was a frankly astonishing admission in an open forum, as it involved not only an actionable, indeed a criminal[29] assault upon the patient but the connivance (some might use the heavier word conspiracy) both to perform the unlawful act and then to cover up the evidence for the sole purpose of concealing from the patient and relatives what had been done. The cover up included the falsification (by omission) of at least fluid charts; forgery of laboratory blood records; and even clinical notes and operation reports. If there had been any adverse consequences of the transfusion, the patient would have been left totally without remedy, and likely without proper diagnosis and treatment, because all trace of the illegal act had been destroyed. A modern Fitness to Practise enquiry today might even have involved the police to investigate potentially criminal conduct and yet that was a senior official in a position of considerable responsibility openly condoning the practice of defying the expressed instructions of the patient and concealing the fact from them.

2.14 Whilst within the UK Raphael Marcus, Jim Watt and Nigel Vukovich, were quietly and unostentatiously pushing back the boundaries of surgery without blood, more open progress was being made in the US and Canada. Those seeking non-blood management in Canada had the undoubted benefit of help from Dr Mervyn Thomas, an Englishman who had trained at Guy's Hospital and then undergone post-graduate training to take his MRCOG (Membership of the Royal College of Obstetricians and Gynaecologists). He emigrated to British Columbia where for decades he provided medical advice

---

[29] See the *dictum* of Lord Donaldson in *re T (Adult: Refusal of Treatment)* [1992] 3 WLR 782 at 787C

and support, working closely with Glen How QC. The growth in non-blood management in Canada and the US was in part due to the much larger numbers of those choosing bloodless treatment in those countries, but perhaps more significantly it was attributable to the wider consumer choice that goes with private health care insurance. Private hospitals are in open competition with one another for the patient's 'business' and so are far more amenable to listening and agreeing to the terms upon which the patient is prepared to entrust himself to their care and pay their bill. And so when patients started asking for non-blood management, the hospitals put themselves out to accommodate them. It was a classic case of trying new techniques and products or expanding the use of existing products off licence, thereby pushing back the boundaries of knowledge and experience of how to manage these cases. The prestigious Englewood Hospital in New Jersey, US is a prime example of the development of non-blood management.

2.15 For the surgeons, it was really back to basics. Firstly, the golden rule with haemorrhage is to identify as rapidly as possible the source of bleeding and put a stop to it to prevent any further blood loss. There is no point in trying to fill the bath with the plug out. In parallel with stemming the bleeding, urgent attention needed to be given to replacing the lost circulating volume. As more than 50% of blood is water, simple and (incidentally) cheap volume expanders such as saline were found to work effectively. Once the bleeding was stopped; the volume replaced and the patient haemodynamically stable, then the patient needed careful monitoring and oxygenation to ensure tissue perfusion but primarily time for the Hb to recover and be brought back up naturally to the pre-blood loss level.

2.16 The second consideration was, in an elective procedure, to try and pre-empt the need for transfusion at all. Sensible planning and pre-operative work-up can often ensure that the patient goes down to theatre with as high a level of Hb as it is practicable to obtain and may obviate the need for replacement. Common sense dictates that if the level at commencement of surgery is only, say, 10 g/dl then the safety margin for acceptable blood loss may be only 3 or 4 g/dl. If however, the pre-operative level is 13 g/dl or higher the margin of safety is inevitably much wider, especially in the case of an unexpected bleed and no blood may need to be given.

2.17 But bloodless surgery primarily involves meticulous surgical technique combined with taking a little extra time and care to avoid any bleed not wholly intrinsic to the particular procedure. Many bloodless surgery patients are taken down to Theatre last in an operating list precisely so that the surgeon can properly take his time without the pressure of other patients backed up waiting. Many senior surgeons and anaesthetists rose to the challenge as did the pharmaceutical industry and the suppliers of surgical equipment and appliances. The range of non-blood volume expanders increased to include, amongst other products, a choice of colloids or crystalloids, each having their own advantages and disadvantages. As experience grew, so the range of procedures widened. It is now common for what were once widely regarded as high blood loss procedures to be performed routinely without blood. For example a top surgeon at the Royal National Orthopaedic Hospital at Stanmore, a tertiary Centre of Excellence, performs many hip replacement procedures, conventionally regarded as high bleed risk, with blood loss as little as half a teacup. At the prestigious St Thomas's Hospital, a top surgeon regularly performs major knee surgery with minimal blood loss. In gynaecology, another eminent London surgeon performs total hysterectomy, sometimes complicated by massive fibroids, with blood loss as little as 30mls.

2.18 A third consideration was the growing awareness of the considerable risks of donor blood and the increasing number of articles in respected professional journals warning of these. A selection of these dangers is discussed earlier but they by no means represent the full out-put of warnings against the over-free use of blood.

2.19 The approval of peers and professional colleagues is a major factor for those prepared to stake their professional reputations on new techniques and practices at the outer edge of current knowledge or practice. One trail-blazer in the US was a senior and respected heart surgeon, Dr Denton Cooley of the Texas Heart Institute. He pioneered techniques of heart surgery without blood and published a report of his work. By 1977 he reported on his 20 years' experience totalling 542 operations on patients without blood transfusion.[30] His figures for mortality and morbidity were in many cases better than comparable procedures where donor blood was given.

---

[30] Cardiovascular Surgery in Jehovah's Witnesses, Denton Cooley—Report of 542 operations without blood transfusion *JAMA* Sept 19, 1977—Vol 238 No. 12 pp. 1256-1258

2.20 The 'Holy Grail' for the pharmaceutical industry is undoubtedly artificial blood—a clinically viable oxygen carrier/haemostatic agent capable of performing the complex functions of allogeneic blood; with adequate half-life *in vivo* and without significant adverse consequences for the recipient. It will be easily stored and transported in conditions that are not so temperature sensitive; will not have the limited shelf life of donor blood products; will be carried for immediate use by military medical teams, paramedics and those first to the scene of an incident or accident and administered without the need for cross-matching in the laboratory. Because there will be no risk of incompatible or contaminated blood; transmission of viral and other infections and the other known complications of allogeneic blood including suppression of the immune system, hospital bed stay will be reduced. But above all else it will eliminate the biggest single source of concern, clearly identified by the Steering Group for SHOT, which is human error in giving the wrong blood to the wrong patient.

2.21 The first pharmaceutical company to achieve this will undoubtedly make a fortune, which is why the Research & Development budgets are so huge, but there is much research ahead. The first generation product *Fluosol*® was found to have the oxygen carrying capacity but its half-life was something of the order of 2 hours so that multiple infusions would be necessary, thereby risking fluid overload. The remarkable Russian experience with the artificial oxygen carrier *Perftoran*® as a second generation perfluorocarbon substance is discussed in chapter 19 but however useful, especially when other treatments are not available, it remains essentially an oxygen carrier only. Similarly, the US experience with haemoglobin based oxygen carrier HBOC-201 is discussed in chapter 20. However, the crucial clotting mechanism and immune response systems of the blood are so complex that replicating them in a recombinant substance is a scientific challenge of the highest order.

2.22 Until a reliable product is developed that will perform all the crucial functions of blood, those managing their patients without blood are not without alternatives. As chapter 4 indicates, there is already a formidable selection available in surgical and anaesthetic techniques and multiple products available in place of donor blood for a significant range of conditions. But first it may be helpful to take a layman's look at the constituents, nature and function of blood.

Chapter Three

A Layman's Guide to Blood

3.1 There are inevitably many textbooks on blood. They range from erudite textbooks, written primarily for consultant haematologists, directors and senior staff of blood transfusion services and others directly involved in clinical practice at an advanced level, to textbooks for medical students and nurses and then for the reasonably intelligent layman.

3.2 This chapter is intended as a fairly basic layman's introduction to blood, its complex nature, components and functions. This book is directed primarily to helping laymen to understand not merely ***that*** non-blood management works but ***how*** it works. It is accordingly important to grasp the basic physiology of blood in certain key areas. These include:

- the importance of the oxygen transport function;
- the four principal formed elements: red cells, white cells, platelets and plasma;
- how red cells are produced (haemopoiesis), their useful life and elimination from the system;
- the need for a sustained level of haemoglobin, in the UK conventionally written Hb and expressed as grammes per decilitre, shortened to g/dl;
- the crucial role of iron;
- the value of nitric oxide;
- the release of oxygen by 2,3-DPG;
- the ratio of formed elements to plasma: the Haematocrit;
- the osmotic balance;
- the balance of alkaline/acidity expressed as pH
- the clotting mechanism including the cascade of Factors leading to formation of a clot and the arrest of bleeding by establishing haemostasis;
- the role of plasminogen and plasmin in dissolution of blood clots; and
- the immune system including defence against invading bodies and infection.

Each of these is considered in turn, although it is the effective combination of all these functions that really matters.

Of the total volume of blood, the formed elements comprise 45% and the plasma 55%. The plasma itself is made up of 91.5% water, so one of the main issues in considering the principles of replacement of blood loss is that more than half of the total content of blood (.536) is water. The capacity of the healthy body to adapt to blood loss is most easily demonstrated by the blood donor. After giving a unit of blood the donor conventionally receives a cup of tea and a biscuit and, after a short rest, goes on his way. This is perhaps the simplest demonstration of the principle of fluid and volume replacement of blood loss.

The importance of the oxygen transport function

3.3 Blood is primarily a transport medium that circulates through the arteries, capillaries and veins, exchanging fluid and gases with the bodily tissues, carrying nutrients in and waste products out. The main nutrient is oxygen, absorbed through the lungs and transported by the red corpuscles to the heart to pump it around: to the brain to control the major bodily functions and to all the bodily tissues to nourish them. Each haemoglobin molecule contains 4 atoms of iron. As each atom can carry one molecule of oxygen, it follows that one haemoglobin molecule can carry up to 4 molecules of oxygen. This is important when it comes to measuring oxygen saturation – when all available binding sites for oxygen are filled and also when only partial saturation is possible.

The major waste product, after giving up the carried oxygen, is carbon dioxide carried back through the venous system to the lungs, where it is exhaled and the whole cycle is endlessly repeated. Other wastes and excesses of cellular activity, including uric acid, are carried to the kidneys, spleen, liver, etc. for selective elimination through the urine and faeces.

Additionally the blood carries:

- hormones secreted by endocrine glands to their target glands and tissues;
- heat generated in more active tissues to other less active tissues;
- antibodies to areas of infection; and
- clotting factors that help blood to coagulate and thereby to minimise its loss from ruptured vessels.

The four principal elements: Red cells, White cells, Platelets and Plasma

3.4 The **Formed Elements** (also called corpuscles) fall into 4 main parts.

a) **Red Cells** or erythrocytes (from Greek ὲρυθμοσ = red and χυτοσ = cell) perform the crucial role as carriers of oxygen. Each is a disk with an average diameter of 7.2 micrometres hollowed out on either surface. It is small enough and sufficiently flexible to pass through the smallest tissue. There are 5 million erythrocytes to a cubic millimetre. Each erythrocyte contains 600 million haemoglobin molecules. So there are 3,000 million molecules of haemoglobin (Hb) per cubic mm.

b) **White Cells** or leucocytes provide defence against any virus, bacteria or other foreign protein substance. There are two basic types—neutrophils and monocytes—that operate by devouring any micro-organisms or foreign protein. Most of us are familiar with pus around an infected wound that is mainly leucocytes that have died combating infection. Lymphocytes provide the immune response.

c) **Platelets** or thrombocytes function in the mechanism of blood clotting, more properly called coagulation. This too is a highly complex process.

d) **Plasma Proteins:**
Within the straw coloured liquid:
- Albumin helps to maintain the osmotic balance
- Globulin contains antibodies involved in the infection fighting mechanism and
- Fibrinogen and prothrombin have a major role in the clotting mechanism.

How red cells are produced (haemopoiesis), their useful life and elimination from the system

3.5 This process begins during the 5th month of foetal life and continues until death. All blood cells originate from undifferentiated cells called *haemocytoblasts*. The blood is a vortex with new cells being constantly created and used cells whose useful life has come to an end being eliminated. Each erythrocyte has a life span of approximately 120 days; 2 to 10 million red cells are destroyed each second. And yet a constant volume/ratio is automatically maintained. And although spent red cells are destroyed and eliminated, by a remarkable process of considerable complexity the crucial iron from the redundant cell is preserved and returned to the bone marrow for re-deployment in the newly emerging red cells.

For the first few years of life, red marrow occupies virtually the entire bone capacity. Over the next 20 years it is gradually replaced by fatty yellow marrow that has no erythropoietic function. In adults erythropoiesis tends to be confined to flat bones, irregular bones and the ends of long bones. The main sites are the sternum, ribs, pelvis and skull.

Red cell production is stimulated by factors that lower the oxygen such as high altitude, nutritional deficiencies, respiratory disturbances and, of course, blood lost from the circulating system. The body has a built in compensating mechanism to bring the level back up to a normal concentration for that individual. The key ingredient *Erythropoietin* (EPO) is secreted naturally by the kidneys & pancreas. However it is now available—like insulin for diabetics—in a synthesised form known as *Recombinant EPO* (r-HuEPO). Its application and benefits, often used most efficiently in conjunction with iron, are a key feature in non-blood management of anaemia (low Hb).

The need for a sustained level of haemoglobin

3.6 The blood of the average healthy human male contains 13 to 18 grammes of Hb per 100 millilitres or 13-18g/dl. In the female it is 12-16g/dl. As to the oxygen-carrying capacity, in round figures each 100ml of blood delivers 5ml of oxygen. A normal healthy concentration is 97%-saturated out from the lungs and 70%-saturated back. However, other than in cases of severe anaemia, there is substantial spare capacity of Hb. Because of the importance of monitoring the concentration of oxygen being transported around the body and of delivery for tissue perfusion, sophisticated measuring devices have been developed, used primarily in operating theatres and intensive care units but with desk-top sets hand-portable for 'near-patient' testing.

The crucial role of iron

3.7 The affinity of oxygen and its capacity to bind with the circulating blood is governed very largely by the iron content of the blood. Iron is stored in two main areas, the primary being the haemoglobin. But additionally there are iron reserves distributed between *myohaemoglobin* (which acts as an oxygen reservoir within the muscle fibres); cytochromes and iron stores in the form of *ferritin* and *haemosiderin*, a protein shell containing iron salts which may be present inside certain cells. Iron also has a function in the formation of many enzymes in the body. The way in which these iron stores can become depleted causing iron-deficiency anaemia and the correction of iron deficiency with intravenous iron forms a crucial part of non-blood management.

The value of nitric oxide

3.8 A lesser known but nonetheless crucial ingredient is *nitric oxide* known as the endothelium-derived relaxing factor or EDRF. In simple terms the endothelium (inner lining) of blood vessels uses nitric oxide to signal to the surrounding smooth muscle to relax, thus resulting in vasodilation and increasing blood flow. In essence it helps to smooth the path of blood flow. The vasodilation does not decrease the volume of blood that the heart pumps but rather it decreases the force the heart muscle must exert to pump the same volume of blood. It has an especial use in paediatric intensive care where nitric oxide/oxygen blends are used in critical care to promote capillary and pulmonary dilation in neo-natal patients. *Glyocarn*® has been used as a nitric oxide stimulant not only benefiting sedentary patients but giving enhanced performance to trained athletes including a reduction in blood lactic acid after strenuous exercise.

Oxygen binding and release by 2,3-DPG

3.9 The role of haemoglobin is primarily to bind oxygen and transport it around the circulation to achieve tissue perfusion. However if that binding were too secure the object would be defeated, as the oxygen would simply remain bound and be carried round and then back through the venous system to be excreted. This does not occur because of a molecule 2,3 Diphosphoglycerate (2,3-DPG) that is produced within the red cell by the metabolic breakdown of glucose. It has the same concentration in red cells as Hb and is bound to it. The function of 2,3-DPG is precisely to allow the Hb to release oxygen to the tissues more easily. By contrast, stored donor blood has very low levels of 2,3-DPG. This is a reversible lesion of blood, which is damage incurred to the blood by the very process of storage. As a result, some recipients of stored blood are compromised because the release of oxygen to the tissues is minimal. Transfused cells depleted of 2,3-DPG can recover only half their normal level within a 24-hour period. In many cases the very need for transfusion is for urgent oxygenation and tissue perfusion and this period may not be rapid enough for a compromised or severely ill patient. Nothing is to be gained by adding 2,3-DPG to stored blood because the red cell membrane is impermeable to this molecule. Although the storage lesion is reversible in the recipient, it takes the one thing the patient usually does not have: time.

The ratio of formed elements to plasma—the haematocrit

3.10 The normal range for healthy blood is composed of 45% formed elements and 55% plasma.

The osmotic balance

3.11 It is precisely because more than 50% of blood is water that osmotic balance assumes such importance. *Osmosis* is the passage of a solvent from a less concentrated to a more concentrated solution through a semi-permeable membrane. In humans, the solvent is water and cell membranes control the passage of water. If excessive water is allowed to pass into tissues, especially such as the chest cavity and the air spaces of the lung, the resulting *oedema* can create considerable problems. Plasma proteins are normally retained within the blood mainly because they are too big to escape through the capillary pores into the tissues. They play a major role in creating the osmotic pressure of blood (normally 25mmHg or 3.3kPa). The danger is that if plasma protein levels fall, osmotic pressure is also reduced enabling fluid to pass into the tissues (oedema) and body cavities.

The balance of alkaline/acidity expressed as pH

3.12 The pH scale ranges from 0 to 14. A pH of 7 is neutral. Less than 7 is increasingly acidic and over 7 is increasingly alkaline. It is important to maintain the balance between the amount of carbonic acid and bicarbonate in the blood which must be maintained at a constant ratio of 1:20 in order to keep the hydrogen ion of the plasma at a constant value (pH 7.4). This is the normal pH of blood. Alteration in this ratio will disturb the acid base balance and potentially lead to acidosis or alkalosis. This can become an especial problem in newborn infants when citrates are used as an anticoagulant to preserve donor blood. Because the newborn's immature liver is minimally capable of metabolizing citrates this can lead to citrate intoxication which manifests itself as alkalosis.

The clotting mechanism including the 'cascade' of Factors leading to formation of a clot and the arrest of bleeding by establishing haemostasis

3.13 The clotting mechanism of blood is the subject of major works by professional haematologists, so to attempt to describe it for laymen whilst retaining sufficient scientific accuracy is a challenge. The starting point is that platelets, also called *thrombocytes*, are part of the formed elements found in blood. *Haemostasis* is the term used for the arrest of bleeding, involving the complex physiological processes of blood coagulation and the contraction and repair of damaged blood vessels. It is also used more generally to include the process of preventing blood loss from the body. In its simplest terms, when the endothelial lining of a blood vessel is cut or traumatised, platelets react to block the site of bleeding by forming a platelet plug and then go on to promote wound healing. Thus, blood coagulation (or clotting) is the process whereby blood is converted from a liquid to a solid state so as to plug a break in the circulatory system. Although the process may be initiated by contact of blood with a foreign surface (*intrinsic system)* that is beyond the scope of this work which concentrates on contact with damaged tissue (*extrinsic system)*.

These systems involve the interaction of a variety of substances known as coagulation factors. They lead to the production of the enzyme thrombin which converts the soluble blood protein fibrinogen to the more stable and insoluble fibrin. It is the *fibrin* as the end product that links up with similar molecules to form a fibrous meshwork that forms the foundation of a blood clot to seal off the damaged blood vessel. Although these coagulation factors have specific names, they are conventionally referred to by a medically agreed set of Roman numerals, for example Factor VIIa; Factor VIII; Factor IX etc.

There are 4 identifiable stages to the process often described as a 'cascade', namely:

- vascular spasm;
- platelet plug formation;
- coagulation factor activation; and
- lysis or the breaking down of the fibrin clot.

Stage 1 Vascular spasm

Sometimes described as *vasoconstriction,* this is a spontaneous reaction to a cut in the endothelial lining of the blood vessel. Muscle and elastic fibres in the wall shrink and constrict thereby slowing the flow of blood and allowing platelets to adhere to the damaged endothelium.

Stage 2 Formation of platelet plug

There are then 4 sub-stages to the formation of the platelet plug:

i) platelets make contact with the damaged endothelium;
ii) in doing so they adhere to it;
iii) platelets increase in size and spread out although the damaged endothelium itself releases a chemical PGI2 to ensure that the platelet plug is confined to the area of the injury and does not spread beyond it causing a blockage superfluous to the injury site;
iv) platelets release a chemical adenosine diphosphate (ADP) the chemical bonds of which store energy needed by the cell to assist the muscle contraction and
v) the platelets form a temporary plug which is then anchored in place by fibrin threads made from clotting proteins to form a more stable plug and thereby arrest the bleeding.

Stage 3 The platelets also interact with the complex coagulation factors circulating in plasma. As the platelet plug develops, platelet membranes expose molecules of a substance PF-3. This provides a surface on which clotting factors interact. Coagulation proteins form the fibrin threads that anchor the platelet plug *in situ*. Then through the wound healing process, molecules and cells trapped within the clot begin to repair the endothelial damage. Once this repair of the vessel is complete, the process of constriction can ease and blood flow through it can resume.

Stage 4 The platelet plug presents an obstruction to blood flow that is no longer required once the injured vessel has healed. The process of *clot lysis* is the reduction of the clot allowing the blood then to flow uninterrupted. It starts with plasmin breaking the fibrin clot apart. Trapped within the clot is a naturally occurring molecule called *plasminogen*. Plasminogen activators are naturally present throughout the body. They break down the plasminogen which in turn accelerates the process of breaking the clot down into small pieces which are then excreted.

The cycle of wound; platelet plug; wound healing; and dissolving and dispersal of the plug is then complete. Self-evidently, anything that interferes with this chain reaction will work against the clotting mechanism. But conversely, anything that accelerates the interaction process such as Recombinant Factor VIIa can work towards coagulation and the achieving of lasting haemostasis.

The role of plasminogen and plasmin in dissolution of blood clots

3.14 If the clot were to remain in place after the damaged blood vessel had healed, it could work as an obstruction against restoring proper circulation. So, once the necessary healing has taken place, this mechanism achieves the controlled dissolution of the fibrin plug that forms the basis of the clot, a process known as *fibrinolysis*. In certain circumstances it may be necessary to interfere with or block this mechanism and tranexamic acid may be encountered as an example of such an antifibrinolytic drug.

The immune system including defence against invading bodies and infection

3.15 This is a highly complex and hitherto little understood mechanism. When a virus, bacteria or foreign protein antigen enters the body, it is immediately recognised. A protein molecule MHC (Major Histocompatibility Complex) on the surface of nearly every cell provides its identity tag which is unique in the strict scientific sense of that much-misused word. The immune system recognises its own cells but attacks, as foreign tissue, any cells displaying different molecules/MHC such as viruses, parasites, fungi and bacteria. For these purposes, allogeneic blood and blood derivatives are foreign tissue and immediately recognised as such. The immune system produces antibodies that destroy or neutralise the invading antigen to make it harmless. Because this response system is triggered automatically, suppression of the immune system can have severe consequences. In organ transplants, the rejection of the donor material by the host is addressed specifically by immune suppressant drugs. In blood transfusion the problem is that allogeneic blood is akin to and often described as a tissue transplant and thus capable of generating a reaction.

Summary

3.16 Blood is a remarkable substance and provided it receives adequate oxygen and nutrients it is entirely self-regulating (principally by homeostatic mechanisms) in spontaneous production and maintenance of:

- Cells;
- Overall volume;

- Haematocrit—the ratio of formed elements;
- Haemoglobin—oxygen carrying capacity;
- Nitric oxide to enhance blood flow;
- Release of oxygen by 2,3-DPG;
- Osmotic balance;
- pH—the balance of alkaline/acidity;
- Immune system and defences against foreign substances;
- Temperature—a self-regulating thermostat;
- Clotting mechanism automatically triggered;
- Elimination of red cells at end of useful life but iron retained; and
- Urgent replacement of red cells when needed.

Even this brief introduction to the complexities of blood gives rise to some fairly basic questions.

Should we be tampering with this highly complex and literally life-sustaining fluid at all?

And if so, should we not be absolutely sure, on a proper scientific basis, that what we are doing is beneficial and not harmful to the patient?

Chapter Four

An Introduction to Non-Blood Management

4.1 This chapter is very definitely not an attempt to tell clinicians how to manage without blood. It would indeed not only be presumptuous, especially for a lawyer, but largely otiose as there already exists the excellent *Manual for Blood Conservation*[31] and other publications some of which are referred to in this work. For those who want to explore the topic in greater scientific depth the *Manual* is strongly recommended reading, especially:

- Chapter 9: Surgical Methods to minimise Blood Loss;
- Chapter 10: Anaesthetic Methods to Minimise Blood Loss;
- Chapter 11: Pharmacological approaches;
- Chapter 13: Transfusion Triggers in Surgical and Critically ill Patients; and
- Chapter 15: Haemostasis for Surgeons and Anaesthetists.

4.2 This work is accordingly an attempt to explain to non-clinicians, lawyers and laymen some of the basic concepts and also techniques and products that go to make up the clinicians' armoury. As declared, the author has no financial interest in any of the products mentioned but writes from his professional experience, as confirmed in some of the case histories, that the specific products and modalities where mentioned have been proved to work effectively in a specific case. The pharmaceutical industry professional association (ABPI) sets out in its Code of Practice[32] a fairly strictly defined prohibition on the commercial promotion of product use that is off licence and not fully reported in peer-reviewed professional literature. There is a wealth of experience of the successful use of many of the products mentioned below but, because it is categorised as merely anecdotal, its official dissemination is very restricted. Hopefully this work may go some way to rectifying that by at least sharing some information about such cases.

---

31 Dafydd Thomas; J. Thompson and B. Ridler 2005—*A Manual for Blood Conservation*

32 Association of the British Pharmaceutical Industry—Code of Practice 2008

General health and the role of nutrition

4.3 The most feasible way to avoid the routine use of blood transfusion is to maintain healthy blood. It is quite remarkable how many people will be fastidious in only putting into their car engine the very best quality of oil and fuel, and yet expect their body's 'engine' to run on junk fuel. Similarly, just as a heavily laden car may labour to get up hill, so the overweight/obese body may struggle with overload. And many householders will be assiduous in putting products such as *Fernox®* into their central heating systems precisely to limit the furring up of the boiler and radiator pipes and yet ingest foods that will seriously clog their heart and arteries. As was mentioned earlier in chapter 3, part of the contents of the blood are the nutrients (principally sugar and proteins) absorbed from food via the intestine and then processed internally by various glands.

4.4 Thus a healthy diet, weight control and some sensible exercise can all help to maintain a balanced iron metabolism and minimise risks. Iron deficiency anaemia is best avoided by eating a healthy, well balanced diet that includes foods rich in iron. Professional nutritionists agree that these include liver, beef, poultry, fish, pork, eggs, vegetables (such as spinach, peas, green beans, and leeks), potatoes and lamb. Iron absorption is increased by being taken on an empty stomach with ascorbic acid so that the intake of certain vegetables, fruits or juices, such as a glass of orange juice with a meal, can double or even treble the absorption of iron. The routine use of the product *Spatone®* can make a contribution to routine maintenance of healthy blood. Conversely (and as a warning to lawyers especially who as a group tend to drink too much coffee), a single cup of tea or coffee taken with a meal can reduce absorption of iron by almost 50%. Good quality unrefined porridge oats have demonstrably helped not merely in general health but in pregnancy and notably where there is Rhesus conflict. In addition to iron, an adequate daily intake of Folic Acid, Vitamin K and Vitamin B12 is also essential.

To the cynics, this may all sound faddish navel gazing but to many it is simple common sense to look after the body's 'engine' and give it the right fuel. The advent of the science of Sports Medicine and the training regime of top athletes in many sports has given a new impetus to healthy nutrition and teams in several sports at national level monitor Hb levels as well as Body Mass Index and other parameters.

4.5 However it has to be faced that, even with a Primary Care system in the UK that far exceeds that available in most Third World countries, we are not good at preventative medicine; at routine monitoring of Hb levels which are often an early warning that something is wrong; or at pre-operative workup for an elective procedure. Near-patient testing devices are commercially available but still seem to be much underused in most GP's surgeries. A blood test is considered to be quite a major undertaking requiring attendance at a hospital clinic for a phlebotomy, which is staff-intensive and therefore costly. When not all of the required elements of the blood are tested at the same sampling, repeated visits may be required. In many cases, all that is needed is a quick, immediate reading that tells the GP the level of Hb to within a reasonable margin of tolerance and blood sugar level as an early warning of potential diabetes. If the reading is within acceptable limits then no harm is done and very little time and expense incurred. If the Hb is low, then a full blood test in the laboratory can be obtained with the complete profile to assist in diagnosis. Such a near-patient testing set does exist.[33] The case of Natalie M, recounted in chapter 15 as one of the Case Histories, should serve as a salutary warning of the risks of undetected anaemia.

For further reading, an interesting article[34] in *Obstetric Anesthesia Digest* describes the use of the near-patient testing device at elective caesarean section.

Some specific products for managing without blood

4.6 The following are some of the main devices, products or techniques which, whether singly or in combination, experience has shown to facilitate non-blood management:

1. Point of care haemoglobin monitoring device *HemoCue®*;
2. Pre-operative work-up of haemoglobin level with r-HuEPO (*NeoRecormon®* Roche) supported by iron supplements as Iron Sucrose (*Venofer®*) or Ferric Carboxymaltose (*Ferinject®* Vifor Pharma), sometimes in conjunction with *Losec®* to counter iron acidity;
3. Perioperative blood flow monitoring by *CardioQ®* (Deltex Medical);

33 *HemoCue®* by HemoCue® Ltd

34 Gupta et al *Obstetric Anesthesia Digest* March 2009 Vol 29 Issue 1 p. 36 Use of HemoCue® Near-patient testing device to Measure the Concentration of Haemoglobin in Suction Fluid at elective caesarean section

4. Perioperative cell salvage by *Cell Saver®/OrthoPAT®* (Haemonetics);
5. Haemostasis management with Recombinant Factor VIIa (*Novoseven®*);
6. *Celox®* bleeding management gel;
7. Intra-operative use of products for major surgical wound repairs in hernia, uterine and colorectal surgery;
8. Modified anaesthetic techniques; and
9. Management of Deep Vein Thrombosis (DVT) with *Innohep®*.

The following is a layman's explanation designed to assist in greater understanding of each item singly and of how they can be used in combination to considerable advantage.

1. Point of care haemoglobin monitoring device—*HemoCue®*

4.7 One of the single most reliable indicators of some underlying health problem is a reduction in haemoglobin level reflecting underlying anaemia. Many GP's appear to be somewhat slow to recognise this and, despite wide use of finger-prick tests to check blood sugar levels, few would regard an Hb reading as a routine test to be done on the spot in surgery. Instead they mostly rely on a full hospital laboratory blood test. This involves a number of factors:

a) the taking of a sample of blood by a qualified phlebotomist in a quantity dictated by the laboratory computerised system in operation in the haematology department to which the sample will be submitted;
b) the provision of a sample container with suitable anti-coagulant to keep the sample viable until it reaches the lab;
c) the careful labelling/bar coding of the sample to avoid the known risks associated with the possible mix-up of multiple samples converging on the lab, often with patients of similar surname;
d) if not taken in hospital, safe refrigerated storage in the GP's surgery pending collection;
e) arranging secure courier or other service to convey the sample to the lab, often not until several days later especially in remote rural practices where the system may only provide for a couple of collections per week;
f) delay while the laboratory staff, usually with a work overload, process the sample, often necessitating a further appointment for the patient to

see the GP when the results are available thus wasting the time and costs of both;

g) return by the lab to the GP of the full printout results (sometimes up to 14 days); and
h) perhaps of greatest significance in an NHS dominated by cost and the requirements of budget holders etc., substantial cost.

4.8 One of the major disadvantages to the patient of a blood sample taken at a hospital out-patients department or blood clinic is the sheer time and expense incurred. There are many anecdotal reports of such wasted time. For example, the blood clinic at a North London hospital operates a ticket system and before 11 a.m. the ticket number can be over 150. At its peak the queue in front can be more than 80 patients. Very few working patients, employed or self-employed, can readily afford the lost productive time to hang around like that. And as a further example at Royal Free at Hampstead, not the most accessible hospital for many by public transport, the car parking charges, if a space is available, are a major deterrent at a phenomenal £3 per hour. Even those in work will be reluctant, in times of job insecurity, to take a day's vacation simply to have a blood test. A near-patient test on the *HemoCue*® at a brief GP visit would in all probability cut down dramatically on the need for a full lab test. And the report would be instantaneous instead of involving a delay of possibly up to 14 days. The benefit to the patient is considerable.

4.9 In the case of *re O* in chapter 15, one of the factors compounding the iatrogenic anaemia of a premature baby was the frequency and size of the sampling. It was made worse by a typical problem of an NHS Trust increasingly geared to a 'Monday to Friday' laboratory service. A sample taken on a Saturday was sent out of the hospital in which the baby was an in-patient where the lab was closed for the weekend to another hospital 10 miles away. Quite simply, the sample was lost and so yet another sample had to be taken from a baby that needed every drop of its own Hb. This is far from the unusual occurrence that many not involved in the system might be led to believe.

4.10 One answer lies in the *HemoCue*® device, or similar. A summary of its features is as follows:

a) size and convenience. The footprint of the device is no larger than a desk-top telephone. It is battery operated and so completely portable for near-patient testing at, for example, home visits by GP or nurse;

b) ease of use. Packs of sterile disposable cuvettes are supplied with it. All that is needed is a tiny pinprick of blood from the patient. This is inserted into the device and in no more than 30 seconds a digital read out of the Hb is available. This is declared to be accurate to +/- .2 g/dl. The memory can be programmed to record the full details of the patient, date etc. Training in the use of the equipment is very straightforward and usually included by the manufacturer/distributor in the price of the set;
c) because the cuvettes are disposable the risk of contamination is so miniscule as to be discounted;
d) the results are immediately available so that the consultation can proceed on the basis of a known Hb and blood sugar level, saving both patient and practitioner the time, trouble and expense of a further appointment;
e) after the £425 initial cost of the device (at the time of printing) which is inclusive of training CD and Manual, it costs out at £99.95 for 200 micro cuvettes, or in round figures a mere 50p per sample; and
f) if, as a result of the reading and consultation, a full haematological profile is considered necessary, a full sample can still be taken by phlebotomy and transmitted to the lab in the usual way.

In a well-run general practice known high risk patients, such as expectant mothers, should be seen by the practice nurse on each ante-natal visit and a quick reading of her Hb taken. Thus when the mother goes in for the consultation with the doctor they already have in front of them one of the key indicators of her general condition. Anaemia in pregnancy is, in many practices and indeed even in some hospital ante-natal clinics, a much under estimated risk. One study found 35% of mothers in the first trimester and a formidable 85% in the third trimester had significant anaemia. Every mother should go down to the delivery suite with a good healthy Hb. An unpredictable but catastrophic peripartum or postpartum bleed is the nightmare of obstetricians and midwives. Common sense suggests that haemorrhage is much more likely to be tolerated without recourse to donor blood, if the starting point of the Hb at labour is high. Also, the high incidence of elective caesarean section suggests even greater priority should be given to ensure admission of the mother with as high an Hb as is reasonably attainable.

4.11 The *HemoCue®* device is referred to in the SHOT report for 2011 at page 15:

> 'Concerns about the reliability of point of care testing for Hb assessments have begun to be addressed by a pilot study undertaken by UK NEQAS (General Haematology). A preliminary study of blood gas analysers and HemoCue® machines has demonstrated a wide variation in results obtained and therefore a need for wider training and QC assessments'.

The report at page 73 further states:

> 'Point of care machines, including blood gas analysers, must be quality-assured regularly as recommended by SHOT by 2009. Blood gas machines are not always reliable for Hb estimation and must be considered a rough guide at best. Dedicated devices such as the HemoCue® are more accurate but should be regularly compared to local laboratory results'.

2. Pre-operative work-up of haemoglobin level with Recombinant Erythropoietin (r-HuEPO) *NeoRecormon®* (Roche) and Iron Sucrose (*Venofer®*) or Ferric Carboxymaltose *Ferinject®* (Vifor Pharma)

4.12 Once a lower than acceptable level of Hb has been diagnosed, whether by near-patient or full lab test, then steps need to be taken to bring the Hb up to an acceptable level. Along with a diet rich in iron there is a place for oral iron supplements although these are usually not capable of delivering the replacement iron within the timescale needed and are often not well absorbed or tolerated. With many patients there is a need for more urgent and effective steps to stimulate the body's natural production of red cells (*haemopoiesis*). There are two non-blood substances currently available that can achieve this, often in the window of opportunity that may be available when elective surgery is planned but within a limited time frame. An increase of Hb of between 0.5g/dl and 1.0g/dl ***per week*** has been reliably reported. Thus if a low Hb is detected even a few weeks before elective surgery or delivery of a baby, there is still time for remedial action to raise the Hb and avoid any perceived need for blood.

The example of *M* in chapter 15 is instructive. She fell through a hole in the monitoring process with her (locum) GP changing her medication from Warfarin to Aspirin, which led to occult blood loss that went undetected over many months. Her Hb was belatedly detected at 7.4g/dl at a routine out-patient check up by the cardiac surgeon. Because of the anticipated blood loss inherent in the planned surgical procedure, he wanted her in theatre starting with an Hb of 15g/dl. Despite much hesitation and delay on the part of paediatric haematologists with apparently very limited experience of this admittedly off-licence non-blood procedure, she was started on a combination of r-HuEPO and *Venofer*® and the surgical procedure was postponed. Within 9 weeks her Hb had exceeded all hospital expectations and stood at 16g/dl, which is about what would be expected of a female athlete in prime condition. So it is verified that the regimen does work.

4.13 One side effect of Iron, whether orally or IV, is acid intolerance. Acidity and alkalinity are measured on the pH scale which ranges from 0 (extreme acidity) to 14 (extreme alkalinity) although in practice in the human body these limits are never reached. A pH of 7 is neutral and healthy blood is slightly alkaline at 7.4. By contrast the pH in the stomach can be as low as 1 or 2. In laymen's terms, we all understand how food left un-refrigerated and exposed to the air will simply go rotten. In the same way food ingested into the stomach would, unless treated, suffer the same fate. That is why the parietal cells (oxyntic cells) lining the stomach are so important. They generate the acids, notably hydrochloric acid that manage the breakdown and absorption of the nutritional elements of the ingested food and the elimination of the waste products. The parietal cells contain proton pumps, an enzyme that causes acid secretion. The process of production of hydrogen ions in exchange for potassium ions is beyond the scope of this work but undoubtedly energy is produced that pumps the H+ ions (protons) out of the parietal cell, an active process. Ingested iron can irritate these cells lining the stomach and not infrequently give rise to acid reflux, discomfort and sometimes even vomiting. To counter this, when IV iron is given it is often beneficial to use one of the proprietary antacid products such as *Losec*® which acts as a Proton Pump Inhibitor (PPI). These are already used for treating gastric and duodenal ulcers and reflux oesophagitis and have been found to alleviate the vomiting, pain and discomfort. They can be taken orally in tablet form but where, for example in cystic fibrosis, *EPO* and Iron have been deployed to address the anaemia and a quicker relief from the acid irritant is required, the PPI has been successfully administered IV. Unfortunately little of this can be found in the professional literature as most clinicians with experience of deploying *Losec*® to counter iron acidity seem to be too busy to write up and submit a single case experience for peer-reviewed publication. The dissemination of such experience as anecdotal and off licence use is further inhibited by the ABPI Code of Practice referred to above. But many involved in providing non-blood management, even in paediatrics, are successfully using these techniques.

4.14 An increasingly important feature of NHS practice is cost and there are undoubtedly cost implications. One of the disadvantages of the original iron product *Venofer*® was that it was restricted to IV in-hospital administration by a suitably qualified nurse. There had to be a test dose administered, with a wait of 15 minutes to observe any adverse reaction to the iron. Then the infusion took a period of time, sometimes extending to hours, during which the patient should be monitored. This is staff intensive and thus costly with the GP/Primary Care Trust for example being billed by the hospital for £414 as a day patient.

The new generation *Ferinject*® has the advantage of a single administration that can be deployed within General Practice. It still needs administration by a suitably trained nurse and there remain some minor concerns about availability of emergency resuscitation in the (admittedly unlikely) event of a serious reaction. The whole basis of Practice Based Commissioning Groups; Tariff Price and Healthcare Resource Groups (HRG) Codes has been driving cost assessments but there are potentially significant cost gains to be made. Additionally, it is of course far more convenient, and thus to the working patient (employed or self-employed) far more cost effective and less time wasting to avoid the need for a hospital appointment and the notorious delays, travel and waiting time that such entail. Many patients are becoming increasingly disenchanted with the delays in out-patients departments, compounded by the very high car parking charges now imposed by many NHS Trusts, and are welcoming the convenience of this treatment at their GP's surgery which can often be arranged by appointment convenient to them and that obviates the need to take time off work.

Thus the discussion, particularly about cost benefit, continues. It is a sad reflection on the economics of the NHS that some major hospital trusts are resisting the change to the use of *Ferinject*® precisely because it is perceived as depriving them of the day case income of £414 per patient which in one major unit with a conscientious iron management programme amounts to over £160,000. And so the 'bean counters' win out over clinical judgment to the possible detriment of the patient.

The whole issue of preoperative diagnosis of anaemia has been the subject of detailed investigation by a team of high powered experts in NATA. Their published article 'Detection, evaluation and management of preoperative anaemia in the elective orthopaedic surgical patient: NATA Guidelines'[35] makes compelling reading. The editor makes 4 key points:

- Preoperative anaemia is a serious but treatable condition;
- Preoperative haemoglobin measurement (28 days) should allow for treatment;
- Abnormalities should be treated before operation; and
- An algorithm to guide management is proposed.

Recombinant Erythropoietin (r-HuEPO)

4.15 This product received its marketing authorisation, valid throughout the EU, as far back as 16 July 1997, so its use is long established. It seems to be, in some units, a much undervalued product in the early and effective treatment of anaemia. And yet it is a fraction of the cost of donor blood transfusion and literally carries none of the risks. The body secretes the hormone EPO naturally from the kidneys and pancreas as part of the process of *haemopoiesis,* namely production of oxygen carrying red cells. An increase in production is triggered automatically in the body as a compensating mechanism for the reduction in the amount of oxygen reaching the tissues. In cases of acute blood loss or malfunction of kidney or pancreas, a form of r-HuEPO is now used to stimulate the process artificially. But as it is a recombinant or non-blood product, its use is both safe and effective and it is also acceptable to those who choose non-blood management. It has a place in preventive medicine, in pre-operative work-up and in pre-delivery obstetrics but unfortunately the culture of the NHS does not yet seem to have come to terms with its use in this way to any significant degree, especially pre-operatively. There have been a number of studies worldwide. For example an in depth study at the Universities of Bonn and Lübeck, Germany of 5 difficult and diverse cases managed without blood reported:[36]

> 'In conclusion r-HuEPO may be a valuable complement in the management of anaemia in patients unable to receive blood transfusions for religious or medical reasons. The findings obtained in the present cases and in the literature suggest that, on a humanitarian basis, the administration of r-HuEPO is justified both in

---

[35] Goodnough L.T. et al—*Br. J. Anaesthesia* (2011) 106 (1): 13-22

[36] *Eur J Haematol* 1997: 58: 154-159 'Perioperative use of recombinant human erythropoietin in patients refusing blood transfusions. Pathophysiological considerations based on 5 cases'

the treatment of preoperative and postoperative anemia caused by surgery related blood loss…'

This was back in 1997 and many uses, mainly off licence, have been reported since then in a range of medical disciplines, including paediatrics and even oncology, with great success.

Iron supplementation

4.16 The use of EPO in isolation is often not entirely effective because the primary ingredient of the oxygen carrying cell is iron. The body of an average healthy adult patient contains 4g of iron, over half of which is in the haemoglobin in the red cells. The rest is distributed between *myohaemoglobin* (helping to provide an oxygen reservoir in muscles), *cytochromes* (an agent in the electron transport chain), iron stores in the form of *ferritin* (storing iron in the tissues) and *haemosiderin*, (a form of iron salts present in certain cells). Having lost red cells, the body needs not merely to stimulate production with EPO but to supplement lost iron.

The stored iron reserves will be drawn down first in this process but additional iron replacement is essential. Traditionally, iron by mouth in ferrous salt preparations is widely used but a significant proportion of patients experience side effects. Within an hour of ingestion of oral iron supplements some patients experience symptoms in the upper GI which can range from mild, with nausea or epigastric discomfort, to severe epigastric pain and even vomiting. Oral iron is not readily absorbed in the gut but generally tends to be excreted with problems of associated diarrhoea. Conversely some patients experience constipation. Also there is a difference in absorption and side effects between iron lactose and iron sucrose. Hence the use of *Losec*® as a Prion Pump Inhibitor mentioned earlier. The most common side effects are gastrointestinal.

4.17 One product demonstrably successful is *Venofer*®. This was originally developed primarily as an adjunctive therapy to address renal anaemia and largely pioneered by Dr Iain MacDougall, a Consultant Nephrologist at Kings College Hospital, London. However, just as with r-HuEPO, the original Product Licence was limited (in that instance to renal cases) but experience off-licence has demonstrated a much wider and effective use.

4.18 Thus the use of EPO in conjunction with *Venofer*® has been successfully extended to a wide range of applications well beyond the original

Product Licences of each, although there is a dearth of reports of formal clinical trials. Nonetheless, a significant Supplement to the *Canadian Journal of Anaesthesia* in 2003 included[37] an article on 'The use of Iron to increase red cell mass'. That author reviewed the topic in depth and analysed the 3 different iron preparations namely:

- Iron dextran complex;
- Sodium ferric gluconate; and
- Iron Sucrose.

The conclusion was:

> 'From the results of the above mentioned studies, we can conclude that iron-dextran complex has the main disadvantage of being allergenic while sodium ferric gluconate is safe but only in small doses. Iron sucrose seems to be the safest iron preparation for producing the greatest red cell mass in the least time and avoiding the occurrence of a functional iron deficiency state when erythropoiesis is stimulated to a maximum by EPO'.

3. Perioperative blood flow monitoring by *CardioQ*® oesophageal doppler monitor (ODM) (Deltex Medical)

4.19 A persistent problem for surgeons, anaesthetists and perfusionists has been accurate monitoring of cardiac output, blood flow and intravascular fluid status during surgery. There have been a range of techniques in use, such as inserting a pulmonary artery catheter or using systems based on pulse contour analysis and dye solution. These are self-evidently invasive procedures with attendant risks. A less invasive but highly efficient product is the *CardioQ*® oesophageal doppler monitor which uses disposable ultra-sound probes inserted into the oesophagus via the mouth or nose to determine the circulating blood volume. In its simplest terms, the device generates a low-frequency ultrasound signal which is reflected by red blood cells travelling down the aorta. A validated nomogram is used to derive volumetric data such as stroke volume and cardiac output. Crucially improved fluid management is guided by use of the device.

4.20 Reduced circulating volume is known as *hypovolaemia* and leads to insufficient oxygen being delivered to the organs. This in turn can cause medical complications including peripheral and major organ failure that can be

---

37 *Can J Anesth* 2003/506/pp. 3-9

fatal. Hypovolaemia, which is akin to severe dehydration, affects virtually every patient having surgery due to a number of factors ranging from:

- the simple fact that patients undergoing general anaesthetic are starved for the immediately preceding 12 hours;
- the impact of anaesthetic agents; and
- the level of trauma from the surgery itself.

4.21 One consultant anaesthetist, involved in the hospital trial, described it thus:

> 'Blood is inevitably lost during major operations and the flow is "topped up" by adding dense fluids, colloidal solutions that mimic the behaviour of blood. But it is difficult to work out exactly how much to add. In times of stress, the body's "fight or flight" response directs the blood to where it is needed most. During operations that means that the gut and liver are deprived of blood. That is why after operations the digestive system takes several days to recover. The problem can be reduced, and recovery speeded, by adding the right amount of fluid during the operation… Before we had this system we used to be frightened that we might give too much fluid and cause heart failure. So the tendency was to give too little'.

Using fluid and drugs guided by the *CardioQ*® to optimise the amount of oxygen in the circulating blood significantly reduces post-operative complications. This allows patients to make a faster, more complete recovery and return home earlier.

4.22 The *CardioQ*® incorporates the manufacturing company's proprietary software and a small diameter, easy to use, minimally invasive, disposable oesophageal probe that is used for transmitting and receiving an ultra-sound signal. By using this technique, the clinicians are provided with the ability haemodynamically to optimise critically ill patients and those undergoing routine moderate to major surgery through the controlled administration of fluid and drugs.

4.23 This procedure has been highlighted in the media, notably because of the perceived financial benefits of reduced bed stay. Early use was featured in an Article published by the European Society of Anaesthesiology.[38] Indeed a major article in *The Times* of London September 23 2004 quoted the hospital

---

38 Benhamou et al *European Journal of Anaesthesiology* (2004), 21: 576-578 Cambridge University Press—'Factors associated with use of regional anaesthesia: a multivariate analysis of seven surgical procedures in France'

trial of 128 patients undergoing bowel surgery in which patients monitored in the control group were back on a full diet a day sooner and ready for discharge a day and a half sooner, a median of 10 days rather than 11.5. They suffered fewer digestive complications, by a factor of more than 5, and over the short period of the trial saved the NHS Trust £24,000 in reduced bed stays. The patients also felt better and did not need uncomfortable nasogastric tubes to drain stomach secretions while the gut was inactive. The economics are interesting. One hospital spent £85,000 on 10 *CardioQ*® monitors and 700 probes and surveyed patients having moderate and major surgery. It found that patients could be sent home 3 days sooner saving at least £620 per patient. That would enable a hospital doing 2,000 operations a year to increase their throughput to 2,500 and potentially save £1.1 million per year.

The hospital's Chief Executive said:

> 'We have used the *CardioQ* in around 200 operations in the last four months and had very good results. It has improved quality of care for patients as they are healthier when they leave theatre, need less post-operative care and get home quicker'.

4.24 In March 2011 the influential National Institute for Health and Clinical Excellence (NICE) issued official Notes for Guidance giving major endorsement to the current use of this equipment and indeed urging expansion. The figures were approximately £11,000 initial cost and the average cost of a probe is £67 for patients undergoing surgery and £118 for patients in the critical care unit. One crucial finding from a range of peer-reviewed studies cited is that ODM reduced:

a) the use of the higher risk central venous catheters;
b) the length of hospital stay by on average 2 days and in some surgery by up to 6 days;
c) the length of critical care; and
d) perioperative complications by more than 50%.

The overall costs saving on bed stay alone are put at £1,100 based on an average 7.5 day hospital stay. Despite these manifest benefits to both patient and hospital the Committee sadly reports:

> '[It] has been available to the NHS for a number of years but, although used routinely in some hospitals, could be adopted more widely. The Committee were

advised that current barriers to wider adoption include financial, training and motivational issues'.

4. Intra and post-operative cell salvage by *Cell Saver*® 5 and *OrthoPAT*™ (Haemonetics)

4.25 The simple principle of cell salvage is to harvest by suction the blood lost by the patient intraoperatively, filter out the gross debris, wash the residue in saline and spin in a centrifuge before passing through a final filter and back into the body. From the point of suction at bleed site to return to the patient the blood may remain in continuous closed circuit and, as it is the patient's own blood, may be acceptable to him. The procedure clearly meets the main principles of blood conservation as it is the patient's own blood. None of the disadvantages of donor blood apply and there is no risk of any contamination or transmission of any of the usual 'nasties' of donor blood. There is thus no increased hospital bed stay.

4.26 As to the cost, the new machines coming on to the market have come down dramatically in price from the early models at £20k. There are two main machines, the *Cell Saver*® *5* and the *OrthoPAT*™. Since 2001 the latter has been one of the leaders which addressed the issue of 'running costs' which were primarily the cost of having a perfusionist trained in the operation of the machine on stand-by in Theatre. Many NHS Trusts solved this problem by training on their own nurses to be able to use the device as and when needed. But the *OrthoPAT*™ has the advantage that it is fully automated and does not require a dedicated operator to monitor its operation. Further, it is portable with battery and vacuum pump so that it travels easily from Theatre to Recovery and on to the ward. The 'dynamic disk' separation chamber is suitable for a wide range of blood volumes including paediatric cases. Further a single disposable set is provided for uninterrupted salvage both intra- and postoperatively. If a machine is used, then the disposables (replacement filters etc.) cost between £100–170 per usage. When compared with the true costs of allogeneic blood units, put by many as high as at least £1,000 per unit and not with the £125 per unit (formerly £140) usually charged to the NHS Trusts, this is almost petty cash. Enlightened accountants and unit managers are putting this into the budgetary equation and, taking the overall view of benefits especially reduced bed stay, are authorising its use. Not every unit has the appliance and some, not having the automated, still baulk at having a trained perfusionist merely on standby when the machine may or may not be used. But granted that most operating theatre lists usually have at least 5 or 6 cases at a session, the benefit (especially to the patient) even then would seem to far outweigh the cost. A poster at a NATA Symposium demonstrated the cost savings for patients undergoing revision of total hip replacement at a major unit.[39]

4.27 The professional body that represents the interests of Anaesthetists in Great Britain and Ireland is known by its initials AAGBI. The use and benefits of Intra-operative Cell Salvage (ICS) have been drawn together in the AAGBI Safety Guide. This represents the authoritative findings of a specialist Working Party of Anaesthetists and has the support of the 8 professional bodies listed on page 1 of the guide. Interestingly, a survey in 2007 showed that 53% of UK hospitals were then using ICS and, as a combination of blood conservation strategies and concerns over donor blood increase, the current figure is believed to be well up on that survey.

Cell salvage in malignancies

4.28 One important feature of the guide is its chapter 6 that deals with 'Special Circumstances'. Early concerns about the use of ICS in malignancies are gradually being addressed as experience progresses. Also bowel contamination is considered, with evidence indicating that wound infection after laparotomy for abdominal injuries is no different for patients receiving allogeneic or cell salvaged blood.

This whole issue was discussed in depth in a paper presented in 2007 to a Conference of Haematologists.[40] The paper had been prepared in conjunction with a high-powered team of experts practising mainly in centres of excellence in the Leeds/Bradford areas and included 21 author references. Their specialities ranged over haematology; critical care anaesthesia; oncology; palliative medicine; radiology and molecular medicine. One of the major concerns with malignancies is the spread of malignant cells (*metastasis*) from the site of origin. The primary routes of such transmission are through the

---

39 S. Ballard et al Oxford Radcliffe Hospitals and Nuffield Orthopaedic Centre: *'The impact of cell salvage technology on patients undergoing revision of total hip replacement'.*

40 Developing a blood conservation care plan for Jehovah's Witness patients with malignant disease. British Society for Haematology 47th Annual Scientific Meeting Bournemouth, England April 2007

bloodstream and the lymphatic system. It was precisely for this reason that ICS was originally perceived as contra-indicated.

However, 3 published papers[41,42,43] referred to in the presentation in 2007 have gone a long way to allaying concerns over the use of ICS in malignancies.

Cell salvage in Obstetrics

4.29 At page 11, the guide addresses the use of ICS in obstetrics. There is a case for having at least one dedicated cell salvage machine on the delivery suite in every obstetric unit. Postpartum haemorrhage is discussed hereafter in chapter 7 and if only one maternal death can be avoided then the cost/benefit would seem to be established. The benefits of its use are undoubted but budgetary constraints had weighed heavily against it. The debate about the use of ICS in obstetrics seems to be resolving more in its favour and the percentage of units reporting its use is continually increasing. Sadly, with an echo of the NICE report on *Delta Q*® above, 80% of maternity units identified lack of training, rather than safety concerns, as the barrier to more frequent use of ICS.

4.30 In addition to the material in the AAGBI Guide, there have been several useful articles over the past 9 years in mainstream professional journals covering different jurisdictions. In November 2006 an article[44] from Nigeria reviewed transfusion practices during caesarean section in a developing country. An audit of 463 consecutive caesarean sections (of which 78 or 67.2% were emergencies) over a 3 year period monitored the incidence of transfusion of blood. A total of 117 out of the 463 cases were transfused, an overall rate of 25.2%. The rate of transfusion for the various indications was:

Malpresentation (excluding breech): 4 out of 6	= 66.7%
Placenta previa: 28 out of 49	= 59.1%
Uterine rupture: 5 out of 9	= 55.6%
Breech delivery: 8 out of 25	= 32%
Obstructed labour: 35 out of 124	= 28.2%
Precious baby: 1 out of 4	= 25%
Previous caesarean section: 24 out of 141	= 17%

41 Hamm R.S. et al. BJU International 2004; 94(4): 485-6 Red cell salvage in urological surgery
42 Davis M et al. BJU International 2003; 91(16): 474-476 The use of cell salvage during radical retropubic prostatectomy; does it influence cancer reoccurrence?
43 Hansen E. Transfusion Alternatives in Transfusion Medicine 2003;5:472-477 Cell salvage in the presence of malignancy
44 Ozumba B.C. et al J Obstetric Gynaecol 2006 Nov; 26 (8): 746-8

Severe pre-eclampsia: 5 out of 45	= 11.1%
Fetal distress: 3 out of 28	= 10.7%
Others: 3 out of 29	= 10.3%

Commenting on these figures, the authors suggested that a blood transfusion rate of 25.2% during caesarean section is high, inferentially unacceptably so. The indications for the caesarean section, pre-operative anaemia and quantity of blood loss during the procedure were significant risk factors for transfusion. The authors then commented:

> 'Efforts should be made to reduce the blood transfusion without reducing maternal morbidity and mortality. This is very important because of rising HIV infection in developing countries and blood borne disease'.

4.31 In 2009 the Department of Anaesthesia at the prestigious Royal Hallamshire Hospital, Sheffield UK published an article[45] entitled 'Introduction of cell salvage to a large obstetric unit: the first six months'. The Abstract reads:

> '*BACKGROUND*: We introduced red cell salvage to our obstetric Unit following a two month period of training and education. We report a service evaluation of the first six months of activity from May to October 2007.
> *METHODS*: The indications for using cell salvage were:
> Placenta previa; suspected placental abruption; multiple pregnancy; multiple repeat caesarean; previous history of postpartum haemorrhage; refusal of blood transfusion; caesarean section at full dilatation; low pre-operative haemoglobin and at the discretion of the theatre team.
> *RESULTS*: The cell saver was used for 46 patients with a blood loss (median range) of 800 (200-2000) mL and a heterologous transfusion rate of 22% (19 cases). Blood was processed and returned in 19 cases of which nine were emergencies and ten elective. The median volume (range) of blood returned was 390 (200-800) ml. For the Unit as a whole the percentage of all theatre cases who received a heterologous transfusion fell from 10.2% for the equivalent time period in the preceding year to 7.9% during the six month period that cell salvage was in use (P=0.126, chi(2)). There were no adverse reactions following the administration of processed blood.
> *CONCLUSION*: We have successfully introduced cell salvage to our Unit in a relatively short period of time and have used it for the largest series of patients reported in the UK'.

45 King M et al *Int J Obstetric Anesth* 2009 Apr; 18(2): 111-7

4.32 This was followed in 2010 by an article from the Department of Obstetrics and Gynaecology at Leicester General Hospital UK entitled 'Cell saver use in Obstetrics'. The main aim of the study was to determine its role in decreasing the need for homologous blood transfusion. A retrospective study (taken from the electronic database) was undertaken of patients identified as being at high risk of massive obstetric haemorrhage at the time of caesarean section over the 3 year period July 2005 to August 2008. 147 cases were identified of which cell saver was used in 77 (52%). A total of 13 units of salvaged blood were re-infused successfully saving approximately £1,800.

Despite this comparative success, the authors note:

> 'Cell salvage in our practice has not been very effective due to non-availability of trained staff in emergencies and unfamiliarity of techniques, leading to poor salvage via suction. Most of our blood loss is swabbed not suctioned and lack of salvaging from swabs is a contributory factor'.

4.33 In 2012 at the NATA conference the stand out hospital was the Royal Cornwall NHS Trust based in Truro. Their Poster Abstract recounted their 10 year experience of patient blood management in 1,400 patients. 'As a strategy to reduce transfusion, Patient Blood Management (PBM) involves identification and treatment of anaemia in patients prior to operation and blood conservation strategies.' The results were impressive. In orthopaedic surgery blood transfusion rates fell sequentially from 58% in 2002 down to 5-6% from 2008-2012. Intervention with intravenous iron was performed in 672 patients and 212 also received EPO. The conclusion was that introduction of PBM reduced blood transfusion in orthopaedic surgery and intervention for preoperative anaemia increased Hb levels. The Abstract concluded by reporting that this model was successfully developed to include other surgical areas.

4.34 The second Abstract from the same hospital addressed the issue of intra-operative cell salvage in obstetrics. There are a number of notable comments. Firstly the use of cell salvage is now routine and they have 14 cell salvage devices on the delivery ward. Blood and amniotic fluid is collected in all deliveries where there is a detectable bleed. In some case the quantity is insufficient for re-infusion and so is discarded. In those cases where it is sufficient, the mother is automatically offered re-infusion with full explanation and counselling for informed consent and, as it is her own blood, many accept. From October 2010 to October 2011 the use of ICS increased from 55% of all maternity intra-abdominal operations to 93%. 152 of the 605 collections had blood processed. 71 women received a re-infusion and were invited to return after discharge from the unit for test of antibody formation. All re-infusions have been given without adverse clinical signs. No antibodies have been detected in the follow up samples. The conclusion is that ICS can be safely introduced into *routine* practice. For those who need evidence based confirmation, two references are cited.[46,47]

5. Haemostasis management with Recombinant Factor VIIa (*Novoseven*®)

4.35 The clotting mechanism has been outlined for laymen in chapter 3. Factor VIIa has a major part to play in the 'cascade' of interactions that leads to the establishing of a fibrin clot and thus to haemostasis. Developed and indeed licensed for haemophiliacs, recombinant Factor VIIa as *Novoseven*® has proven efficacy within its Product Licence. However its off-licence use has widened dramatically with successful treatment of apparently intractable haemorrhage in a variety of settings.

4.36 At an early NATA conference, a presentation was made by the Chief Trauma Surgeon of the principal hospital in Jerusalem. Because of the on-going armed conflict in Gaza, he and his colleagues have a high incidence of major wound cases and have had to adapt to them. He recounted a case history involving an Israeli soldier who had taken a high velocity bullet in the thigh. Rushed into the unit, he was suffering massive blood loss that they were attempting to staunch but not making real progress. They were literally squeezing the blood bags to get rapid blood into him and he had received a phenomenal 107 units but was still losing ground. As a desperate last resort they used the (then untried) *Novoseven*® and were astonished when they achieved haemostasis in 7 minutes.

This was in the very early days of the product coming on the market and the commercial implications are extreme. A product will only be protected by Patent for a limited number of years. Huge sums have often been invested in the research and development (R & D) and that was true of *Novoseven*®. And so

---

46 Ralph CJ et al. Intraoperative cell salvaged blood as part of a blood conservation strategy in caesarean section: is fetal red cell contamination important? *BJA* 2011; 107: 404-408

47 Sullivan I et al. Is red cell contamination in obstetric cell salvage an important consideration? *Transfus Altern Transfus Med* 2010; 11 S2: 27

the marketing pharmaceutical company have to price the product at such a level that they both recover their R & D and make a sensible return on investment, all within the fixed period that the product remains protected by patent. Once it is out of patent protection, then it becomes effectively a free-for-all and competitors, who have not had the R & D costs, can start to replicate the product and make a much quicker profit. That explains why *Novoseven*® was at that time costing $US5,000 per usage.

4.37 The Israelis are nothing if not pragmatic. They looked at the costs and weighed them against the costs of losing a trained soldier. The two main cost factors are the pension provision for the widow and children and the cost of training on a replacement soldier. These are the quantifiable costs in addition to which there are the unquantifiable that include loss of morale to a unit of the death of a colleague whose life might or could have been saved by appropriate treatment. In the scale of things, the cost of *Novoseven*® was a good investment and its almost routine use is now authorised in that and other Trauma Units.

4.38 Unfortunately a bizarre accounting and budget system has worked its way into some NHS Trusts whereby blood is a central resource effectively 'free' to each department. But non-blood alternatives have to be specifically authorised by a consultant haematologist (who may or may not be readily available, especially at evenings and weekends) and more pertinently, the cost will be debited against that department's budget. Not unreasonably questions are asked about a system where the less expensive and often more cost-effective alternative treatment is constrained in such a way to the detriment of the patient.

6. *Celox*® haemostatic agent

4.39 This is a remarkable and innovative product developed primarily for military use in treating battle casualties who have sustained major penetrating wounds from gunshot and explosive devices but is now increasingly deployed in civilian hospitals. The following, taken from the manufacturer's published material, may be helpful in gaining a basic understanding of how it works so effectively. *Celox*® granules are actually very high surface area flakes. When they come in contact with blood, *Celox*® swells, gels and sticks together to make a gel-like mass. It stops bleeding by bonding with red cells and gelling with fluids to produce a sticky pseudo-clot. This clot sticks well to moist tissue to plug the bleeding site. *Celox*® does not set off the normal clotting cascade, it only clots the blood with which it comes directly into contact. Its mode of action has a number of considerable benefits:

- Its clotting ability has been proven to work in the presence of common anti-coagulants such as *warfarin* and *heparin;*
- It rapidly clots hypothermic (cold) blood, which may be lifesaving in many conditions of Medevac use in extreme cold such as mountain rescues;
- It is made with *chitosan*, a natural polysaccharide that has a known metabolic pathway. That means that any remaining is broken down by the body's normal enzymes and converted into materials normally present, any excess being excreted naturally. In contrast to some other similarly-acting agents it does not use or release non-degrading procoagulant minerals or alumina based clays such as smectite or kaolin which will remain in the body indefinitely.

Celox® has now been developed into a dressing that stops even severe arterial bleeding. The granules are bonded onto the surface of a stable gauze that will not compact under pressure, so that a single pack is capable of packing more than twice the wound volume of some other products. Its natural formula works independently of the body's normal clotting mechanisms to act even where normal clotting is slow or impaired, as explained above. It has repeatedly shown itself quickly and reliably to stop even deep arterial bleeds. The level of its clinical efficacy is demonstrated by the award of the prestigious European Class III CE mark of quality. After a thorough review of the available technologies, *Celox®* is now the UK Ministry of Defence product of choice as a haemostatic agent for the treatment of battlefield injuries and was deployed in Afghanistan. Its use in NHS hospitals is hitherto largely anecdotal and little in the way of peer-reviewed material seems to have been published to date in the UK. It would seem to have great potential for every patient but especially the patient who chooses non-blood management.

7. Biologic Implant surgical wound pads

4.40 Innovations in this area of surgery are also surging ahead. A technique has been developed that in effect uses a collagen gauze-type pad to assist in major wound closure, especially hernia repair. The pad is of a material that is left *in situ;* absorbed into and becoming an integral part of the body tissue surrounding the wound. The integrity of the collagen graft lasts through the body's wound healing process. It requires no rehydration or refrigeration and so is ready to use whenever needed, and it is dimensionally stable. It has been proved to be effective in sustaining wound closure following major invasive surgery especially hernia repair, uterine and colorectal surgery. Although still at the stage of recovering the R & D costs this product has been used extensively in NHS surgical practice. One advantage is that it is supplied in a wide range of sizes that eliminate the need for suturing multiple pieces together. Despite the cost, it has been demonstrated to be cost effective in certain otherwise intractable and potentially life threatening cases involving closure of major surgical wounds and potentially leads to shorter bed stay with fewer complications. Again it is the patient who benefits.

8. Modified anaesthetic management

4.41 Whilst much emphasis is inevitably placed on surgery, the teamwork with the anaesthetist is crucial. A good example of deploying a range of techniques is in an article on the anaesthetic management for ascending aorta replacement in a patient who refused autologous transfusion for religious reasons.[48] Firstly, any surgery involving the ascending aorta represents a major challenge in itself. Secondly, this was a patient aged 69. Thirdly, at the time of presentation and the decision for elective surgery her Hb was 11.7 g/dl, and the clinicians considered that this level did not provide sufficient margin of safety for bloodless surgery of this magnitude. Following the recommendations from 2005,[49] as part of a planned pre-operative work up the patient underwent a course of recombinant erythropoietin 3 times per week together with parenteral iron. In 7 weeks the Hb level rose from 11.7g/dl to 15.4 g/dl. On the recommended transfusion threshold of 7 g/dl, that gave her a margin of over 8g/dl before transfusion would normally even be considered and nearer 10 g/dl before she dropped into the high risk zone. The article describes in technical detail the various modifications made to both surgical and anaesthetic techniques and the discussion concludes:

> 'This management resulted in a successful outcome, but adapting the operational procedure requires careful consideration in each case based on the patient's condition'.

---

48 Shinju Obara et al; *J Anaesth* (2009) 23:436-438 Anaesthetic management for ascending aorta replacement in a patient who refused autologous transfusion for religious reasons

49 Gohel MS et al. *Ann R Coll Surg Engl.* 2005; 87: 3-14 How to approach major surgery where patients refuse blood transfusion (including Jehovah's Witnesses)

9. Management of Deep Vein Thrombosis (DVT) - *Innohep*®

4.42 This is an area of increasing concern. It can be a life threatening condition, particularly if a clot becomes detached from its site of formation and is carried in the blood to lodge in another part (embolism). In an increasingly cost-conscious NHS, it is an expensive side effect leading especially to prolonged bed stay, which is a major factor in all treatment costings. As always, prevention is likely to be better than cure, and the product *Innohep*® has been found to alleviate the risk considerably. One objection (as usual) is that it is far from cheap but its therapeutic properties are well attested. Its published literature[50] demonstrates:

> 'Innohep® offers a reduced risk of bleeding complications (risk reduction = 91%) and death (risk reduction = 51%) when treating patients with proximal DVT compared to UFH'.

An additional benefit is the significant reduction in the number of hospital admissions avoided by treating DVT in an outpatient setting to the mutual benefit of patient and hospital. Ante-natal specialists will be aware of the beneficial effects of this drug in high risk pregnancies.

Iron supplement by mouth

4.43 It is reliably estimated that every year 35% of pregnant women become iron deficient in their 1st trimester and 85% will have become deficient by their 3rd trimester. Iron deficiency is especially common in women carrying twins and those having pregnancies close together. Whilst the recommended daily intake of iron for a healthy adult woman is about 1.5–2mg of iron per day, in pregnant women this can increase to 2–4mg in the 2nd trimester and 3–6mg in the 3rd trimester. That is almost triple the needs of a non-pregnant woman.

4.44 The practice of oral iron administration by tablet is well established although tolerance is sometimes a problem. Additionally *Spatone*® Iron-Plus[51] is a naturally occurring mineral water which contains approximately 0.3mg of iron per ml as ferrous sulphate. Basically it derives from naturally iron-rich spa water from the mountains of Snowdonia. It works more slowly and at a less dramatic level than other iron products but is nonetheless a contributor, even to

---

50 *Current Clinical Evidence for Innohep*®, LEO Pharma Dublin October 2008

51 Worwood M et al; 'Iron absorption from a natural mineral water' (Spatone Iron +) *Clin Lab. Haem* 1996. 18. pp. 23-27

a limited extent, to maintaining a healthy level of iron in the blood and of restoring lost iron naturally. It is marketed in sachets that can be then mixed with orange juice to provide the ascorbic acid to assist absorption, especially if taken on an empty stomach. Major blood loss will usually need more concentrated iron, as outlined above but *Spatone*® has some contribution to make to maintenance of healthy iron levels. In at least one progressive maternity Unit known to the author, *Spatone*® is used in the post-delivery Unit for those mothers who have sustained moderate-to-brisk loss of blood either peri- or postpartum. These mothers are usually breast feeding yet, because of continuing anaemia, sometimes feel faint when standing and find considerable benefit from taking iron in this natural form. These are patients who cannot be discharged home because of sub-optimal levels of Hb. Given the significant costs of even a single day's occupation of a hospital bed, as a matter of simple cost/benefit it would be interesting to see a study of earlier discharge rates if products such as *Ferinject*® were to be used to speed up the process of restoring lost iron. But yet again it is the patient who would benefit.

4.45 These products described are available and, where necessary, licensed for use within the UK NHS, but it would be wrong to omit the remarkably effective Russian experience with an artificial oxygen carrier *Perftoran*® described in more detail in chapter 19. This is licensed in Russia, Kazakhstan, Ukraine and Mexico. Also the US research into haemoglobin based oxygen carriers (HBOC-201) described in chapter 20.

4.46 This chapter has included a brief narrative explanation of some of the specific techniques and products used for non-blood management either alone or in combination. Whole textbooks are devoted to this topic but the following largely self-explanatory list may be a helpful summary to give the layman an overview.

Surgical devices to minimise blood loss

4.47 Electrocautery/Electrosurgery
Laser Surgery
Argon beam coagulator
Stereotactic radiosurgery
Microwave coagulating scalpel
Ultrasonic scalpel

Techniques and devices for controlling bleeding and shock

4.48 a) Bleeding

- Direct pressure
- Ice packs
- Elevate body part above level of heart
- Haemostatic agents (see below)
- Prompt surgery
- Tourniquet
- Controlled hypotension

b) Shock

- Trendelenburg/shock position (patient supine with head lower than legs)
- Medical Antishock Trousers (MAST)
- Appropriate volume replacement after bleeding controlled

Surgical and anaesthetic techniques to limit blood loss

4.49

- Hypotensive anaesthesia
- Induced hypothermia
- Acute normovolemic haemodilution
- Hypervolemic haemodilution
- Intra-operative/post-operative blood salvage
- Laparoscopic (keyhole) surgery
- Reduce blood flow to skin
- Meticulous haemostasis
- Arterial embolisation
- Pre-operative planning:
    - Enlarged surgical team/Minimal Time
    - Surgical positioning
    - Staging of complex procedures

Devices and techniques that limit iatrogenic blood loss

4.50

- Transcutaneous oximeter
- Pulse Oximeter
- Microsampling equipment
- Essential tests only
- Multiple tests per sample
- Smaller samples (paediatric sized tubes)

Volume expanders

4.51 Crystalloids
- Ringers Lactate
- Normal saline
- Hypertonic saline

Colloids
- Pentastarch/hetastarch
- Gelatine
- Dextran

Haemostatic agents for bleeding/clotting

4.52 Topical
- Surgical adhesives
- Haemostatic swabs
- Fibrin sealants

Injectable
- Tranexamic acid
- ε-Aminocaproic acid
- Desmospressin
- Vitamin K

Other agents
- Aprotinin (*Trasylol*® Bayer)
- Conjugated oestrogens
- Vasopressin
- Cryoprecipitate
- Recombinant Factor VIIa

Therapeutic agents and techniques for managing anaemia

4.53 Stop any bleeding
- Oxygen support
- Artificial oxygen carriers when available
- Maintain intravascular volume
- Haemanitics (iron, folic acid, Vitamin B12
- Erythropoietin (r-HuEPO)
- Nutritional support
- Immunosuppresive agents if indicated
- Hyperbaric oxygen therapy
- Tolerate lower degree of normovelic anaemia (10/30 Rule has no scientific basis)

4.54 Most of these techniques, products and procedures are discussed in more detail in context in other parts of this book. For those who seek scientific source material, the Clinical Strategies produced by the Hospital Information Services of Jehovah's Witnesses are meticulously researched. This body monitors over 3,000 professional journals published worldwide and extracts up to date material helpful for non-blood management. Their protocol relating to surgical management cites 181 source references and to obstetrics and gynaecology a formidable 219. The NICE guidelines published in December 2014 cover place of birth, care throughout, the different stages of labour, pain in labour and monitoring during labour. The RCOG welcomed these revised Intrapartum Care guidelines. They are a vital source of information for healthcare professionals involved in the care of women and their babies. The Management of Emergency Treatment (MOET) Course Manual 3rd edition 2014 is readily available from the College.

4.55 What may put the effectiveness of these techniques into perspective are the findings in professional journals researching the comparison in outcomes between blood and non-blood. In 2003 a retrospective cohort study of 556 patients compared the risks of death after major trauma for Jehovah's Witnesses and other religious groups. There was no significant difference in mean injury severity score identified among religious groups nor any statistically significant associations between religion and injury severity score. Significant predictors of mortality were the usual factors:

- age;
- systolic blood pressure upon admission;
- Glasgow Coma Scale Score; and
- type of trauma.

Taking all these factors into account, the authors of that study concluded that in choosing non-blood management Jehovah's Witnesses had no increased risk of death after major trauma compared with other religious groups.

4.56 Several further studies, making due allowance for pre-operative risk factors, have confirmed this finding in non-trauma settings, citing no difference in operative morbidity or mortality in patients undergoing:

- cardiac;[52,53,54]
- neurologic;[55]
- urologic;[56]
- orthopaedic;[57,58] and
- major gynaecologic and obstetric[59] surgery.

The comparative rarity with which Jehovah's Witnesses die from severe anaemia after major elective surgery as reported in these studies is reinforced by figures suggesting that transfusion may actually contribute to an adverse outcome.[60]

4.57 In September 2015 the British Committee for Standards in Haematology published guidelines 'The Identification and Management of Pre-operative Anaemia'.[61] As in the PREVENTT study referred to earlier, the distinguished authors bring together substantial expertise and cite a formidable 74 authoritative references. The guidelines include 2 specific recommendations:

> 'Where transfusion avoidance is desirable (e.g. in patients who refuse blood or those with complex alloimmunisation), erythropoiesis-stimulating agent (ESA) therapy may be indicated to treat pre-operative anaemia.
>
> When ESA therapy is indicated pre-operatively it should be given with iron supplementation to maximise its efficiency'.

---

52 Ott D.A. and Cooley D.A. *JAMA* 1977; 238: 1256-1258 Cardiovascular surgery in Jehovah's Witnesses. Report of 542 operations without blood

53 Rosdengart et al *J Am Coll Surg.* 1997;184: 618-629 Open heart operations without transfusion using a multi-modality blood conservation strategy in 50 Jehovah's Witness patients: implications for a 'bloodless' surgical technique

54 Stamou et al. *Am J Cardiol.* 2006;98: 1223-1225 Comparisons of Cardiac surgery outcomes in Jehovah's (sic) versus non-Jehovah's Witnesses

55 Suess et al. *Neurosurgery* 2001; 49: 266-272 Neurosurgical procedures in Jehovah's Witnesses: an increased risk?

56 Roen et al. *NY State J Med* 1972; 72: 2524-2527 Extensive urologic surgery without blood transfusion

57 Bowen et al *Clin Orthop relat Res* 1985: 284-288 Posterior spinal fusion without blood replacement in Jehovah's Witnesses

58 Nelson et al. *J Bone Joint Surgery Am.* 1986; 68: 350-353 Total hip arthroplasty in Jehovah's Witnesses without blood transfusion

59 Bonakdar et al, *Obstetr Gynaecol.* 1982; 60: 587-590 Major gynaecologic and obstetric surgery in Jehovah's Witnesses

60 Vincent et al, JAMA 2002; 288: 1499-1507 Anaemia and blood transfusion in critically ill patients

61 *British Journal of Haematology*, 2015, 171, 322-331

Chapter Five

Blood Conservation—The Way Forward?

5.1 The known and accepted hazards of donor blood described in the previous chapters are such that there is now a compelling ethical and, since the case of *Montgomery*, legal argument for an explicit duty to warn every patient of the risks. If consent to treatment were to be at a level that the patient has the opportunity of evaluating the risk/benefit equation—*i.e.* truly informed consent—then there would seem to be such a duty to warn. The legal consequences of the decision in *Birch v UCH* [62] are discussed below as the forerunner to the settled law now laid down in *Montgomery* and considered in more detail in chapter 9.

5.2 Taken one stage further, the controversial question arises as to whether the time has now come to reverse the burden of choice from opting out to opting in. At present there is a presumption that an unconscious patient would consent to blood transfusion in his best interests. Those who choose non-blood treatment (principally although not exclusively Jehovah's Witnesses) carry an Advance Decision document expressly informing the treating team that they do not consent and specifying whether this decision stands in situations when life is, or may be, at risk. Similarly they have to sign a modified consent form for elective procedures.

5.3 Do we in the UK have something to learn from the Paul Gann Blood Safety Act of California? Paul Gann was a senior and respected politician in California who had stood as a candidate for the Senate of the US. In 1987 at age 75 he became infected with HIV as a result of a contaminated blood transfusion. Knowing that he had a limited life expectancy, he courageously devoted the short remainder of his life to campaigning for a change in the law, a campaign taken up and acted upon by the State legislature. The California Health and Safety Code provided that the risks and benefits of donor blood and possible alternatives must be discussed with the patient before he makes an informed choice *to accept*.

[62] *Birch v University College Hospital NHS Trust* [2008] EWHC 2237 (QB)—Cranston J.

5.4 In 2002 there were published some important comments about the need for change in UK practice:

a) 'To put these changes into effect in the United Kingdom will require a cultural shift among clinicians, managers and policy makers. No longer should clinicians prefer the convenience and immediate benefits of allogeneic transfusion over more troublesome but safer alternatives...

   Although it may turn out to be more expensive to use blood sparingly in the short run, lower consumption of allogeneic blood will both minimise the danger from variant Creutzfeldt-Jakob disease and alleviate the growing problem of recruiting loyal volunteer donors. If the threat of variant Creutzfeldt-Jakob disease transmitted by transfusion materialises it will be hard to defend the casual practices in the use of blood that linger from an era when it was believed that British blood was by definition safe. The remedy is not to wait for the arrival of yet another screening test but to bring allogeneic blood use under firm control now'. [63]
b) 'The dangers of blood transfusion make it desirable to consider alternative measures whenever possible'. [64]
c) 'Moreover, Jehovah's Witnesses present acceptable medical arguments to justify their refusal, such as the risks of infection as well as the immunological and non immunological risks that are associated with blood transfusions'. [65]

In that same year the *BMJ* published an article by Dr Ivor Cavill,[66] a practitioner with considerable experience of the role of iron in health and disease and especially of the use of iron in conjunction with r-HuEPO. The very title emphasises professional thinking in reducing blood transfusion and the more positive approach of improving the patient's own ability to make own blood.

5.5 Over the next few years there were several relevant citations:

---

[63] Making Blood Safer—Stricter vigilance and fewer transfusions are the way forward, *BMJ* (Editorial) 2002; 325:400-1 Philip Mortimer, Director, Sexually Transmitted and Bloodborne Virus Laboratory, Central Public Health Laboratory, London NW9 5HT

[64] *Code of Practice for The Surgical Management of Jehovah's Witnesses*, The Royal College of Surgeons of England, 2002; p. 6

[65] Comite Consultatif de Bioéthique de Belgique, *Opinion No. 16 of 25 March 2002 concerning the refusal of blood transfusions by Jehovah's* Witnesses, p. 19

[66] Cavill I. Senior Lecturer in Haematology, University of Wales College of Medicine, Cardiff, Reducing blood transfusion. Focus should be on improving patient's ability to make own blood. *BMJ* 2002; 325 (7365): 655

a) 'In all twenty studies, the level of recurrence of infections was significantly high (up until ten times more) in the group of transfused patients than in the non-transfused ones'. [67]
b) 'Many of the techniques developed for use in Jehovah's Witness patients will become standard practice in years to come in an effort to conserve blood stocks and reduce the need for transfusion'. [68]
c) 'Implementing the principles of bloodless surgery requires a co-ordinated team approach, across all phases of peri-operative care. Already standard in many centres across the world, these principles are likely to become increasingly prevalent in UK surgical practice'. [69]

Between a rock and a hard place

5.6 In December 2002 came disclosures[70] that raised significant doubts about the claimed superior safety of blood used in the UK. If there are two lessons to be learned from the contaminated blood scandals described in chapter 1 they are:

a) that experience has shown overwhelmingly that harvesting blood from voluntary donors in the UK whose current health and lifestyle has been disclosed and checked as carefully as practicable (donor de-selection or self-referral) is far safer than harvesting from paid providers from abroad who, in order to effect the sale, may be less than forthcoming (or like the Texas donor in some cases downright dishonest) about disclosure of risk factors; and
b) that a government-run service funded solely by the taxpayer and excluding any incentives for financial gain leads to greater professional integrity and safety. Commercial operations are inevitably driven by profit motive and there will always be the temptation, in the interests of the shareholders' bottom line, to compromise safety

---

67 Hill G E, Fralley W H, Griffith K E et al, Allogeneic Blood Transfusion Increases the Risk of Postoperative Bacterial Infection: A Meta-analysis, *The Journal of Trauma, Injury, Infection and Critical Care*. May 2003, (translation) pp. 908-914

68 Milligan L.J., Ballamy M.C Anaesthesia and critical care of Jehovah's Witnesses, *Continuing Education in Anaesthesia, Critical Care & Pain*, 2004; 4:35-39

69 Gohel MS; Bulbulia R.A; Slim F.J at al How to approach major surgery where patients refuse blood transfusion (including Jehovah's Witnesses), *Annals of Royal College of Surgeons of England* 2005; 87: 3-14

70 '50m deal ensures safe blood from US', *The Times* 18 December 2002 Nigel Hawkes Health Editor

against profit. The Arkansas Prison Scandal and the Canadian and French experiences demonstrate this quite clearly.

5.7 Despite this, those responsible for blood distribution in the UK at the end of 2002 faced a major dilemma—a shortage of plasma and yet the increasing awareness of vCJD for which there were no reliable tests and no effective sterilisation treatments. Plasma is the fluid in which red and white cells circulate. It contains numerous components such as albumin, immunoglobulin, blood clotting factors and antibodies. Every year the NHS used 5,000kg of albumin for tens of thousands of patients treated for burns, shock and major trauma, 2,000kg of intravenous immunoglobulin for immune disorders and for unborn children and 400,000 bottles of Factor VIII to treat 3,000 haemophiliacs. The global shortage of plasma is caused principally by the increasing use of immunoglobulins for immune diseases and the fact that, ironically due to advances in medical knowledge, haemophiliacs are living far longer.

The 'rock' of harvesting blood for payment

5.8 The US collects 60% of the world's plasma and supplies up to 45% of the European market. Seeing the profitable prospects of this market shortage, it is scarcely surprising that the major plasma companies have been bought up by multi-nationals who would seem to be more interested in profit than patients. The NHS originally owned Bio Products Laboratory (BPL) of Elstree, Herts where plasma was processed into a range of products, especially cryoprecipitate. This organisation used to buy significant quantities of plasma from a US company, Life Resources Inc. of New York, a company founded in 1977, not by haematologists or other medical specialists but by 3 commercial entrepreneurs. It has been highly successful to the point that it operates 24 harvesting centres across the US where it buys plasma from paid donors. BPL had contracts to buy in plasma from Life Resources but the US Company warned BPL that its contracts were not going to be renewed. This created the very real possibility that BPL would have gone out of business by 2004. The UK government ordered a financial evaluation from the major accounting firm KPMG who advised that purchase of the US Company was the most cost effective way of ensuring continuity of supplies. There does not seem to be any public report of the risk evaluation from a medical standpoint, but the outcome was that the Department of Health spent £71million to acquire Life Resources Inc.

Thus, the NHS continued to import into the UK extensive quantities of US blood products (notably plasma) harvested from paid donors on commercial terms. The figures make interesting reading. Those selling their blood in the US are allowed to provide plasma 8 times a month and sell up to 60 litres a year—4 times as much as the World Health Organisation recommends. The typical payment is between $US15 and $US20 per sale. Those with rare antibodies can be paid as much as $US50 per sale. So the financial inducements are considerable. But the whole transaction casts an interesting light on the risk evaluation of vCJD, namely that buying in plasma from paid US providers with its known risks is considered a lower risk than that posed by vCJD.

The final step in the abrogation by the government of control over the supply of plasma was the highly controversial sale in 2013 of its 80% shareholding in BPL, the primary plasma processing facility in the UK, to a US private equity fund Bain Capital. The price was a mere £230 million with a condition that the purchasers fund a £50 million renovation of the aging plant and equipment at the processing centre at Elstree. The retention of a minority 20% holding seems to have been no more than mere tokenism. Many powerful voices were raised against the proposed sale including the well-respected Dr David Owen. He speaks with triple authority as a doctor, a former Minister of Health, and a distinguished member of the House of Lords.

In a personal letter to the then Prime Minister he set out cogent and compelling arguments for preserving proper control over plasma and ensuring that it was harvested from unpaid UK donors. He highlighted the known risks of imports from paid providers in the US from whom plasma was commercially harvested and with a frequency substantially exceeding the WHO recommendations.

Sadly his arguments went unheeded as did those of many others equally well-informed and vehemently opposed to the sale for sound medical reasons.

The 'hard place' of vCJD

5.9 Creutzfeld-Jakob Disease is a fatal brain disease first recognised in the 1920's. What was not fully understood for many years was the transmission of the 'slow virus' which causes the disease, from human growth hormone (hGH), the practice being to extract the hormone from the pituitaries of cadavers.

Between 1959 and 1985 almost 2000 children were treated with hGH but had later developed CJD. The treatment with hGH had originally been a clinical trial under the auspices of the Medical Research Council but subsequently became a treatment programme for which the Department of Health was responsible. The various families came together in an action group *The Creutzfeld-Jakob Disease Litigation, Plaintiffs v United Kingdom Medical Research Council.*[71] Since 1985, 16 of the recipients had died of CJD and a further 3 were expected to do so. The surviving claimants were divided into 2 groups. In Group A, 11 claimants had developed CJD as a consequence of receiving hGH contaminated with the CJD virus. A further 87 claimants in Group B had received hGH but had not, as yet, been diagnosed with CJD.

The trial judge, Morland J, found that because of the emerging evidence about the transmission of slow viruses, the treatment programme should have been at least partially suspended from 1st July 1977. He held that the defendants had been negligent in permitting the programme to continue, because information about the risk of low virus infection was conveyed in a cursory manner. In concluding that the Department of Health had been negligent on the basis of its lethargy in carrying out enquiries and research into the risk of slow virus transmission, once it had been alerted to that risk, the judge stated a number of general principles. First, the question of negligence has to be assessed on the basis of the standards and knowledge which could reasonably have been expected at the time of the alleged negligence. Secondly the risks of the programme had to be weighed against the benefits:

> 'Many advances in medicine carry with them a risk. A risk may be, from a scientific point of view, theoretical and may never become a reality. A risk may be a real risk, but, weighed against the benefit of the drug or treatment, a risk upon careful consideration worth taking, but the risks of a drug or treatment need constant review in the light of expanding knowledge and experience'.

A pause may be appropriate to consider the implications of that judgment in the context of non-blood alternatives. The risk involved in the non-blood option, weighed against the now known risks of allogeneic blood and blood components, may be a real risk but 'a risk upon careful consideration worth taking'. The important question remains as to who evaluates the risk and more

---

[71] (1996) 54 BMLR 8; [1996] 7 Med LR 309

especially who takes the final decision. Is it not the right of the competent patient to decide whether or not to take that risk?

In 1996 doctors reported a variant of the disease, thought to be associated with consumption of beef contaminated with bovine spongiform encephalopathy (BSE) and consequently at considerably, if not uniquely, increased risk in Britain. The year 2004 saw the emerging problems of transmission of the Variant (vCJD) in blood highlighted both in an article in the Journal of Pathology and a front page article by the normally non-emotive Health Editor of *The Times*[72] under the headline 'Thousands carrying hidden CJD time bomb'. He wrote:

> 'Britain is facing a vCJD time bomb with research published today suggesting that thousands of people across the country unknowingly carry the killer disease. In the largest study into potential effects of vCJD, scientists predict that up to 4,000 people may be infected by the agent responsible for the degenerative brain disease, which is the human form of mad cow disease. Some may already be passing it on through blood transfusions and contaminated surgical instruments so that the disease may continue to kill for decades. Last night experts gave warning that the government-funded study, published today in the Journal of Pathology, might even have underestimated the threat. Pathologists who examined more than 12,500 specimens of tonsils and appendix removed in operations found evidence in three cases of the prion protein responsible for vCJD. If that proportion is repeated across the country, about 3,800 people would be carrying the infective agent–far more than the 141 who have died of it so far. The samples were anonymous, so it is impossible to identify the three who tested positive. Most came from people aged between 20 and 29, the peak age for developing vCJD...That people may be unwittingly carrying vCJD infection does not mean that they will get the disease. But even if it remains permanently in a sub-clinical state, there are alarming implications for surgery and blood transfusions'.

5.10 At a more formal and professional level, the serious threat of vCJD is monitored by a joint UKBTS/NIBSC Professional Advisory Committee. The following are some extracts from their Position Statement dated 11th March 2010:[73]

> 'To date there have been definite and probable cases of vCJD:

---

[72] *The Times* No. 68081 May 21 2004—Nigel Hawkes Health Editor

[73] Joint United Kingdom Blood Transfusion Services and National Institute for Biological Standards and Control Professional Advisory Committee

> 170 cases in the UK, 25 cases in France, 4 cases each in the Irish Republic and Spain, 3 cases each in the US, 2 cases each in Portugal and Italy and 1 case each in Canada, Saudi Arabia and Japan.
>
> The eventual number of individuals within the UK population likely to develop vCJD remains uncertain and it is similarly uncertain how many current or past blood or tissue donors could be incubating the disease.
>
> In December 2003 the first probable transmission of vCJD by blood transfusion was described. The transfusion occurred in 1996, the blood donor at the time was well but went on to develop symptoms of vCJD in 1999. The recipient was diagnosed in 2003.
>
> The second transmission leading to clinical disease was reported in February 2006. The patient developed symptoms about 8 years after receiving a blood transfusion from a donor who developed symptoms of vCJD about 20 months after donating blood.
>
> A third transmission leading to clinical disease was reported in January 2007 in a patient who developed symptoms just over 8 years after receiving a blood transfusion from a donor whose symptoms of vCJD appeared about 17 months after donating this blood.
>
> A further transmission of vCJD was described in February 2009. The patient suffered from haemophilia and had received batches of Factor VIII to which a donor who subsequently developed vCJD had contributed plasma. The patient died of other causes but was found to have evidence of prion accumulation in his spleen. Further details are awaited…
>
> 18 people who later developed vCJD have been traced as blood donors and gave blood donations that were transfused to recipients…
>
> 11 blood donors have contributed to 25 plasma pools from which 191 plasma batches have been manufactured'.

In summary, the incubation period seems to be 7 to 8 years from symptom-free donor to diagnosis of clinical disease in the recipient.

As to policy, the Position Statement makes it very clear:

> 'Blood, plasma, cell and tissue products should only be given when they are essential to the quality of life, health or survival of the patients…It is a priority for the UK Chief Medical Officers and the medical community in the UK to ensure that patients are treated with blood or tissue products only when there is real clinical need…

There is increasing use in the NHS of techniques that can, for some patients, reduce the need for transfusion of donor blood or avoid it altogether'.

5.11 In April 2004 there was implemented the exclusion of whole blood donors who state that they have received a blood component transfusion in the UK since 1st January 1980. This resulted in the self-deferral of 3-5% of blood donors. It was extended in November 2005 to transfusions anywhere in the world. And later this deferral criterion has been extended to blood donors who are unsure whether they received a transfusion. As mentioned, this resulted in the partly foreseen fall in the donor pool and caused a serious re-evaluation of the transfusion threshold. The Chief Medical Officer for England then firmly proposed a threshold of 7g/dl. In the peer reviewed article 'Guidelines on the management of massive blood loss'[74] the view was repeated from 2001 'Red Cells are rarely indicated when the haemoglobin concentration is >10 g/dl but almost always indicated when it is <6 g/dl.' The author was involved in a case when an expert witness for the patient had this threshold of 6g/dl put to him forcefully in cross-examination. His succinct answer was 'The expression *almost always* clearly envisages circumstances when transfusion is not given, principally when the patient, as here, does not want it.'

5.12 However for years one particular group of patients for reasons of religious conscience have not been prepared to accept allogeneic blood under any circumstances. Jehovah's Witnesses are in practical terms the only group whose Hb level has been allowed to drop below 5g/dl without transfusion of donor blood. The experience of the medical profession in treating this large group (now over 8 million members worldwide) with non-blood management was evaluated in 1994 in another peer-reviewed article entitled 'What can we learn about the need for transfusion from patients who refuse blood? The experience of Jehovah's Witnesses'.[75] There was extensive reporting of survival at levels well below 5g/dl. Table 2 in the article reports 27 cases of patients who survived at Hb levels below 5g with ages ranging from 78 years to 20 years; 8 survived at under 4g/dl, 3 under 3g/dl, and 2 at under 2 g/dl. In one exceptionally skilful piece of intensive care reported by a District Hospital Unit in Sheffield,[76] they successfully pulled back a patient from a phenomenal 1.8 g/dl. Whilst no patient or clinician would choose unnecessarily to push the

74 *British Journal of Haematology*—2006 135, 634-641
75 Viele & Weiskopf—*Transfusion* Vol 34, No. 5—1994
76 Howell & Bamber: *Anaesthesia* 1987, Vol 42 44-48

boundaries to these levels, the clinical facts show that survival is possible. That case was in 1987 and major advances have been made in non-blood management over almost 30 years. The overwhelming conclusion has been that there has been no significant effect on morbidity or mortality in treating without blood and indeed there is a move for blood conservation and to try and achieve non-blood management as the gold standard as envisaged:

> 'Bloodless surgery has come to represent good practice, and in the future, it may well be the accepted standard of care'. [77]

5.13 One problem area is that non-blood management has now become so routine with many specialists that it is scarcely considered worth the time and effort to write up an individual case for publication in a peer-reviewed professional journal. But one such case was reported in an Abstract at the 2011 Conference of NATA in Dublin by Dr Stone of the Dudley Group of Hospitals NHS Foundation Trust.

> 'Introduction: A Jehovah's Witness patient was admitted for left percutaneous nephrolithotomy (PCNL) with a preoperative haemoglobin of 15.3 g/dL. The patient had confirmed preoperatively that he would not accept any of the primary blood components but would accept plasma derivatives.
>
> Methods: During the procedure significant bleeding from the PCNL tract occurred. This was controlled but continued postop and the haemoglobin dropped to 7.2 g/dL. The patient was given 2 doses of recombinant factor VIIa, aprotinin and tranexamic acid in an attempt to stop the bleeding. The patient was taken back to theatre and an emergency nephrectomy for continued bleeding from the PCNL tract was performed.
>
> Results: Following the procedure the patient's haemoglobin was 5.3 g/dL. 2 days postop the patient was taken back to theatre for cystoscopy and evacuation of blood clot with the haemoglobin falling further to its lowest level of 3.2 g/dL. Following discussion with a Haematologist, the patient was prescribed 20 mg iron sucrose daily and 25,000 units EPO 3 times per week. 10 days later the haemoglobin had risen to 6.7 g/dL and the patient was transferred to a ward from the intensive care Unit. The patient was discharged 15 days postop with haemoglobin of 7.1 g/dL. EPO injections were continued for a further 7 days at which point the haemoglobin had reached 10 g/dL.

---

77 Adelola O A, Ahmed I, Fenton J.E 'Management of Jehovah's Witnesses in Otolaryngology, Head and Neck Surgery' *American Journal of Otolaryngology—Head and Neck Medicine and Surgery*; 29 2008 270-278

> Conclusion: We have demonstrated the efficacy of EPO and IV iron in salvaging a patient from life-threatening anaemia. We have gone on to produce a protocol for use in similar situations in the future'.

This case would seem to be a classic example of a patient admitted with an acceptably high Hb level and the surgical team then encountering a significant bleed resulting in his being taken back to theatre for emergency nephrectomy and then again for evacuation of a clot. The non-blood management, intra-operatively and post-operatively, has been exemplary, especially considering the undoubted pressure on clinical, nursing and ICU staff caused by a drop in Hb to a low of 3.2g/dl.

5.14 As to risks, there is a significant body of peer-reviewed medical literature (some of which is cited in this work) that identifies current risks including:

- The not infrequent mistake of giving the wrong blood;
- Contaminated blood;
- Transfusion reaction;
- Suppression of the immune system; and
- Transmission of viral and other infections including hepatitis; HIV and CJD.

5.15 Transfusion Related Lung Injury (TRALI)

One of the very serious complications justifies some comments on its own. Firstly is the very nomenclature, the condition prefaced by 'Transfusion related', which tells its own story. It is defined as 'an acute lung injury that is temporally related to a blood transfusion in that it must occur within the first 6 hours following a transfusion.' It is characterised by the acute onset of non-cardiogenic pulmonary oedema.[78] A major problem for researchers seeking to eliminate the condition is that the aetiology is currently not fully understood although it is thought to be immune mediated. Some specific antibodies directed towards Human Leukocyte Antigens (HLA) or Human Neutrophil Antigens (HNA) have been implicated and this bears directly on the exclusion of one identified group of donors. Women who are multiparous (have had more than one child) develop these antibodies through exposure to foetal blood. As a

[78] Toy P. et al Transfusion-related acute lung injury: definition and review. Crit Care Med. 2005 Apr; 33(4): 721-6

result, transfusion of blood components harvested from these donors is thought to carry a higher risk of inducing immune related TRALI.[79]

5.16 Whilst TRALI is typically associated with plasma products such as FFP, it can also occur in recipients of packed red blood cells due to the residual plasma present in the unit. As an indication of the gravity of the consequences, the immune-related form of TRALI is reported[80] as occurring in the US once in every 5,000 transfusions and has a mortality of 6-9%. The risk to neonates, especially pre-term and ELBW, with immature lungs, is self-evident.

5.17 Additionally there is reference to TRALI in the report (cited in *A.C. v Manitoba*) of an International Consensus Conference on Transfusions and Outcomes[81] that included the following:

> '...there is little evidence to support a beneficial effect from the greatest number of transfusions currently being given to patients. The vast majority of studies show an association between red blood cell transfusions and higher rates of complications such as heart attack, stroke, lung injury, infection and kidney failure and death'.

As one spokesman put it: 'The results of the conference firmly establish the view that, rather than being a benign procedure, blood transfusion is associated with increased risk of medical complications.'

5.18 Another interesting suggestion is that due to a declining donor pool leading to blood becoming a scarce resource, its use should be limited to those who really need it as a life-saving procedure and want it to the extent of being an informed patient willingly accepting any risks involved. In England and Wales, despite extensive advertising and urging, only 3% of adults are currently blood donors and 50% of these give 75% of the total donations. A further 6% of donors lapse each year, far exceeding new donors coming forward to replace them and so the diminishing donor pool is causing increasing concern. It is almost inevitably providing momentum for non-blood alternatives.

---

79 Muller JY, TRALI: from diagnosis to prevention. *Transfus Clin Biol*. 2005 Jun; 12(2):95-102

80 Transfusion-related acute lung injury (TRALI): a serious adverse event of blood transfusion. *Vox Sang*. 2005 Jul;89(1):1-10

81 Blood transfusions and outcomes, *Medical News Today*, 23 April 2009

The Archer Inquiry

5.19 The victims of the contaminated blood scandals of the US, Canada, France and Ireland recounted above were at least afforded the dignity of a major Public Inquiry and awarded compensation. The *Krever Report* in Canada is held up as a model of its kind. In Ireland, following a similar Tribunal of Inquiry, *ex gratia* awards of compensation were the sterling equivalent of £750,000 for those infected with hepatitis and £101,000 for HIV. By contrast, the government in the UK has maintained a consistent denial of liability, originally offering a mere £6,400 *per annum,* grudgingly increased under pressure of public outcry to £12,800. Finally a group of Law Lords combined to establish their own Inquiry chaired by an eminent lawyer, Lord Archer QC, former Solicitor General. It was denied public funding, had no Standing Counsel to assist it and, being non-statutory, did not have the powers to compel the attendance of witnesses or the production of documents. The experience of most lawyers acting for patients and surviving relatives in these cases is that they are not primarily motivated by compensation. More than anything else they want the truth, answers to important questions as to how the disaster was allowed to happen, explanation of what safeguards are now in place to prevent the same thing happening to others, hopefully an apology or some expression of regret and (perhaps an illusory expectation) some accountability. The refusal of co-operation by the Department of Health to assist the Inquiry to achieve these ends borders on the shameful. Perhaps the nadir was reached when, as the Report records,[82] officials were only allowed to meet the Inquiry Panel in 3 'private, informal and un-minuted meetings'. Despite what many victims doubtless regarded as these blatant attempts at non-cooperation and non-disclosure, the report unearthed some significant information. It found that 4,670 haemophiliacs were infected with Hepatitis C, of whom 1,243 were also infected with HIV. By May of 2009 almost 2,000 people had died as a result of this contaminated blood and £142 million had been paid to victims. The Inquiry then went on to look at the level of compensation paid out by the government of Ireland where those who contracted Hepatitis C were paid on average £750,000 and those infected with HIV £101,000. It recommended that comparable compensation be paid to the UK victims. The government refused, arguing that the Irish compensation levels were based on the proposition that

---

82 *Report of the Archer Inquiry* 2009 at p. 9

the Blood Transfusion Service was found to be at fault, which was not the case in Britain.

5.20 One aggrieved victim, Andrew March, an award winning composer, took a case on Judicial Review. In the course of the hearing, the evidence of the senior civil servant from the Department of Health was that the estimated annual cost in 2010 of the proposals actually announced by the government would be £3.8 million. A system similar to the Irish system was never fully costed but a rough costing of a comparable system was £3–3.5 *billion*. On 16 April 2010 Holman J., an experienced judge of the Family Division sitting to hear the case in the Administrative Court, in a neat judicial aphorism ruled that the UK government's approach 'has been, and remains, infected by error.'[83] The limited newspaper report after the case merely stated that 'The Department of Health said it would consider the position arising from this decision.' The blunt reality seems to be that the Department and the cash-starved Treasury have neither the money nor the will to pay on the more generous scale applicable in Ireland. The consequence was a Private Members Bill Contaminated Blood (Support for Infected and Bereaved Persons) Bill sponsored by Lord Morris of Manchester. It was introduced in the House on 26th May 2010; completed its passage through the Lords but made no progress in the Commons as the parliamentary session prorogued. Reintroduced in the Lords it made its laborious way again to the Commons. However it was not moved for debate on 20th January 2012 and so the order to read the Bill a second time lapsed. The website stated 'There is no indication when the Bill will progress further'.[84] It seems to be a not unreasonable inference that fears are indeed coming to pass that the government is deliberately delaying and will do what it can to avoid paying. As the Chief Executive of the Haemophilia Society justifiably commented, those infected and the bereaved relatives are understandably rightly aggrieved. But perhaps more compellingly the refusal of the state to accept liability or to pay adequate compensation for transfusion of contaminated blood provides a powerful argument in support of those who choose, albeit for other primary reasons, to stand firm on their choice of non-blood alternatives. If they are given blood and anything goes wrong, they will only get a much reduced *ex gratia* payment at the discretion of the department

[83] *The Queen (on the application of Andrew Michael March) v Secretary of State for Health* [2010] EWHC 765 (Admin)

[84] www.dodslegislation.com/bill/2010-11—contaminated blood support for infected

and not the proper compensation as an order of a judge that they would receive if legally entitled.

5.21 *New Scientist* is a long-established and very well-respected journal not usually given to emotive headlines. Its published materials are thoroughly researched and peer-reviewed at a very high level and it has a well-deserved reputation for scientific objectivity. It is that very scientific integrity that makes all the more compelling the articles published in an edition in 2008.[85] The full texts are worth reading but the following extracts (hopefully not unfairly taken out of context) highlight some of the serious reservations in the scientific community:

5.22 'An act of faith in the operating room'

> 'A series of studies suggest [it] may increase the risk of death in all but the most serious cases of anaemia and people suffering a catastrophic loss of blood. It appears that this damage is done not by infectious agents in the transfused blood but by the blood itself—possibly because of chemical changes that have a deleterious effect on the recipient's immune system. The precise mechanism is still unclear and every effort should be made to uncover it so that surgeons can be made aware of all the risks involved'.

5.23 'Blood doesn't always save lives'

> 'As long as surgeons use special techniques, Jehovah's Witnesses can have surgery—including operations with the greatest potential for blood loss such as open heart surgery—without ever receiving a drop of someone else's blood. Now some surgeons and anaesthetists are questioning whether every patient shouldn't get the same treatment. Over the past decade a number of studies have found that, far from saving lives, blood transfusion can actually harm many patients…
>
> For almost 9,000 patients who had heart surgery in the UK between 1996 and 2003, receiving a red cell transfusion was associated with three times the risk of dying in the following year and an almost six fold risk of dying within 30 days of surgery compared with not receiving one. Transfusions were also associated with more infections and higher incidence of stroke, heart attack and kidney failure—complications usually linked to a lack of oxygen in body tissues'. (Circulation, Vol 116 p.2544)

5.24 In the same year, the professional journal of those engaged in critical care where, almost by definition, the use of blood and blood products features

[85] *New Scientist*—26 April 2008 pp. 5, 8-9.

prominently, published a high-powered review of the literature on the efficacy of red cell transfusion of the critically ill. In addition to including in the text the comment 'In the vast majority of studies, the risks associated with blood transfusion outweighed the benefits,' the conclusion states with stark simplicity: [86]

> 'Despite the inherent limitations in the analysis of cohort studies, our analysis suggests that in adult, intensive care unit, trauma, and surgical patients, RBC transfusions are associated with increased morbidity and mortality and therefore, current transfusion practices may require re-evaluation. The risks and benefits of RBC transfusion should be assessed in every patient before transfusion'.

5.25 In 2009 there was a shift of emphasis in the UK to acknowledge the greater role of anaesthetists in avoiding blood transfusion. An article by two senior and well-respected anaesthetists at Leeds General Infirmary set out in the opening Abstract the following: [87]

> 'Clinical strategies to avoid blood transfusion are now considered a routine part of the peri-operative management of any patient presenting for major surgery. The universal introduction of pre-assessment clinics in the UK and the increasing acceptance of the need for multidisciplinary team (MDT) meetings mean that anaesthetists now play a major role in reducing the need for peri-operative transfusion'.

The authors list a range of pre, peri and postoperative techniques including:

- Intra-operative strategies to avoid transfusion;
- Patient positioning;
- Ventilation;
- Controlled hypotension;
- Antifibrinolytic agents;
- Acute normovolaemic haemodilution (ANH);
- Cell salvage;
- Normothermia; and
- Reinfusion of blood from wound drains.

They conclude with a simple statement on transfusion threshold:

---

86 Marik et al, Efficacy of red blood cell transfusion in the critically ill: A systematic review of the literature. Crit Care Med 2008 Vol 36 No. 9 pp. 266

87 'Clinical strategies to avoid blood transfusion', J.R.Cole & M.H.Cross *Anaesthesia and Intensive Care Medicine* 2009 11:2 47-49

'Undoubtedly the most significant reductions that have been made in avoiding transfusion over the past 10 years have been due to the education of doctors that a reduced transfusion threshold of 8-9g/dL is safe'.

5.26 In January 2010 the US government instituted a $US4.7 million programme for the extensive re-training of its military doctors, surgeons, anaesthetists and paramedics in haemovigilance, blood conservation and the techniques of non-blood management. The training school is the prestigious Englewood Hospital, New Jersey, which has been in the forefront of advancing the use of techniques and medication to try wherever possible to avoid donor blood. A major reassessment of cost in the US has given cause to re-think. Thus, however belatedly, (at least in the US) there is finally an acknowledgement of the risk/benefit evaluation and a major shift in policy (and finance) at the highest level away from the liberal use of donor blood to the benefit of at least the patient in the armed forces.

5.27 Further impetus was given to non-blood management by the publication in January 2012 of an article which specifically addressed the outcomes in patients who receive small amounts of intraoperative blood transfusion. Its particular value is that it examined a large sample of patients from 173 hospitals throughout the US. The details are worth reading but the conclusions state with simplicity:

'There is a dose dependent adverse effect of intra-operative blood transfusion. It is likely that a small, possibly discretionary amount of intraoperative transfusion leads to increased mortality, morbidity and resource use, suggesting that caution should be used with intraoperative transfusions for mildly hypovolaemic or anaemic patients'.

5.28 Hopefully we may see the Department of Health, the BMA and the Medical Defence Societies taking positive steps in this direction from a liberal to a conservative approach. In California they changed the law to reverse the presumption of consent. In the UK that should not be necessary. The legal status of Department of Health Circulars and the issuing of 'Best Practice' directives from the profession would almost certainly suffice to change existing practice equivalent to the force of law.

5.29 In the UK even if the climate amongst practitioners is not yet ready for the major change to a policy of opting in rather than opting out, the cumulative effect of this evidence suggests that no patient, of whatever age, should ever be forced or coerced by medical paternalism or court process to accept an unwanted transfusion of donor blood.

Conclusion

5.30 Drawing all this together, in some respects blood donated in the UK is now safer as a result of improved sterile harvesting, processing, leucodepletion, testing, storing and distribution. But there remain very serious concerns about the risks inherent in giving donor blood to any patient, especially adult blood to neonates.

5.31 The balancing of demand and use of donor blood is well summarised in an article in a leading journal[88] under the heading 'Challenges of meeting the future blood transfusion requirement in England and Wales'. Three quotes from the conclusion seem relevant:

> 'Each and every donation is a precious commodity and should be treated as such. It should not be given as therapy without clear evidence of its benefits and clear understanding of its risks…
>
> All patients should be managed in a more evidence based and holistic manner to reduce the likelihood of transfusion. For instance treatment of iron deficiency anaemia with iron therapy rather than transfusion could reduce the need for a significant proportion of RBCTs…
>
> There is need to reduce the growth in demand for blood products. We must accept the challenge that growth cannot continue at the present rate and take real steps to ensure that any growth reflects real evidence based clinical need and is not driven by historical practice'.

5.32 What is required is recognition of the scale of the problem and the will to implement the necessary changes. However H. G. Wells summed up nicely the English approach to change:

> 'In England we have come to rely on a comfortable time-lag of fifty years or a century intervening between the perception that something ought to be done and a serious attempt to do it'.

---

[88] Osaro et al *Transfusion alternatives in Transfusion Medicine:* 11, 72- 81

Chapter Six

Is there an evidenced based threshold for transfusion?

6.1 The medical profession rightly insists on a proper scientific evidence base for any particular practice. And yet at the same time initiative would be inhibited and new developments stifled at birth if there were not those prepared to expand the boundaries of knowledge and indeed to try and manage patients who choose treatment beyond those boundaries. That inevitably sets up a potential for conflict between those who feel that until there is an evidence base for a new procedure it should not be implemented for patients and those who are convinced that the boundaries are set too narrowly and should be pushed back.

6.2 This is in reality the situation that has developed in the profession over the issue of the threshold (or trigger) for transfusion of allogeneic blood or blood products. The earlier chapters of this work recount, primarily in chronological order, the events surrounding the development of transfusion practice and some of the major setbacks that have been encountered along the way. This chapter extracts and draws together (citing where appropriate some of the previous references) the main events and issues that bear more directly on this specific but professionally contentious issue of transfusion threshold or trigger.

6.3 The starting point is the implementation of transfusion as an acceptable medical technique as far back as 1942 [1.38]. There seems to have been no serious scientific or evidenced based evaluation of the practice as such but merely concentration on the development of the techniques for its practical application. An arbitrary threshold of 10g/dl was arrived at and adopted generally by the profession. It could have been fixed at 11-12 g/dl or at 7-8 g/dl and 10 g/dl seems to have been arrived at for no better reason than it being a nice round number. As was stated in evidence to the Krever Inquiry in Canada, [1.15]:

> 'The aetiology of this requirement is cloaked in tradition, shrouded in obscurity and unsubstantiated by clinical or experimental evidence'.

That would seem to many to provide a rather shaky 'evidence base' for a procedure that was to be adopted so enthusiastically by practitioners and developed to the present level of extensive practice.

6.4 Some 18 years later a well-reasoned and compelling article by a Canadian doctor [1.12] drew attention to the way in which medical practice develops and how 'the accepted treatment of today was risky yesterday and will be obsolete tomorrow'.

6.5 In 1967 the Sainsbury Inquiry into the Thalidomide disaster [1.6] addressed the issue of effectiveness of pharmaceutical products generally and the ensuing legislation simply accepted, without further question or evidence, the validity of blood transfusion and elevated its status to a statutory 'medicine'.

6.6 It was thus not until 1975, 33 years after the adoption of blood transfusion as an approved practice, that a serious evidence base in professional journals started to be created. The persuasive editorial in the professional journal *Anaesthesia* [1.16] urged what in modern parlance would be described as a 'Conservative Strategy' in the use of allogeneic blood and blood products.

6.7 In the 1970's Dr James Watt, with a pre-operative Hb of 6.5g/dl. successfully underwent major surgery performed by Mr Marcus and without transfusion. That case never made its way on to any evidence-based database and so does not feature in any statistics but it was a clear, if early, demonstration that bloodless surgery can be successfully carried out at that lower level of Hb. The key seems to have been exemplary surgical technique in maintaining haemostasis combined with top quality anaesthesia.

6.8 In 1987 there was published, again in *Anaesthesia,* a report from a hospital in Sheffield UK of a case involving patient survival at a mere 1.9g/dl that does not seem to have received the wide attention that it deserved. Firstly this was not a major research centre, teaching hospital or ranked as a Centre of Excellence with the special level of funding and equipment that goes with such status. It was however, as the work of its ICU demonstrated, a very good quality District Hospital within the NHS. Secondly as the date indicates, this preceded by many years the discovery and development of the many weapons in the non-blood armoury that are now taken almost for granted. There was no EPO, effective IV iron such as *Venofer*® *or Ferinject*® nor had Intraoperative

Cell Salvage or many of the sophisticated anaesthetic techniques of either pre-operative or post-operative monitoring in ICU been developed. As the authors of the article very modestly stated, the patient 'owed her survival to simple intensive care management'.

Here one might have thought was some more firmly based evidence for the effectiveness and success of non-blood management but it seems to have passed almost unnoticed. Perhaps it was too far outside main-stream practice of the time which was still to transfuse at 10g/dl.

6.9 However by 1994 more serious consideration was being given to the known and developing hazards of allogeneic blood. At the conference of the Royal College of Physicians held in Edinburgh there was discussed the relevant question:

> 'How did we get a "Magic Number" for pre-operative haematocrit or haemoglobin level?'

The subject was picked up and developed in an article in *The Lancet* the whole of which is worth reading but one paragraph of which is of particular relevance to this topic of transfusion threshold or trigger:

> 'Despite more than five decades of established practice, doctors still do not agree about precisely when and why they should transfuse red cells and how efficacy can be assessed...One message was clear, the traditional transfusion trigger—i.e. the critical haemoglobin value justifying transfusion intervention - needs to be considerably revised...And despite the diversity of views, there was little dissension from the idea that a therapy that costs so much...deserved to be put on an altogether more substantial scientific basis'.

6.10 The same year 1994 saw the publication of the significant study by *Viele & Weiskopf* into outcomes in the UK involving Jehovah's Witnesses, the principal but not only group of patients who choose not to accept transfusion of allogeneic blood whatever their level of Hb. This is one of the few evidence-based studies of outcomes in managing what conventional practitioners would regard as unacceptably low levels of Hb for surgical intervention. The very nature of the study means that the numbers are of necessity restricted but it does provide some firm evidence worthy of consideration.

The main piece of evidence is that it reports 27 patients with ages ranging from 78 years to 20 years who survived at Hb levels of below 5g/dl. The lower age level reflects the current ambiguous state of the case law in England and Wales. A mature minor can choose to accept treatment at any age at which he can meet a very mild test of competence. On the other hand no patient under 18-years-of-age can, on a strict interpretation of the law, refuse treatment and the court will give the NHS Trust that applies for it a permissive order to transfuse. Thus England & Wales lag behind other common law jurisdictions such as Canada (an age of 16 and even below if competence is established) and Ireland where they have been for a long time considering change in the law to age 16. Elsewhere in Europe it is mainly 15 years except The Netherlands where it is 12 years.

Eight patients survived at under 4g/dl; 3 at under 3g/dl and 2 at under 2g/dl. One of these was the survivor in the Sheffield hospital mentioned above at 1.9g/dl. So, contrary to popular understanding, there is evidence-based finding that survival is not merely possible in theory but demonstrated in practice. Critics will doubtless point to the limited number in the study but may wish to consider how else figures can be obtained. In the very nature of things there can only be a retrospective study as it would be unacceptable to many Ethics Committees to permit any randomised trial that allowed Hb to drop to such levels without clear, informed and legally binding consent. That is highly unlikely to be given except by those who formed the basis of the particular study and who had a genuine conscientious objection to allogeneic blood as a matter of principle.

6.11 Events moved on very slowly in terms of official recognition of a restrictive transfusion regime although individual practitioners are known to have been practising non-blood management – they were just too busy to write about it in the medical journals. However in 2003 the Chief Medical Officer, Professor Liam Donaldson, in his official Annual Report entitled 'On the State of Public Health', stated that he believed too many unnecessary blood transfusions were being given in England. He added:

> 'The gift of blood is too often squandered by unnecessary and inappropriate use'.

He expressed concern at the fall in the donor pool (down by one fifth in 4 years). He further suggested that transfusion is unnecessary unless the haemoglobin falls below 7g/dl. He also proposed that only consultants, and not junior staff, should be allowed to order blood and blood products.

Some may find this compelling evidence coming from such a source representing the UK Department of Health under whose supervision or control medical practitioners in the NHS are engaged.

AAGBI produced a Protocol for the Management of Anaesthesia for Jehovah's Witnesses in which these comments of Professor Donaldson were reported. The same report appeared in the second edition published in November 2005. Again it seems not unreasonable to suggest that such authorities represent cogent 'evidence' of at the least the official position of both the Department and the professional body of anaesthetists on this issue of 'threshold'.

6.12 In 2009 a case came before the Canadian Supreme Court concerning the right of a mature minor to take her own decision not to accept allogeneic blood. In the course of a lengthy judgment that runs to over 80 pages the court cited the report of an International Consensus Conference on Transfusions and Outcomes that included the following: [89]

> '...there is little evidence to support a beneficial effect from the greatest number of transfusions currently being given to patients. The vast majority of studies show an association between red blood cell transfusions and higher rates of complications such as heart attack, stroke, lung injury, infection and kidney failure and death...
> The results of the conference firmly establish the view that, rather than being a benign procedure, blood transfusion is associated with increased risk of medical complications'.

6.13 In March 2010 the gravity of the threat to health posed by vCJD was referred to by a joint UKBTS/NIBSC Professional Advisory Committee. The following are some extracts from their Position Statement:[90]

> 'Blood, plasma, cell and tissue products should only be given when they are essential to the quality of life, health or survival of the patients...It is a priority for the UK Chief Medical Officers and the medical community in the UK to ensure that patients are treated with blood or tissue products only when there is real clinical need...
>
> There is increasing use in the NHS of techniques that can, for some patients, reduce the need for transfusion of donor blood or avoid it altogether'.

---

89 Blood transfusions and outcomes, *Medical News Today*, 23 April 2009

90 Joint United Kingdom Blood Transfusion Services and National Institute for Biological Standards and Control, Professional Advisory Committee Report, 12 March 2010

6.14 The scale of the perceived problem is perhaps best demonstrated by the resources allocated. The Department of Health, in conjunction with the Scottish Government Health Department, has set up the National CJD Research and Surveillance Unit (NCJDRSU). It is based at the Western General Hospital in Edinburgh working in conjunction with the university. Its 23rd Annual Report 2014 includes data up to May 2015 and is available online at cjd.ed.ac.uk. Its function is CJD surveillance in the UK and it is impressively staffed with 3 professors, 11 doctors in varying specialties and a further 18 research and support staff.

In summary, their assessment of vCJD is that the peak has passed 'but may increase again particularly if differing genetic sub-groups with lower incubation periods exist'. At paragraph 2.5 under Transfusion Medicine Epidemiology Review it confirms that 4 instances of probable transfusion transmitted infection have been identified. It concludes that the identification of these cases together with the fact that 2 of the cases were associated with a common blood donor 'establishes beyond reasonable doubt that blood transfusion is a transmission route for vCJD'.

6.15 At the 2011 NATA Conference in Dublin, Dr Stone of the Dudley Group of NHS Hospitals submitted a compelling poster relating to surgery on a patient who had a healthy pre-operative Hb of 15.3g/dl which should have given a wide margin of safety for that particular procedure. The operating team ran into serious trouble with a major bleed and then a further operation for evacuation of a clot resulted in a drop of Hb to a mere 3.2g/dl. However this was successfully treated with a regimen of iron and EPO and she was salvaged from what had been a life-threatening situation. That report provides another piece of evidence-based data on transfusion thresholds.

6.16 At the 2012 NATA conference in Copenhagen, there was a spirited discussion demonstrating the two extremes on this crucial issue of transfusion threshold. On the one hand was a presentation from a well-known practitioner from the US, a country where the practice of medicine is a multi-billion dollar operation with virtually every known treatment modality available (albeit at a price). He cited references from professional journals and his very strong emphasis was on 'evidence-based medicine'. He was prepared to accept a conservative transfusion regime that provided for a threshold of 8g/dl and in extreme cases 7g/dl but was scathing of and totally resistant to any suggestion that a patient could or should be treated at a level any lower without transfusion of allogeneic blood.

6.17 At the other end of the spectrum there was firstly a poster from practitioners at two state hospitals in Nigeria entitled 'The challenges of meeting the future of blood transfusion requirements in Sub-Sahara Africa: the need for developments of alternatives to allogeneic blood'. The following extracts are of particular relevance:

> 'This paper focuses on challenges of meeting the future blood transfusion requirements in Africa, a continent associated with the predominance of family replacement and commercially remunerated blood donors rather than regular benevolent, non-remunerated donors who give blood out of altruism…
>
> Concerns about adverse effects of allogeneic blood transfusion should prompt the review of transfusion practices and justify the need to search for transfusion alternatives to decrease or avoid the use of allogeneic blood. These strategies should include the correction of anaemia using pharmacological measures, use of antifibrinolytics to prevent bleeding and the use of erythropoietin, oral and intravenous iron to treat anaemia and use of non-pharmacological measures; preoperative autologous donation and perioperative red cell blood salvage and nomothermia to reduce blood loss in surgical patients. This will help optimize the use of the limited blood stocks'.

The second part of the discussion came from a Nigerian surgeon who was advocating precisely that which the poster had summarised: the avoidance of the use of allogeneic blood. He went further and argued cogently for avoiding having an arbitrary or fixed transfusion threshold but allowing the Hb to drop to any level so long as there were vital signs of the patient responding to treatment. It was not unknown for patients to walk into clinic and their Hb later to be established at 3.5-4g d/l. Regrettably his logical arguments, based on practical experience in a difficult medical environment presenting challenges of patients with levels of Hb almost unheard of in the US, were treated with derision and disdain as not being 'evidence-based'.

6.18 The post script to this discussion was provided at an informal meeting after the formal sessions of the conference had closed. An experience was related of a female patient aged 31 in a European country who returned to have her second baby at the hospital that had safely delivered her first child. Post-delivery she had placenta problems, started to bleed and her Hb dropped to 5g/dl. On the 8th day post-delivery she sustained a massive blood loss. Her Hb dropped to 2.4g/dl, and within a couple of days further dropped to a level that could not even be measured. In the meantime there had been a change of doctor in the ICU who was willing to consult with a professor from Australia who had extensive experience in non-blood management. The same day the patient was started on EPO and high dose *Ferinject*®. Her Hb recovered sufficiently that 23 days later she was discharged home with an Hb of 7.2g/dl having received no blood. She made a full recovery.

6.19 Unfortunately the findings of the *Viele & Weiskopf* study of 1994 and single case reports such as this do not fit the preconception of evidence-based medicine which looks for studies based on large numbers. But the fact remains that there does exist a substantial body of evidence (some professionally documented and some admittedly anecdotal) of survival well below what are regarded in western countries as conventional thresholds for transfusion.

6.20 Thus there does not appear to be any firmly established evidence-based threshold, recognised as such by the profession, at which transfusion *must* be performed for survival.

Chapter Seven

Obstetrics

7.1 It may well be stating the obvious but it is important to bear in mind in the context of non-blood management, that pregnancy is not of itself an illness but a natural function of procreation by women of child-bearing age who should usually be in very good health. However most young married men and expectant fathers were probably unaware of just how risky a process pregnancy and childbirth is capable of becoming, especially *peripartum* or *postpartum* haemorrhage.

7.2 Maternal deaths are closely monitored (Confidential Enquiries into Maternal Deaths – CEMD) and it is readily acknowledged by all, professionals and laymen alike, that the loss of even one mother in childbirth is one too many. However there are those mothers who, even in pregnancy and childbirth, hold firm to their conscientious beliefs and choose non-blood management. Obstetricians, obstetric anaesthetists, haematologists and midwives are accordingly increasingly coming to terms with managing these cases without resort to donor blood. Their collective experience is being gradually accumulated and recorded in professional journals.

7.3 Until 2007 there had, so far as can be established, only been two published series in the world literature on the obstetric outcomes of Jehovah's Witnesses and these evaluated maternal morbidity in 332 and 33 women who delivered respectively in New York and Detroit. Due to the paucity of similar data in the UK a group of specialists in obstetrics and gynaecology, based primarily at the North Middlesex Hospital in North London but working with others from the Royal Free and the Stirling Royal Infirmary, decided to 'review the demographics and obstetric outcomes of Jehovah's Witness women in an inner city hospital and to evaluate the effect of refusal of blood on morbidity and mortality in those with peripartum haemorrhage'. The results of their research were published in an obstetric journal in May 2007[91] and are worth studying in detail. There is a strong emphasis on pre-delivery monitoring of Hb

91 'Obstetric care of Jehovah's Witnesses: a 14-year observational study' *Arch Gynaecol Obstet* (2007) 276: 339-343

levels and for remedial action to bring them up to acceptable levels to withstand a peri- or postpartum bleed; the benefits of good preparation including having cell salvage immediately available to meet the speed with which obstetric haemorrhage can occur as well as the potential for underestimating blood loss; and the need for urgent consultant input. The conclusion summarises the findings thus:

> 'Women who are Jehovah's Witnesses have a higher risk of maternal death from obstetric haemorrhage. However their refusal to accept blood transfusion or primary blood products must be treated with respect and dignity even if this decision may result in death. The antenatal care of these women requires a multidisciplinary approach, which includes effective communication, optimisation of predelivery haemoglobin, involvement of senior obstetricians and early aggressive treatment of haemorrhage'.

7.4 The article also sets out as an Appendix the Royal College of Obstetricians & Gynaecologists pragmatic *Care Plan for Women in Labour Refusing a Blood Transfusion.*[92] This offers serious, scientifically based guidance on a range of techniques and products all intended to assist a safe delivery of a healthy baby without resort to donor blood. For additional material on the broader welfare of mother and baby, the book 'Humane Perinatal Care' is strongly recommended reading. It is the joint work of Professor Beverley Chalmers who works at the Centre for Research in Women's Health at Sunnybrook and Women's College Health Science Centre at the University of Toronto, Canada. The other author is Professor Adik Levin who was formerly head of the Neonatal and Infants' Department at Tallinn Children's Hospital in Estonia. It was he who cared for the baby whose case history is recounted in chapter 15. He has since been a temporary adviser for the World Health Organisation; has lectured in more than 25 countries and published many articles and books. His humane and caring attitude to his patient and his unbiased professional conduct and evidence in the witness box in that case in Tallinn were impeccable and his views command respect.

Of perhaps even greater assistance to practitioners is the 3rd edition of the Managing of Obstetric Emergencies and Trauma (MOET) course manual published in June 2014.[93] This really sets the 'gold standard' in managing such

---

[92] *Royal College of Obstetricians and Gynaecologists (RCOG)* News October 2000

[93] *Managing Obstetric Emergencies and Trauma: The MOET Course Manual*, 3rd Edition, Sara Paterson-Brown and Charlotte Howell

emergencies and is recommended reading for all involved but especially for those about to undertake the MOET course itself.

7.5 This chapter addresses issues of general application to obstetrics and the specific problem of postpartum haemorrhage. It is important to recognize the priority of trying to avoid haemorrhage and its consequent anaemia rather than having to react to controlling it after blood loss has started. First and foremost is the role of healthy nutrition in pregnancy. The foetus is being nourished across the placental cord by the mother and so healthy blood in the mother will be reflected in healthy nourishment and growth of the baby. The importance of diet and especially adequate iron is dealt with in detail in chapter 4 but of all those most in need, expectant mothers are probably top of the list of priorities and natural oral iron should be a routine part of ante-natal care. Again the lack of monitoring of Hb levels is a profound weakness in many parts of our system of ante-natal care and experience suggests that too many mothers suffer from some level of anaemia, often undetected until they go down to the Delivery Suite and some crisis erupts.

7.6 One study already cited found 35% of mothers in the first trimester and a formidable 85% in the third trimester had significant anaemia. The role of the 'near-patient' testing device *HemoCue®* has already been discussed and the progressive development is recorded in an article in 2001[94] so it is by no means a new or experimental technique. The use of r-HuEPO in conjunction with Iron supplementation has also been discussed.

The simple objective is to ensure that, whether it is to be a natural birth or an elective (or especially an emergency) caesarean section, the mother starts with as high a level of Hb as is reasonably attainable given that she is additionally nourishing the foetus.

Sadly, this is an area in which many GP's and ante-natal clinics fall short of the ideal. However a number of NHS Trusts have begun to address the problem and have established, or are in the process of establishing, a Protocol for early monitoring for anaemia and action by EPO/Iron to raise Hb levels before admission for delivery.

---

[94] *Clin. Lab. Haem* 2001. 23. 91-96 Use of a new *HemoCue®* system for measuring haemoglobin at low concentrations

Delayed cord clamping

7.7 Even in a normal delivery, there are procedures that can provide extra sustenance to the new born. One study[95] at a progressive maternity unit identified the advantages of delayed clamping of the placental cord. The technique involves no more resources than time (which admittedly to the busy midwife may be scarce) and gravity. Immediately upon emerging from the birth canal the baby is held below the level of the mother for a short while (professional experience ranges up to 120 seconds) to enable the residual foetal blood to drain naturally from the mother through the cord into the baby before the cord is clamped. The process can be accelerated by what has become known as 'cord milking'. The concept of delayed cord clamping is simplicity itself but adds to the vital foetal haemoglobin of the newborn upon which it will exist until the process of haemopoeisis (or production of its own blood) commences naturally. Given the comparatively small circulating volume of the average neonate, this small but significant quantity of additional placental blood can fortify the oxygen carrying capacity, the clotting mechanism and the immune system; and justifies that little extra care being taken in delayed cord clamping.

The RCOG statement on the updated NICE guidance *Intrapartum Care* of December 2014, has given further emphasis to the length of delayed cord clamping:

> 'The guidelines also give clear advice on cord clamping and timing. RCOG guidelines state that the cord should not be clamped earlier than is necessary based on a clinical assessment of the situation. Delayed cord clamping may benefit the neonate in reducing anaemia and particularly the preterm neonate by allowing time for transfusion of placental blood to the newborn infant'.

RCOG Guidelines

7.8 Green Top Guideline No. 47 'Blood Transfusion in Obstetrics' is the second edition and replaces that of 2007. It is the defining source material on this topic and should be required reading for all those involved in obstetric practice and especially risk managers and hospital lawyers.

---

95 Wardrop et al. University of Wales, College of Medicine. *J Perinat Med* 1995; 23(6): 443-51 The roles and vital importance of placental blood to the newborn infant

Maternal deaths

7.9 The CEMD reports perform a valuable function in providing a focus for reporting and in collecting and collating information about maternal deaths. They are used to examine what went wrong and to make recommendations to avoid similar tragedies.

Additionally another research group, Mothers and Babies Reducing Risk through Audits and Confidential Enquiries across the UK (MBRRACE-UK) has taken the process a stage further and conducts a Maternal, Newborn and Infant Clinical Outcome Review Programme. The report dated December 2014 entitled 'Saving Lives, Improving Mothers' Care – Lessons learned to inform future maternity care from the UK and Ireland CEMD 2009-2012', provides helpful information.

In opening, it states:

> 'Obstetric haemorrhage is a leading cause of maternal mortality worldwide accounting for up to 50% of maternal deaths in some countries, while in the UK it accounts for approximately 10% of all direct maternal deaths…In England the recorded incidence of PPH has nearly doubled from 7% of all maternities in 2004/5 to 13% in 2011/13 (Health and Social Care Information Centre 2012)'.

7.10 The report sets out in some detail an analysis of various aspects of the problem and at §4.4 includes an overview of care and lessons to be learned that includes the following:

> '…In all the maternal deaths due to haemorrhage reviewed, potential improvements in care were identified which may have made a difference to the outcome. Improvements are most needed in clinical recognition of the severity of the problems and resuscitation techniques. In five deaths (28%) the administration of excessive uterotonics was identified as a key contributory factor'.

Surprisingly, the report displays one serious lack of perception, empathy or perhaps understanding. At §4.3 under the sub-heading 'The mothers who died' it says:

> 'Two mothers were Jehovah's Witnesses'.

7.11 This raises several questions, firstly as to why it was thought appropriate to identify two such deceased mothers by their religion when neither the religious beliefs, nor lack of them, was mentioned in respect of any of the others. Do their beliefs in fact add anything to what is supposed to be a clinical review?

Secondly it might have presented a more balanced and complete reporting if it had also mentioned that in both cases the ultimate findings were not merely that each had received sub-optimal care, but that the deficiencies amounted to clinical negligence. In each case the surviving widower sued for bereavement and loss of the wife and mother and their claims were both settled by the NHS LA with damages of several hundred thousand pounds for manifest and uncontested negligence. It would seem that one lesson to be learned is the timely provision of adequate senior and competent staff matched by adequate resources to manage such extreme cases properly.

7.12 A more recent report dated May 2016 is the Perinatal Mortality Surveillance Report to which the observations above in 7.8 equally apply.

Postpartum haemorrhage

7.13 This is probably the most alarming event for obstetricians and midwives, and all those working on the delivery suite. An early CEMD report in 2001 stated that, statistically, massive obstetric haemorrhage occurs in 6.7 per 1,000 deliveries. The difficulty is in trying to identify in advance which mothers comprise that 6.7 per 1,000. The pregnant woman who would be thought to be at the greatest risk is the one who is obese, often grossly so, smokes and drinks to excess throughout the pregnancy and takes minimal fresh air or exercise. Yet frequently she is the one who sails through delivery like shelling peas. By contrast, an expectant mother who is health conscious, watches her weight, does not smoke, limits her alcohol intake to an occasional glass of wine and takes regular exercise may turn out to be the one who sustains a peri or post-partum haemorrhage, often with perineal tears that need surgical intervention to stem the blood loss.

7.14 What has proceeded as an apparently normal delivery by the birth canal can, in literally seconds, turn into a life-threatening emergency. The mother sustains one or more tears and the blood literally gushes out at a truly frightening speed. The immediate priorities are to obtain clinicians of the greatest seniority and experience as can be made available (preferably consultants) to deal simultaneously with:

a) identifying the source of the bleeding and immediately suturing; packing and maintaining pressure on the site of the bleed;
b) the early use of a haemostatic agent Factor VIIa such as *Novoseven®* as appropriate;
c) immediate and urgent replacement of the volume of fluid assessed to have been lost;
d) if practicable and the mother consents, (or hopefully has consented in anticipation) the cell salvage and re-infusion into the mother of as much of her own lost blood as can reasonably be salvaged; and
e) the commencement of the process of restoration of the lost red blood cells with adjunctive therapy such as r-HuEPO and iron.

7.15 The key to this, confirmed in a succession of CEMD reports, is quality preparation, especially in the deemed high risk patient who has elected to sign a consent form that precludes the administration of donor blood. In the best units, these mothers have been identified early in their pregnancy so that even their ante-natal care is supervised by a consultant. In addition to procedures identified in the article from the North Middlesex Hospital referred to above, in at least one unit in an NHS hospital known to the author, a consultant obstetric anaesthetist assumes this role and whenever practicable is on duty for the delivery, in anticipation of this very risk. She ensures that full resources of non-blood management are readily available especially immediate volume replacement with the product of choice, whether colloids or crystalloids, simple saline, Hartmann's solution or Ringers Lactate. Additionally *Novoseven*® Factor VIIa as a haemostatic agent in available, if judged clinically appropriate in a given case. The third piece of equipment is the cell salvage machine with staff trained in its use if the model available so required. The benefits of cell salvage during caesarean section have been discussed in a professional journal[96] as far back as 1998 so again this is not some new or untested procedure. The routine use of cell salvage at the Royal Cornwall Hospital at Truro is but one example of best practice.

7.16 To many overworked and harassed obstetricians and midwives on a delivery suite in the NHS this combination of consultant input and resources

---

[96] A Rebarber at al. *American Journal of Obstetrics and Gynaecology* 179 September 1998 715-720 The safety of intraoperative autologous blood collection and autotransfusion during cesarean section

may seem to be the *Nirvana* of delivery management but it represents best practice and should be the aim. However, they should all read and be familiar with the cited article 'Obstetric Care of Jehovah's Witnesses: a 14 year observational study'.[97] This study was undertaken at the hospital in North London that is believed to have the highest rate in the UK of deliveries of high risk patients choosing non-blood management.

7.17 As a classic of its kind, the immediate emergency management of the patient *K*[98] in the case in Ireland stands as a model. Although most of the media attention to the case concentrated on the almost bizarre (and probably unrepeatable) circumstances leading up to the postpartum emergency and the arguably inappropriate legal process and manoeuvrings thereafter, the actual medical response was exemplary.

7.18 Firstly the consultant obstetrician moved rapidly to suture the significant tears from which the blood had flowed so profusely. He did this with great speed and skill, suturing the various layers, and then inserted a vaginal pack to maintain pressure on the sutured sites. To that he then added manual pressure that, in an outstanding commitment to his patient, he maintained for an hour. Simultaneously his consultant anaesthetist colleague administered volume replacement and Factor VIIa *Novoseven*® achieving haemodynamic stability in a very short time. In this case there was no cell salvage machine available and so the two consultants between them had to manage with what they had. Gradually what had undoubtedly been a life-threatening emergency passed and the patient's condition stabilized but at an Hb level of 5g/dl. This is where the medical opinion diverged. The consultant obstetrician, after nearly an hour of maintained pressure and no sign of continued or renewed bleeding, told the birth companion (who was also translating for the patient whose native language was French):

> 'You can tell your friend that she will be alright now. She will not need blood unless she has another bleed'. [99]

---

[97] N Massiah et al, *Arch Gynaecol Obstet* (2007) 276: 339-343 Obstetric Care of Jehovah's Witnesses: a 14 year observational study

[98] *Fitzpatrick & another v K*, High Court, Dublin Laffoy J. (unreported) Trial transcript and see chapter 17.

[99] *Fitzpatrick & another v K* op cit

7.19 At that stage it appeared that the combined and skilled efforts of the two consultants had achieved haemostasis; there was no sign of continuing bleeding; nor any clinical indication that she was likely to sustain another bleed. The immediate (and literally hands on) treating consultants believed that the critical life-threatening emergency had passed and that with further quality management no donor blood need be given. However, the Master, as the senior clinician in the hospital with ultimate responsibility, took a different view on the immediacy of the need for blood support; overrode his treating consultants and brought in hospital solicitors who instituted the court process that led to the non-consensual administration of donor blood.

The case of Emma

7.20 The tragic death of Emma after successfully giving birth to healthy twins inevitably attracted a great deal of media attention. Some of the reporting was measured and balanced but much of it emotive and some even bordering on the hysterical. The opportunity of castigating Jehovah's Witnesses for what was seen to be and reported as the wholly unnecessary death of a beautiful young wife and mother was apparently too good for some sections of the media to resist. 'Door stepping' and lying in ambush with long lens cameras to take pictures of the father and those caring for the surviving twins caused massive intrusion into the privacy of the grieving families.

7.21 Many of the key medical facts that emerged in the Inquest did not fit the emotive headlines or the way that the story was run and so never were reported. The old journalist's adage 'Never let the facts get in the way of a good story' is still apparently alive and well. Thus the record is somewhat different from the public perception.

7.22 Emma, aged 22, was a member of a large extended family of Jehovah's Witnesses. In October 2007 she was admitted, in good health in her first pregnancy, to the consultant unit of her local NHS Hospital. However as she was expecting twins it was a delivery that should have rated as high risk and been planned accordingly and been at least adequately supervised (if not actually conducted by) an obstetrician of consultant status. After an instrumental delivery carried out by a registrar of only one year's seniority, the same registrar undertook sutures for repair of an episiotomy and other lacerations.

7.23 Emma then developed a postpartum haemorrhage, causing a large haematoma to accumulate in the rectal area with significant pain. Only at that stage was the (locum) consultant called in. Taken to theatre for evacuation by him of the haematoma and repair of the residual bleeding points, she bled profusely down to an Hb of 2.2g/dl. In ITU this dropped to 1.6g/dl which was for all practical purposes on the facts of the case non-survivable and she died the following morning of cardiac arrest.

7.24 The following specific areas of concern emerged at the Inquest, summarised as follows:

a) Management of delivery of a known high-risk case by a registrar obstetrician of only one year's seniority;
b) the undertaking of an instrumental delivery (with its known increase of risk) by such registrar without immediate consultant supervision;
c) suturing of episiotomy and associated lacerations by such registrar again without any consultant input or supervision;
d) failure to put in place any or any sufficient monitoring of Emma on her return to the general ward despite the registrar noting (and signing) in her Operation Report 'concerns over haematoma developing';
e) delay of over 2 hours between first complaint of rectal pain (indicative of the development of haematoma) at 02.00 hours to obtaining the consultant on call and getting Emma down to Theatre and finally under general anaesthetic at 04.06 hours;
f) inadequately equipped theatre; for example a diathermy kit was not immediately available, compounding delay;
g) prolonged operation time extending the level of risk;
h) failure to use haemostatic agent recombinant Factor VIIa (Novoseven® available but not used) to assist in stemming the haemorrhage and establishing haemostasis; and
i) failure to manage the anaesthesia in theatre on both occasions at other than registrar level with no apparent consultant input.

7.25 Two significant matters emerged in evidence. To the astonishment of most of those present in court, the registrar obstetrician, when pressed in cross-examination about her own recorded note 'concerns over haematoma developing' and the acknowledged failure to put in place monitoring of Emma, resiled totally from the note. Although it appeared immediately above her authenticating signature, she claimed it was made in error and did not accurately reflect her ***then*** concerns over a haematoma developing, even though that was precisely the condition that developed and set in train the events that led to Emma's death. She offered no explanation of how such an error came to be made.

7.26 Secondly, the opinion of an independent expert had been sought by the coroner and the very senior and experienced consultant gave measured and balanced evidence. His main point was that the decision surgically to evacuate the haematoma was only one option. The alternative, and indeed his professionally preferred option, albeit coming to the case after the event, would have been to treat conservatively. Manage the pain; leave the haematoma undisturbed to contribute to the achievement of continuing haemostasis; then let the haematoma dissolve over a period of time. Given the need to avoid donor blood, the choice of the conscious and competent patient, it was the less invasive and the lower risk option.

7.27 There was also a legal point. The less invasive conservative option was never offered to Emma when signing the form of consent to the surgical procedure although the law, as now clarified by *Birch,*[100] says that the failure to offer it and to discuss the relative risks and benefits was of itself capable of being a negligent breach of duty. For the objective reader these facts may assist in putting the media reporting of this case into perspective.

7.28 However perhaps the final vindication of Emma is the outcome of the litigation. After several years, in early 2012 when the twins were nearly 5-years-of-age, the NHS Trust, after a number of expert reports into the overall treatment, finally admitted liability. They stood firm on the earlier events but ultimately conceded that it was the decision to take Emma down to theatre and attempt an evacuation of the haematoma where things had gone wrong. It was conceded that the procedure should have been discontinued much earlier and on that basis liability was admitted. The widower received appropriate damages but the primary outcome was the payment of significant damages to be put in Trust for the children. Regrettably the ultimate admission of liability and payment of damages and costs received nothing like the original publicity that caused so much distress to the families.

[100] *Birch v UCH NHS Trust supra*

Maher deceased v Pennine Acute Hospitals NHS Trust[101]

7.29 The case of Emma was followed in July 2011 by a case that bore remarkable similarities. The difference is that this case went to trial and resulted in a judicial award of damages of £375,000 against the NHS Trust. The headline to the case report reads 'Trust liable for death of Jehovah Witness despite refusal of blood transfusion.' The death occurred on 2 April 2004 and, for reasons never satisfactorily explained, the case did not conclude until 23 June 2011.

7.30 Mrs Maher was admitted to the maternity unit of her local hospital and was safely delivered of a healthy girl just before 6 a.m. on the 31st March 2004. The delivery was by caesarean section and the wound was closed with no awareness of the remaining haemorrhage. It was from a rupture in the posterior wall of the uterus due to a contraction against obstruction whilst the baby was still *in utero*. It was conceded by all concerned that the haemorrhage could not have been noted at the time of closure even with the exercise of reasonable skill and care. Thereafter, however, blood loss continued and went unnoticed. The records showed that whilst the transfer to the post-natal ward took place at 06.50, no member of staff checked the patient for 1 hour 20 minutes between 07.25 and 08.45, which the judge, Mr Recorder Hinchcliffe QC, held 'on any view amounted to an extraordinary lack of care.'

7.31 By 08.45 the patient was examined and noted to be 'extremely pale' and by 08.50 staff were concerned at the falling blood pressure. At 08.57 Mrs Maher was in pain and had operated her PCA (Patients Controlled Analgesia) 297 times with 22 effective doses. At 09.15 abdominal pressure resulted in a gush of blood from the vagina. The consultant obstetrician was notified of the situation at 09.15, but did not arrive until 10.25. Meanwhile a decision to transfer to theatre was taken at 10.15 and the transfer effected at 10.30. Even at this point Mrs Maher was able to give clear instructions that she did not wish to receive blood. Although she survived the operation she died on 2 April 2004 of multi-organ failure arising from severe blood loss.

7.32 Inevitably much of the claim turned on the midwifery and medical evidence. The judge preferred that of the midwifery expert called for the

---

[101] *Maher v Pennine Acute Hospitals NHS Trust (unreported)* Clinical risk 2011 Vol 17 No. 5 pp. 206-208

claimant. She suggested that medical staff should have been summoned by 08.21 at the latest. This was largely because the *Dynamap*® reading at this time was alarming since pulse had increased to 140 and BP had declined to 107/174. Staff should have realised by 08.21 at the very latest that a life threatening situation had potentially arisen. It was known that Mrs Maher was one of Jehovah's Witnesses and would not accept blood or blood products. The Trust's own Protocol stated that time was of the essence in such cases.

7.33 It was agreed by the expert obstetricians that from commencement of anaesthesia to stopping the bleed would have taken about 35 minutes. There were disagreements in the other expert medical evidence but the judge found that had a crash call been made, the latest realistic time for the emergency team to arrive would have been about 08.25. On balance, had the surgery commenced at 08.40 resulting in stopping the bleeding by 09.15, Mrs Maher would have had a slightly better than even chance of survival.

7.34 In addition to disputing the medical evidence, the Trust argued (unsuccessfully) that the deceased's refusal of blood broke the chain of causation. Neither counsel had discovered any civil authority on the point although there was a criminal case, *R v Blaue*[102] where one of Jehovah's Witnesses was an innocent victim who had been stabbed by the defendant and had died after refusing a blood transfusion. On appeal against his conviction for manslaughter, the Court of Appeal had held that no break in the chain of causation arose when the victim died as a result of such a refusal. Lawton LJ. in that case did not suggest that matters would be different in a civil claim.

7.35 In the course of his judgment Lawton LJ. had said:

> 'Counsel for the appellant … submitted that the jury should have been directed that if they thought the girl's decision not to have a blood transfusion was an unreasonable one, then the chain of causation would have been broken. At once the question arises—reasonable by whose standards? Those of Jehovah's Witnesses? Humanists? Roman Catholics? Protestants of Anglo-Saxon descent? The man on the Clapham omnibus? But he might well be an admirer of Eleazar who suffered death rather than eat the flesh of swine or of Sir Thomas More who unlike nearly all his contemporaries was unwilling to accept Henry VIII as Head of the Church in England. Those brought up in the Hebraic and Christian

[102] *R v Blaue* [1975] 3 All ER 446 at p. 450b—d and in Archbold Criminal Pleading and Practice 2015, Sweet and Maxwell

> traditions would probably be reluctant to accept that these martyrs caused their own deaths.
> As was pointed out to counsel for the appellant in the course of argument, two cases each raising the issue of reasonableness because of religious beliefs could produce different verdicts depending on where the cases were tried. A jury drawn from Preston, sometimes said to be the most Catholic town in England, might have different views about martyrdom from one drawn from the inner suburbs of London'.

7.36 In the case of Mrs Maher the judge held that, given that she was one of Jehovah's Witnesses, it could not be said that she was acting unreasonably in refusing a transfusion. The Trust knew of her religious belief and knew that she would refuse a transfusion even if the treating team were of opinion that her life depended upon it. The Trust had a Protocol to deal with the situation. Whilst the defendants were not responsible for causing the blood loss, they were responsible for allowing it to continue for such a time that the patient died. This conduct was a substantial and proximate cause of death. In the absence of a blood transfusion, death was inevitable. The Trust knew that no transfusion could take place. Accordingly there would be judgment against the defendants for the agreed sum of £375,000 plus costs.

7.37 The facts and legal issues were remarkably similar to those of the Inquest into the death of a patient who was one of Jehovah's Witnesses that occurred on 10 March 2009. It was not an obstetric case but the patient underwent, under local anaesthetic, a pleural aspiration by insertion of a needle between ribs. The treating doctor made 4 unsuccessful attempts at the procedure. In so doing he managed to puncture the spleen and left kidney but the internal abdominal bleeding went undetected. After a series of largely unexplained delays, compounded by poor note-keeping and an inadequate response to clearly expressed nursing concerns, an emergency developed and the patient underwent urgent surgery. By that time it was effectively too late and, although she survived the attempted remedial surgery, she died 3 days later.

7.38 At the Inquest in 2010, the coroner's findings included:

- 'a significant error in misjudging the site of the aspiration;
- elements missing from Dr X's notes including timings;

- nursing notes failed to note that the patient's blood pressure was dropping;
- a higher level of monitoring should have been established due to her beliefs;
- no hourly observations when the blood pressure fell to 90/47;
- delay in obtaining the attendance of a more senior colleague;
- survival chances would have been improved by appropriate management of her treatment and if action had been taken without the delays evidenced; and
- questioning the need to await the results of a CT scan before proceeding to emergency surgery'.

Although admitting negligence and liability, the NHS Trust tried, despite the decision in *Maher v Pennine Acute NHS Trust* cited above, to advance the unattractive mitigation that the patient was effectively responsible for her own death by refusing a transfusion.

Risk Management

7.39 An interesting starting point for risk management is the former practice in Babylon under the Code of Hammurabi c. 1772 BC. The consequences for the medical practitioner were in direct proportion to the outcome. Whilst there were substantial rewards for success, whether by appointment to a prestigious position or financial or both, there were severe consequences for an adverse outcome and on a sliding scale dependent on the social status of the patient.

7.40 Although unworkable in modern medical practice, it would undoubtedly concentrate minds and hopefully lead to the exercise of even greater care and provision of additional resources. The current figures for clinical negligence in obstetrics are less than encouraging. The NHS moved from Professional Indemnity Insurance, for which the individual practitioners formerly paid the premiums, to a centralised fund for meeting claims. It now has a Litigation Authority which maintains its own risk management team and accordingly keeps fairly detailed statistics. In the period from April 1995 to 31 July 2012, just over 17 years, there were 8,311 claims in obstetrics in the UK. Nearly 39% of these claims have been successfully resisted without any damages being paid. Conversely, 41.6% of such claims resulted in payments of damages. Unlike some other jurisdictions the '*loser pays the costs*' rule inevitably inflates the total paid out but to July 2012 the total sum of damages and costs exceeded a formidable £743 million.[103]

7.41 Averages can be notoriously misleading especially where a couple of major but disproportionate claims significantly inflate the majority of smaller claims but, even allowing for that possibility, they do give an overview of the problem. Even working in round figures it suggests an average payout of the order of £9 million. The irony is that 40 or 50 years ago many of the babies would not have survived at all or not for very long. It is the very advances in critical and intensive care, both equipment and skilled staff, that is now giving life expectancies that can be measured in decades rather than in days or months. The consequences of longer life expectancies feed through into the awards of damages as the biggest single item for a seriously damaged baby is likely to be long-term 24 hour medical and nursing care.

7.42 What may perhaps make startling reading for many is the sheer scale of the problem. The figures are equivalent to approximately 478 claims per year. That is 1.3 claims per day or 1 obstetric claim every 18 hours. These sad figures convert to a claim in excess of a staggering £117,000 per day.

Taking at random one particular kind of injury, cerebral palsy, demonstrates the problem. The conventional way of assessing damages in these cases is to arrive at a lump sum up to the date of award or settlement. In 3 recent awards the lump sum ranged between £2.8 million, through £3 million to £3.875 million making an average of £3.2 million. There has evolved a scale of periodical payments that is stepped in line with increasing age and therefore costs of increased care. The lowest was £142.500 per annum to age 19 and £190,000 thereafter. The highest was £268,000 to age 11; £321,000 between 11 and 18; £370,000 from 18 to 21 and £387,500 thereafter. Assuming that child survives to 40 years of age, a prospect by no means fanciful despite the level of impairment, the total cost to the NHS is likely to be of the order of £19 million.

7.43 The common-sense question immediately arises:

> Does it not make simple economic sense, quite apart from common humanity, to increase massively the resources devoted to obstetrics and pay some part of these huge sums to the enhanced training and

[103] Figures provided by The NHS Litigation Authority

employment of obstetricians and midwives and the provision of state-of-the-art equipment that they need?

7.44 The most recent and authoritative decision is that of *Montgomery* discussed in more detail in chapter 9. In a case of threatened shoulder dystocia no advice was given to a vulnerable mother to elect caesarean section and such failure vitiated the mother's consent to a normal delivery by the birth canal. It rendered the treating hospital liable to damages for the catastrophic injuries sustained by the baby.

7.45 Sooner rather than later, someone at the top of the organisation may have to come to grips with a financial situation that appears to be no longer sustainable.

Summary

7.46 These reports from CEMD, MBRRACE-UK and others are carefully considered by the RCOG and recommendations set out for the profession. The Green Top Guidelines represent the most recent thinking of the RCOG and are authoritative documents.

The underlying problem however remains not with the recommendations themselves but whether the necessary funding can be made available to implement them.

Chapter Eight

Low Birth Weight Infants and Anaemia of Prematurity

Anaemia of prematurity

8.1 This is a difficult and indeed emotive area for non-blood management but, as in all other cases, it turns on the specific facts of each individual condition. The underlying problem is that precisely because of the prematurity, the baby's bone marrow has not yet reached the stage where it can replace natural wastage of red cells, especially when exacerbated by iatrogenic losses incurred through multiple sampling. Further, the baby's lungs have not developed to the point where it can sustain pressurized ventilation for prolonged periods. Although the use of surfactant and other adjunctive therapies has been tried successfully, it is frequently the case that the treating team will feel driven to override the parental choice of non-blood and therefore seek an order from the court. As the case histories in chapter 15 show, judges have traditionally granted leave to transfuse in these cases. On the other hand, the risks inherent in transfusing adult blood or blood products (especially plasma imported from paid donors in the US) into a neonate with potential suppression of the immune system are increasingly being recognized and the more progressive neo-natal consultants are more amenable to considering and attempting non-blood management in appropriate cases. The severe problems of TRALI are discussed in chapter 4 but they are made much worse when a pre-term or low birth weight baby is concerned, owing to the especial vulnerability of the under developed lungs.

Delayed Cord Clamping

8.2 The role of delayed cord clamping has already been briefly discussed in chapter 7. It is by no means a novel concept, as the leading study[104] in the UK goes back to 1995. In 2000 a team from the Children's Hospital in Munster,

104 Wardrop et al—University of Wales College of Medicine. *J Perinat Med* 1995; 23(6): 443-51 The roles and vital importance of placental blood to the newborn infant

Germany reported[105] a 'Randomised controlled trial of delayed cord clamping in very low birth weight preterm infants.' Their conclusion was:

> 'Delayed cord clamping of 45 s[seconds] is feasible and safe in preterm infants below 33 weeks of gestation. It is possible to perform the procedure at caesarean section deliveries and it should be performed whenever possible. It reduces the need for packed red cell transfusions during the first six weeks of life'.

8.3 Four years later a 'Cochrane' Review[106] reported:

> 'Delayed cord clamping for babies born early improves their health. In the womb, blood flows to and from the baby and the placenta bringing oxygen to the baby from the mother's blood. If the cord is left unclamped for a short time after birth, some of the baby's blood from the placenta passes to the baby to help the flow of blood to the baby's lungs. In the review of studies on babies born prematurely, delaying cord clamping for just a very short time helped the babies to adjust to their new surroundings better. Further studies are needed on longer delays to see whether this brings even more benefit'.

Also that author's conclusions:

> 'Delaying cord clamping by 30 to 120 seconds, rather than early clamping, seems to be associated with less need for transfusion and less intraventricular haemorrhage. There are no clear differences in other outcomes.'

8.4 In 2008, a report[107] of further development of umbilical cord milking of infants born at less than 29 weeks gestation concluded:

> 'The initial mean haemoglobin value in the milked group was significantly higher than in the control group…Milking of the umbilical cord is a simple and cost-free method that reduces the number of neonatal blood transfusions'.

8.5 In 1996, consideration was already being given to the (off licence) use of recombinant EPO in premature infants and discussed in a leading journal.[108] The topic was re-visited and approved in 2002.[109]

---

105 *Eur J Pediatr* (2000) 159; 775-777 A randomized controlled trial of delayed cord clamping in very low birth weight preterm infants

106 Rabe H et al. *Cochrane Database of Systematic Reviews* 2004 Issue 4 July 2004 Early versus delayed umbilical cord clamping in preterm infants

107 S. Hosono et al *Arch Dis Child Fetal Neonatal Ed* 2008; 93; F14-F19 Umbilical cord milking reduces the need for red cell transfusions and improves neonatal adaptation in infants born at less than 29 weeks gestation: a randomized controlled trial

108 *Archives of Disease in Childhood* 1996; 75: F65-F68 Blood transfusions and human recombinant erythropoietin in premature infants

Iatrogenic anaemia

8.6 In conjunction with the use of EPO, the concept of blood conservation to try and avoid transfusing premature infants led to greater awareness of the importance of preserving so far as possible the infant's own blood. The condition of iatrogenic anaemia became more clearly identified. That is where it is the actions of the very treating team that are inducing or aggravating the anaemia.

8.7 The first issue was the size of the sample being drawn off the infant for analysis. The standard haematology lab is computerized and the earlier system required a sample of a minimum size appropriate to adults. This was one of the problems in the *Baby O* case described in the case histories. Whilst the premature infant needed every drop of its own Hb, large quantities were being drawn off for each sample for analysis, despite the protestations of the parents. As early as 1991 the problem was being discussed by concerned professionals.[110] The answer was micro-sampling, described in a journal in 1998.[111]

8.8 Reducing the size of the sample was only one step. Reducing the interval between samples was another important factor. Even the simple step of sampling every 8 or 12 hours instead of 6 or 4 hourly can make a significant difference. The problem is to find the right balance between the treating team having the information obtained from sampling to enable them to address and adjust the treatment plan and, on the other hand, the need to preserve every possible drop of the infant's own blood.

8.9 An additional weapon in the armoury was the development of the new *HemoCue*® system for measuring Hb at low concentrations together with pulse oximeters and bedside gas analysers. One inevitable problem is financial but it is vital to ensure that every premature baby unit has these necessary resources. Just as important is the culture or attitude of being constantly aware of the need to preserve the baby's own blood.

---

109 *Transfusion Alternatives in Transfusion Medicine* Vol 4 No.1 February 2002 pp. 14-19 Management of the anaemia of prematurity using recombinant erythropoietin

110 *British Journal of Intensive Care*, July/August 1991 104-105 Anaemia due to blood sampling in critically ill children

111 *Bloodless Surgery Update* Vol 3 No 1 p. 4 Microsampling

8.10 Two studies one in Europe in 2000 and one in the US in 2005 highlight the benefits and techniques in reduction of red cell transfusions. In the first[112] the report from Denmark found:

> 'In our group of extremely early born infants we found a strong correlation between the volume of blood drawn and the volume transfused during the first three months of life...
>
> We found an acceptably low frequency of samplings, analyses and transfusions...From 1994 our NICU has carried out continuous registration of all iatrogenic blood losses in every individual infant. General awareness of this fact may indeed have diminished blood losses further'.

8.11 In 2005, a US study[113] reported:

> 'The mean volume of RBC transfusions decreased by 43% with use of the POC analyzer...The use of a bedside gas analyzer is associated with clinically important reductions in RBC transfusions in the ELBW infant during the first two weeks of life'.

Exceptionally low birth weight infants—ELBW's

8.12 Two outstanding examples are quoted (from among many) of what can be achieved given a competent team motivated to achieve non-blood management in low birth weight neonates. The first, back in 1998, is the case[114] of Chantelle Reyes. Born at 23 weeks and weighing a mere 1.1 pounds, the report described how she 'beat the odds and survived a premature birth without the routine blood transfusion doctors prescribed.' The use of micro-sampling and EPO featured prominently in the non-blood management of what is believed to be one of the youngest pre-term babies to survive in Canada and without blood.

The second case is that of *Baby C* described in more detail in the chapter on Ireland. In summary, the baby was born at 24 weeks and 5 days gestation and weighed only 750 grammes. The hospital sought and was granted a permissive order to transfuse but a highly skilled ICU team gradually pulled him through without blood being transfused. After 11 weeks in ICU he was finally

---

[112] L.P. Madsden et al—*Scand J Clinic Lab Invest* 2000; 60; 125-132 Impact of blood sampling in very preterm infants

[113] A. Madan et al, *Journal of Perinatology* 2005; 25: 21-25 Reduction in Red Cell Transfusions using a bedside Analyzer in extremely low birth weight infants.

[114] *'The Winnipeg Sun'* May 19 1998

discharged home and no blood was given. He is now thriving and catching up on weight with his contemporary full term babies.

Rhesus incompatibility

8.13 Although the use of anti-D in western medical practice is reducing the incidence of Rhesus incompatibility, when this does arise the complications to the foetus can be significant and even fatal. There are still reported cases of severe complications not merely of raised bilirubin levels but even of *hydrops foetalis.*

The basic concept is the incompatibility of the Rhesus positive and negative factors between the mother and father that sets up potential conflict between mother and foetus. The key consequence is the raised level of bilirubin in the child's blood, known as *hyperbilirubinaemia.* It is this raised bilirubin level that creates the jaundice and the very real fear is of kernicterus—a staining and consequent damage of the brain by the bile pigment bilirubin. Immature brain cells in the basal ganglia are affected, usually irreversibly. As brain development progresses a pattern of cerebral palsy emerges, usually at about 6 months of age. This results in uncoordinated movements, deafness, disturbed vision and feeding and speech difficulties. The advanced stage includes *hydrops foetalis,* which is likely to be fatal. Bilirubin can be tolerated up to a known level in the newborn but, once the level crosses a certain predetermined level, the practice had been to carry out exchange transfusion.

The most effective treatment is ultraviolet phototherapy which speeds up the process of breaking down the bilirubin and excreting its detritus through the gut. This has now been developed to multi-lamp procedures whereby virtually the entire body of the infant is continuously exposed to the lamps. It has also been demonstrated that charcoal by mouth can be beneficial, as it binds to the bilirubin and expedites its excretion. The technique of plasmapheresis has also been developed to deal with the more severe and intractable cases.

8.14 Many of the technical aspects of managing this condition are outside the scope of this work. Suffice it to say that non-blood management of the condition in babies of parents who choose such treatment is established. The case histories recount the successful treatment of the baby born to the mother whilst awaiting trial in Estonia for allegedly causing the death of her earlier baby, a charge of which she was ultimately acquitted. Also, the case in Dublin where a precautionary court order was obtained but no transfusion ever used.

Chapter Nine

The Right of the Competent Patient

A paradigm shift from medical paternalism to informed choice

'The greatest dangers to liberty lurk in insidious encroachment by men of zeal, well-meaning but without understanding.'[115]

9.1 The right of the competent adult patient to exercise choice in medical treatment has over many years increasingly engaged medical practitioners, ethics committees, risk managers, lawyers and the courts. In Part A of this chapter the author identifies the fundamental principles of the right to choose how we live, the legal status of patients and their right to choose their treatment options in those countries whose jurisprudence is based on the common law. Similarly, he reviews the basic principles discernible in the European systems of codified law and the common ground throughout the 47 Member States who are now High Contracting parties to the European Convention on Fundamental Rights and Freedoms (the Convention). In Part B he outlines the paradigm shift on disclosure that has taken place from medical paternalism to informed patient choice

Part A: The early position at Common Law

9.2 The common law approach has always been that man is born free and entitled to hold any beliefs and engage in any conduct subject only to the constraints placed upon him by such laws as are necessary for the common good in a civilised society.[116] This philosophy finds its overt expression in the common law approach to and regulation of the rights of the patient compared with the duties and responsibilities of the medical profession.

9.3 The broad expression of freedom referred to above was confirmed by the eminent Professor Glanville Williams QC, Professor of Criminal Law at Cambridge University who wrote:[117]

---

[115] *Olmstead v US* 277 US 472 at 479 (1927) *per* Justice L Brandeis
[116] *Entick v Carrington* (1765) 19 St TR. 1030
[117] Glanville Williams, *Textbook on Criminal Law*

'The general principle of English law is that things may not be done to a person without his consent merely on the ground that they are done for his benefit: we are to be protected from busybodies who think they know what is good for us better than we ourselves. In adopting this principle the law is simply giving effect to the libertarian philosophy expounded by John Stuart Mill:

> "The sole end for which mankind are warranted, individually or collectively, in interfering with the liberty of action of any of their number, is self-protection ... The only purpose for which power can be rightfully exercised over any member of a civilised community, against his will, is to prevent harm to others.
>
> His own good, either physical or moral, is not a sufficient warrant. He cannot rightfully be compelled to do or forbear because it will be better for him to do so; because it will make him happier; because, in the opinion of others, to do so would be wise or even right. These are good reasons for remonstrating with him, or reasoning with him, or persuading him, or entreating him, but not for compelling him, or visiting him with evil in case he do otherwise. To justify that, the conduct from which it is desired to deter him must be calculated to produce evil to someone else.
>
> The only part of the conduct of anyone, for which he is amenable to society, is that which concerns others. In the part which merely concerns himself his independence is, of right, absolute. Over himself, over his own body and mind, the individual is sovereign...
>
> The only freedom which deserves the name is that of pursuing our own good in our own way so long as we do not attempt to deprive others or impede their efforts to obtain it. Each is the proper guardian of his own health, whether bodily, or mental and spiritual"'.[118]

9.4 Some 73 years ago a judge of the Supreme Court of one of the States in the US in a case involving freedom of conscience and worship said:[119]

> 'Freedom of conscience is much older than the Declaration of Rights or the common law. Peter and John first invoked it when they were commanded by the High Priest and the Roman rulers to speak and teach no more in the name of God. (Acts 4:17-21). So the soil from which it springs like many other cherished precepts of the common law reach back to Hebrew origin and historically reveal why a free press, speech and religion are in a preferred class, protected by the State and Federal Constitutions and immunized from charge by the State'.

---

[118] *On Liberty* [1859] Chapter 1 Everyman Edition pp. 72-73; 75
[119] *Singleton v Woodruff, Chief of Police* 153 Fla. 84, 13 S. 2d 704 1943

9.5 The choice of non-blood treatment as made by Jehovah's Witnesses and others is, accordingly, primarily a matter of religious conscience. It is this freedom of conscience, firmly founded in the Judeo-Christian and humanist traditions, to choose how we live that has driven the law and the common law judges when the issue of patient choice in medical treatment has come before them.

9.6 However, in the jurisprudence the starting point for most common lawyers is the classic dictum of Cardozo J. in a US case as far back as 1914:[120]

> 'Every human being of adult years and sound mind has a right to determine what shall be done with his own body; and a surgeon who performs an operation without his patient's consent commits an assault for which he is liable in damages'.

9.7 The more generous tort litigation culture in the US means that the medical negligence cases are brought there with jury awards in what would be regarded in the UK as massive sums, including punitive damages, disproportionate to the actual negligence or loss. Grisham's writings are not all fiction. Medical litigation in the UK has been much more conservative. The most blatant and indefensible claims were usually settled discreetly by the medical insurers, often with a confidentiality clause to protect the reputation of the doctor and hospital. Others were fought with the full range of medical and legal expertise available to the defendants through bodies such as the Medical Defence Union or Medical Protection Society. Later for the NHS that responsibility was taken over by the NHS Litigation Authority (NHSLA).

Fundamental principles of consent

9.8 Dr Leahy Taylor, the very experienced former Secretary of the Medical Protection Society, in his seminal work 'The Doctor and the Law' published in 1982 expressed the principles with clarity and simplicity:

> '... it is an assault to carry out any examination or treatment which involves laying a finger on the patient without consent...'.[121]

[120] *Schloendorff v Society of New York Hospital* [1914] 105 NE 92 at p. 93

[121] Leahy Taylor, J. MB, BS, DMJ, MRCGP (Secretary of The Medical Protection Society) *The Doctor and the Law* (1982) 2nd Edition—Pitman

Notably, such consent was not qualified by any requirement for the secondary consent of a relative or proxy. The competent patient alone had the right to decide. That has been the official view of the MPS for the past 34 years.

Legal right to patient autonomy and bodily integrity

9.9 The starting point for consideration of the legal relationship between doctor and patient and the principles of consent must surely be the Hippocratic Oath and especially the guiding principle *Primum non nocere.* As the great nurse Florence Nightingale so famously wrote in 1859:

> '[...] a Hospital [...] should do the sick no harm'. [122]

Harm in this context may mean amputating the wrong limb; removing the sound instead of the diseased organ; sewing up and leaving clamps or swabs inside the patient; giving the right treatment but to the wrong patient or the right drug in the wrong dosage; and similar obvious harm which is well documented in the medico-legal case law. But harm can extend beyond those examples. Treatment without consent, of a kind to which the patient objects and finds repugnant to his/her conscience, is capable of causing egregious harm.

9.10 As Binnie J. an experienced judge of the Supreme Court of Canada said in a leading case [123] involving a mature minor:

> 'Forced medical procedures must be one of the most egregious violations of a person's physical and psychological integrity against the will of an individual...'

9.11 The definitive judicial ruling stated above came in the US in 1914, now over 100 years ago. The cumulative case law in England and elsewhere has reasserted these principles summarised by Butler-Sloss LJ in the leading case of *MB* in 1997:

> 'A mentally competent patient has an absolute right to refuse to consent to medical treatment for any reason, rational or irrational, or for no reason at all, even where that decision may lead to his or her own death'. [124]

9.12 It is important not to confuse a patient's decision that the doctor may personally think is irrational with a clinical diagnosis of lack of capacity. Many authorities have pointed out that doctors generally (and paternalistically) view a

---

122 *Notes on Hospitals*—Florence Nightingale 1859
123 *AC v. Manitoba* (2009) SCC 30—6 June 2009
124 *re MB (Medical Treatment*) [1997] 2 FLR 426 per Butler-Sloss LJ at 432

patient's agreement with their recommendations as demonstrating capacity, and only question capacity in the event of refusal. For example Devereux, Jones and Dickinson writing in the BMJ in 1993 observed:

> 'Many medical ethicists have commented wryly on the catch 22 by which patients whose competence is in doubt will be found rational if they **accept** the doctor's proposal but incompetent if they **reject** professional advice ...'.[125, 126]

The fundamental premise is that treatment recommended by a doctor is *prima facie* in the patient's best medical interests, and therefore in his best interests judged objectively. It is then posited that a competent patient will consent to whatever is in his objective best interests. Devereux, Jones and Dickinson continue:

> 'This assumes two debatable points: that the doctor is right about what is in the patient's best interests and that treating the patient even without the patient's consent will still help the patient.'[127] Such assumptions, in effect, allow practitioners to do whatever they wish to an unresisting patient, irrespective of his true capacity to make decisions, or lack of it. It is submitted that such a position is unwarranted when patients may lawfully refuse treatment "for reasons which are rational, or irrational, or for no reason"'.[128]

As it was put by one judge in the leading case on Advance Directives:[129]

> 'The patient has the right to be wrong'.

The Protocol issued by the Royal College of Surgeons specifically says regarding one group of patients who choose non-blood management:

> 'This is a deeply-held core value and they regard a non-consensual transfusion as a gross physical violation'.

The scope of consent

9.13 The case of *re C* in 1994 shows how even a psychiatric patient detained in a Special Hospital such as Broadmoor and *prima facie* lacking psychiatric

---

125 See, for example, Devereux, Jones & Dickenson 'Can Children Withhold Consent to Treatment?' (1993) 306 BMJ 1459

126 The matter of a manifestly incompetent but compliant patient was considered in *R v Bournewood Community and Mental Health NHS Trust ex parte L* [1998] 3 WLR 107 (HL)

127 *ibid*

128 *Sidaway v. Governors of Bethlem Royal Hospital* [1985] AC 871 *per* Lord Templeman at 904 F, compare *In re T (Adult: Refusal of Treatment)* [1992] 3 WLR 782 (CA) at 786 note above

129 *Malette v Shulman* 1990 67 DLR (4th) 321: Supreme Court of Ontario

competence may nonetheless have capacity to choose his treatment in certain circumstances. He was aged 69; undoubtedly a dangerous schizophrenic, having stabbed his former girlfriend which led to his detention in a secure hospital. He suffered, amongst other psychiatric symptoms, florid delusions that he was an eminent world class surgeon of exceptional and outstanding ability. In evidence to the Judge he expressed the grandiose delusions of an international career in medicine during the course of which he had never lost a patient.

Many readers may be familiar with some surgeons like that - far from being detained in a psychiatric institution, they are busily engaged in operating theatres in hospitals around the country, firmly convinced that they are surgeons of exceptional and outstanding ability!

In a case in 2007 challenging the Medical Defence Union[130] over refusal to continue insurance cover, a very experienced judge referred to some such doctors thus:

> '... the so-called benign incompetents (long on bedside manner, charm and communication skills but short on clinical skills) ...'

The reader can rest assured that the medical profession is not alone in having 'benign incompetents'. We at the Bar have our share and some are even Judges!

Part B: The progression of the law on the duty of disclosure

9.14 So having set the scene on consent generally, it might be helpful to consider consent and disclosure, as now decided by *Montgomery*, in its context, taking a brief look at where the law started, some of the significant cases along the way; then look in more detail at the decision in *Montgomery;* and finally some thoughts on its practical impact and how it may affect the work of clinical negligence claimant lawyers and NHS defence lawyers.

The case law shows just how far there has been a progressive yet paradigm shift from medical paternalism (*Doctor knows best*) to patient choice. This has mainly involved a progressive development of the law on the duty on the treating doctor to make full, frank and honest disclosure to the patient of relevant information as to risks and benefits and also available alternatives so

[130] *J v Medical Defence Union* [2007] EWCA Civ 262

that the patient has the fullest available information upon which to base his or her choice.

9.15 A starting point is a little known case from 1954,[131] reported only in *The Times* of London but not in the official law reports, that sets the scene. The patient brought a claim against her surgeon and the prestigious Barts' Hospital, based on negligence, alleging additionally absence of true consent and therefore non-consensual and actionable medical intervention. The patient was a person to whom self-evidently her voice was of crucial value and was diagnosed with a goitre for which surgery was recommended.

In a pre-operative consultation with a very eminent surgeon, in response to a direct question from her about risk, the surgeon simply lied to her about the risk of the procedure to her vocal cords. When the risk did in fact materialise at operation, resulting in quite serious paralysis of the left vocal cord, the patient (not unreasonably) claimed that such conduct by the surgeon in telling her a deliberate lie vitiated any purported consent. At trial the doctor admitted he had lied but purported to justify it as 'he did it for her own good because it was of vital importance that she should not worry'. Surprisingly to many the claim was dismissed. This was clearly medical paternalism personified and an early attempt at what is now known as the 'therapeutic exception' that would be highly unlikely to meet the criteria for that exception today.

9.16 In those far off days medical cases in the UK were heard by juries. Following a forceful direction from the judge, who was manifestly against such a claim and remarkably deferential to the medical profession, the jury dismissed the claim.

This was Denning J. sitting at first instance, the same judge who in that same year had made the comments in *Roe v Minister of Health*[132] effectively deprecating and positively discouraging the bringing of complaints and claims against medical practitioners save in the most egregious and blatant circumstances. He had said:

> '...we should be doing a disservice to the community at large if we were to impose liability on hospitals and doctors for everything that happens to go wrong. Doctors would be led to think more of their own safety than of the good of their

[131] *Hatcher v Black and Barts' Hospital The* Times July 2nd 1954 QBD
[132] *Roe v Minister of Health* [1954] 2 QB 66 at p.86

> patients. Initiative would be stifled and confidence shaken. A proper sense of proportion requires us to have regard to the conditions in which hospitals and doctors have to work'.

9.17 Later, as M.R. in the criminal appellate jurisdiction, he was incredulous and refused to believe that officers of the West Midland Regional Crime Squad could have fabricated evidence on such a vast scale to convict four alleged IRA bombers in what became known as the 'Birmingham Four'. They served many years in prison before having their convictions finally quashed. But Denning obviously thought that it would be something approaching the end of civilisation as we know it for the court to believe the allegations of the defendants against the establishment.

This case of *Hatcher* probably represents the high water mark of judicial deference shewn to the doctor, the medical profession and the establishment generally and the low water mark of the patient's right to have all relevant information before making a choice.

9.18 It was followed 3 years later in 1957 by the landmark case of *Bolam.* The unfortunate patient in a well-known mental hospital in Friern Barnet, North London, submitted to electro convulsive therapy (ECT) which he alleged was negligently administered without due medication safeguards against the known risk of involuntary muscular spasm. He was quite severely injured.

The legal tide was still running in favour of the doctors as demonstrated by the classic direction (still to a jury) given by McNair J. the trial judge:

> 'The true test for establishing negligence in diagnosis or treatment is whether he had been proved to be guilty of such failures that no doctor of ordinary skill would be guilty if acting with ordinary care. A doctor is not negligent if he was acting in accordance with a practice accepted as proper by a responsible body of men skilled in that art, merely because there is a body which takes a contrary view'.

The court clearly placed the opinion of 'a responsible body' of the medical profession as overriding the right of the patient to be fully informed. Thus if the defendant doctor could round up enough fellow practitioners to say that what he did was acceptable practice in a significant body in the profession, he could be absolved from responsibility.

9.19 By 1960 the issue of actions for professional negligence, and its concomitant response of the medical profession in 'Defensive Medicine' was discussed in a pithy article by a Canadian doctor entitled '*Why do people sue their doctors?*' [133] He wrote in the Canadian Bar Journal:

> 'First and foremost is the very nature of medical practice itself. In a field of rapid discovery, the accepted treatment of today was risky yesterday and will be obsolete tomorrow. During the period of yesterday, the treatment was new and hazardous, perhaps experimental in the eyes of the court and few doctors would come to its defence. During the period of tomorrow it is obsolete, antiquated, proven to be wrong, condemned in the witness box and accepted as negligent by the court. It is only during the period of today that the treatment is right and proper and this period is made ever shorter by the rate of discovery'.

The practice of medicine in the UK had for years been conducted very largely on the basis of standard practice as laid down in *Bolam* but those wise and sensible observations from Canada do not seem to have had any serious impact.

9.20 In 1985 the then House of Lords carried out an extensive review of the doctor's duty of disclosure of risk in what became the leading case of *Sidaway.* They rejected negligence based on a failure to disclose a 1% risk. Scarman LJ's classic dissent is a masterpiece and has now proved to be not only correct but years ahead of its time. There followed a succession of cases, principally:

Chester v Ashfar, [134] mainly concerned with causation but contains observations about the duty of the doctor to warn of risks (in that case put at 1% - 2%) that the operation might lead to 'serious adverse result';

Pearce v United Bristol Healthcare Trust, [135] where the baby was over term; the consultant decided against a C-section preferring to 'let nature take its course' and await a normal delivery, but the baby died *in utero;* and

Birch v UCH Hospital NHS Trust where in a centre of excellence the standard diagnostic procedure was a catheter angiogram and there was a failure to advise or to offer the less invasive alternative of an MRI scan. Serious damage resulted from a stroke caused by the foreseeable dislodging of a blood clot. Quantum was agreed at £621,000. The claimant succeeded.

Each case was moving, however slowly, towards informed consent.

---

[133] *Why do people sue their doctors?* (1960) 3 Canadian Bar Journal, 222

[134] *Chester v Ashfar* [2004] UKHL 41; [2005] 1 AC 134

[135] *Pearce v United Bristol Healthcare Trust* [1999] PIQR p.53

9.21 In the meantime other well-respected common law jurisdictions were moving much faster than the UK in support of patient autonomy and the right to be informed before making a choice and giving valid consent.

i) United States

As mentioned earlier in the case of *Schloendorff* in 1914, the court had ruled in favour of the right of the patient 'to determine what shall be done with his own body'.

9.22 Nearly 60 years later (1972) in *Canterbury v Spence*,[136] the US court again had to consider the right of the patient to disclosure of information to enable him to reach an intelligent decision:

> 'The root premise is the concept...that every human being of adult years and sound mind has a right to determine what shall be done to his own body...true consent to what happens to oneself is the informed exercise of a choice, and that entails an opportunity to evaluate knowledgably the options available and the risks attendant upon each. The average patient has little or no understanding of the medical arts and ordinarily has only his physician to whom he can look for enlightenment with which to reach an intelligent decision. For me it is almost axiomatic that from this consideration springs the need, and in turn the requirement, of reasonable divulgence by physician to patient to make such a decision possible...
>
> Due care...may oblige the physician to advise the patient of the need for or the desirability of any alternative treatment promising greater benefit than that being pursued. Just as plainly, due care normally demands that the physician warn the patient of any risks to his well-being which contemplated therapy may involve'.

Notably the judge, in finding for the patient, said that it was 'almost axiomatic' that the patient should be given the information needed to reach such a decision.

ii) Canada: Reibl v Hughes[137]

9.23 In 1980 the patient underwent surgery that carried a known risk of stroke put at 10%. When that materialised, she claimed successfully against her doctor. The court drew a distinction between whether the doctor carried out the professional activities by reference to the applicable professional standards,

[136] *Canterbury v Spence* (464) F.2d 772) 1972
[137] *Reibl v Hughes* [1980] 2 SCR 880

which is a matter for expert medical evidence. By contrast, the real issue in the case was the patient's right to know the risks and that was not a matter for doctors' evidence:

> 'Expert medical evidence is, of course, relevant to findings as to the risks that reside in or are as a result of recommended surgery or other treatment. It will also have a bearing on their materiality, but this is not a question that is to be concluded on the basis of expert evidence alone.
>
> The issue under consideration is a different issue from that involved where the question is whether the doctor carried out his professional activities by applicable professional standards. What is under consideration here is the **patient's right to know** what risks are involved in undergoing or foregoing certain surgery or other treatment.' [Emphasis added]

iii) Australia: Rogers v Whittaker [138]

9.24 Ms Rogers was a teacher who had very deficient eyesight in one eye to the extent that she was almost wholly dependent for her vision on the sight in the good eye. It was accepted by the experts that, for the contemplated surgery to try to improve the bad eye, there was a risk of blindness of 1:14,000 and by conventional medical standards of that time considered an improbable eventuality. The patient asked about risks but was kept in ignorance. She underwent surgery to the deficient eye that not only failed but also caused her to lose her sight in the good eye on which she was dependent, rendering her blind. Had she been informed of the risk, she would not have had the operation.

At trial in 1992 it was shown that a very substantial body of responsible eye surgeons world-wide also would not have disclosed that risk. But the court held that for that patient it was a **material risk** which it was essential, as a matter of law, for the doctor to disclose. Her claim succeeded.

Gaudron J. said:

> 'Whether the position is considered from the perspective of the individual patient, or from that of the hypothetical prudent patient, and unless there is some medical emergency or something special about the circumstances of the patient, there is simply no occasion to consider the practice or practices of medical practitioners in determining what information should be supplied'.

9.25 The majority opinion of the court included the following:

[138] *Rogers v Whittaker* (1992) 175 CLR 479

> 'There is a fundamental difference between, on the one hand, diagnosis in treatment and on the other hand the provision of advice or information to a patient. In diagnosis and treatment the patient's contribution is limited to the narration of symptoms and relevant history; the medical practitioner provides diagnosis and treatment according to his or her level of skill.
>
> However except in the cases of emergency or necessity, all medical treatment is preceded by the patient's choice to undergo it...but the choice is, in reality, meaningless unless it is made on the basis of relevant information and advice. Because the choice to be made calls for a decision by the patient on information known to the medical practitioner but not to the patient, it would be illogical to hold that the amount of information to be provided by the medical practitioner can be determined from the perspective of the practitioner alone, or for that matter of the medical profession...
>
> Whether a medical practitioner carries out a particular form of treatment in accordance with the appropriate standard of care is a question in the resolution of which responsible opinion will have an influential often decisive role to play; whether the patient has been given all the relevant information to choose between undergoing and not undergoing the treatment is a question of a different order...'.

9.26 In 2003 Sedley LJ. in *Wyatt v Curtis,*[139] had to consider a case involving non-disclosure of a risk of around 1% that chicken pox during pregnancy might result in significant brain damage. He said:

> '...there is something unreal about placing the onus of asking upon a patient who may not know there is anything to ask about...an approach which requires the patient to question the doctor disregards the social and psychological realities of the relationship between a patient and her doctor, whether in the time-pressured setting of a GP's surgery, or in a hospital. Few patients do not feel intimidated or inhibited to some degree'.

At a recent medico-legal seminar chaired by an eminent LJ., he was somewhat critical, even dismissive, of the Australian ruling in *Rogers v Whittaker.* During the discussion that followed, a leading Silk got to his feet and said that, although it was not common knowledge, he had a glass eye. He would not contemplate surgery on the good eye even if the cited risk was as far out as 1 in a ***million***. Perhaps that puts in perspective how the individual patient approaches risk. It is a very subjective test.

---

[139] *Wyatt v Curtis* [2003] EWCA Civ 1775

The law of informed consent in *Montgomery* v *Lanarkshire* as decided by the UK Supreme Court

9.27 With the notable exception of the dissenting speech of Scarman LJ. in *Sidaway*, the UK clearly lagged behind the three other comparable common law jurisdictions quoted above. However the concept of medical paternalism overriding patient choice has now been rejected and finally laid to rest in the landmark case of *Montgomery v Lanarkshire Board of Health* decided by the UK Supreme Court in March 2015. The court upheld the right to autonomy and to patient informed choice. It set out clearly the duty of disclosure of risks and benefits and of alternatives.

This case brought to an end the 'paradigm shift' from medical paternalism (enshrined in the decision in *Bolam*) to the doctrine of informed consent. It has been a long haul and has had to work through several phases. *Sidaway* marked a turning point although (Scarman dissenting) the House of Lords still supported the doctor and not the patient on the right of the patient to information upon which to make the choice; *Birch* took the right of the patient a major step further in requiring disclosure of less invasive and therefore less risky alternatives; and now *Montgomery* has finally declared the law to be that of informed consent.

The Facts

9.28 The facts are instructive. It is well known in obstetrics that pregnant mothers who are insulin-dependent diabetics tend to have babies whose heads are of normal size and capable at delivery of passing naturally through the birth canal and the pelvis. But because of an exceptional build-up of tissue/muscle caused by the mother's diabetic condition they do tend also to have unusually wide shoulders so that, even if the head will pass, the shoulders frequently will not. A not unusual complication is the condition of *shoulder dystocia,* when the shoulder is too wide to pass and the baby becomes wedged. One consequence of this may be that the umbilical cord becomes trapped and compressed, thereby cutting off the vital maternal blood supply with disastrous and possibly fatal consequences for the baby.

It was described in the case by one expert witness (§9 of the judgment) as 'a major obstetric emergency associated with a short and long term neonatal and maternal morbidity [and] an associated neonatal mortality'. That description was entirely consistent with guidance from RCOG. Maternal morbidity is also increased: statistically in 11% of cases of shoulder dystocia there is postpartum haemorrhage and in 3.8% fourth degree perineal tears. The guidance advises that help should be summoned immediately when shoulder dystocia occurs. When the mother is in hospital this should include assistance from midwives, an obstetrician, a paediatric resuscitation team and an anaesthetist.

9.29 Hence on pre-delivery consultation with diabetic mothers it is fairly common practice for the consultant obstetrician to recommend delivery by caesarean section for the undoubted benefit and safety of both baby and mother. From a reading of the full judgment in the Supreme Court (which is available online on www.bailii.co.uk and highly recommended) it appears from several comments that the treating consultant may have been reluctant to advise caesarean section as she seems to have preferred professionally to achieve delivery in the normal fashion by the birth canal. There is additionally an inferential disapproval of those mothers who are sometimes described (often unfairly or inaccurately) as 'too posh to push!'

9.30 The mother came from a family with medical background where both her mother and her sister were doctors and she herself had attained a BSc. in molecular biology. She had worked for a pharmaceutical company as a hospital specialist and was described by the Lord Ordinary as 'a clearly highly intelligent person'. The importance of that background was that, had the true nature of the risks been adequately explained to her, she would have been quite capable of grasping the full significance and the medical implications and almost inevitably, in the interests of the baby, have asked for a caesarean section. But the same principles of supplying sufficiently intelligible information upon which to base an informed decision should have applied to a patient of little or no education or intelligence.

In addition to being a diabetic, she was only 5 feet in height and of fairly petite build. Even to a layman those simple facts start alarm bells ringing when considering a normal delivery. Additionally the consultant placed some considerable importance on the 'probable' weight at delivery. Ultrasound scans, from which the prospective weight is estimated, are notoriously unreliable, being only assessments of likely birth weight known to be accurate to plus or minus 10%. It is not a numbers game.

Another factor pleaded in the claim was the failure adequately to respond to cardio-tochograph (CTG) readings of foetal distress.

9.31 As Lady Hale said at §112 of the judgment:

> 'It was well recognised in 1999 that an insulin dependent diabetic mother could have a larger than average baby. This brings with it a 9 to 10% risk of 'mechanical problems' in labour, either that the baby's head will fail to descend or, worse still, that it will descend but the baby's shoulders will be too broad to follow the head through the birth canal and will therefore get stuck'.

As events turned out, (§22) 'during the 12 minutes between the baby's head appearing and the delivery, the umbilical cord was completely or partially occluded, depriving him of oxygen'. The consequence was catastrophic injuries including cerebral palsy and Erb's palsy with a significant claim for both the immediate damage and life-time care.

The Legal Arguments

9.32 The legal niceties turned on the extent to which there was a duty on the treating obstetrician to volunteer to the mother the nature of the risks of shoulder dystocia and to make a positive recommendation for a caesarean section. Clearly there had been some quite extensive discussion between the mother and obstetrician and the latter was aware of her well-established professional duty to give truthful answers to questions if asked. However, absent a **direct** question from the mother along the lines of 'Do you advise that I should have a caesarean section?' the court of trial and the appellate court had held that there was no positive duty to **volunteer** the advice.

At §58 the Supreme Court cited with approval the comments of Sedley LJ. in *Wyatt v Curtis* already quoted.

The Supreme Court Judgment

9.33 In reviewing extensively the development of the law on patient choice, the court considered in depth (§43-§49) the three leading cases already cited from the US, Canada and Australia. The court came down fairly firmly in favour of the right of the patient to have sufficient information to make an 'informed' choice and indeed a duty on the treating doctor to provide sufficient information to enable such a choice to be made.

The relevant core of the judgment is from §74-§93. At §81-85 the judgment makes some compelling points:

> '§81. The social and legal developments which we have mentioned point away from a model of the relationship between the doctor and the patient based on medical paternalism…'

At §89-90 the court makes 3 specific points:

i) whether a risk is material cannot be reduced to **percentages;**

ii) the doctor's advisory role involves **dialogue** with the patient. 'The doctor's duty is not therefore fulfilled by bombarding the patient with technical information which she cannot reasonably be expected to grasp, let alone by routinely demanding her signature on a consent form'; and

iii) the court specifically said that the '**therapeutic exception** should not be abused'.

9.34 The conclusion of a detailed and well-reasoned judgment is encapsulated in §87:

> '…An adult person of sound mind is entitled to decide which, if any, of the available forms of treatment to undergo, and her consent must be obtained before treatment interfering with her bodily integrity is undertaken. The doctor is therefore under a duty to take reasonable care to ensure that the patient is aware of any material risks involved in any recommended treatment and of any reasonable alternative or variant treatments. The test of materiality is whether, in the circumstances of the particular case, a reasonable person in the patient's position would be likely to attach significance to the risk, or the doctor is or should reasonably be aware that the particular patient would be likely to attach significance to it'.

There of course remains available the defence of the 'therapeutic exception' under which, in the reasonable exercise of medical judgment the treating doctor decides (exceptionally) that it would be detrimental to the health of the especially vulnerable patient to make disclosure to that patient, but as the court said very firmly at §85 that it 'cannot provide the basis of the general rule'.

9.35 In passing, it is interesting to note that the full court concurred in the leading judgment which runs to 105 paragraphs. In marked contrast, Lady Hale, with her usual crisp precision, in her concurring judgment reaches the same conclusion in a mere 11 paragraphs.

One telling finding is the interchange between obstetrician and patient at §114 from which Lady Hale suggests that there was a **moral** element in the decision of the treating doctor when it should have been a simple medical judgment:

> 'Whatever Dr M may have had in mind, this does not look like a purely medical judgment. It looks like a judgment that vaginal delivery is in some way morally preferable to a caesarean section: so much so that it justifies depriving the pregnant woman of the information needed for her to make a free choice in the matter…'

She then quotes with approval the *St George's* case and adds:

> 'She [the patient] cannot force her doctor to offer treatment which he or she considers futile or inappropriate. But she is at least entitled to the information which will enable her to take a proper part in that decision'.

Perhaps the judge's most powerful expression is:

> 'Gone are the days when it was thought that, on becoming pregnant, a woman lost not only her capacity but her right to act as a genuinely autonomous human being'.

Those are compelling words in support of patient autonomy and informed choice that should resound not merely around the world of obstetrics but throughout medical treatment generally.

9.36 Two points of comment. Because this was an appeal against dismissal of the claim on liability, there are no figures given for quantum. But for a damaged birth with injuries of this severity to the baby needing life-time care and not inconsiderable suffering by the mother, it must be a significant claim.

The second point is the quite astonishing delay. It is not of the magnitude of Dickens' fictional *Jarndyce v Jarndyce* but 16 years from the negligent management of delivery to the judgment of the Supreme Court seems manifestly excessive. Maybe they do these things differently in Scotland but it does seem a huge delay when the mother needed the money as soon as possible to provide proper care and facilities for her much damaged baby.

9.37 A further comment on the applicability of the GMC guidelines of 2013.[140] Additionally the NICE guidance of 3 December 2014 *Intrapartum*

[140] *Consent: patients and doctors making decisions together*—GMC 2013

Care: care of healthy women and their babies during childbirth includes the following:

> 'The revised guideline places a greater emphasis on patient choice creating a culture of respect. Putting patients at the centre of their care is of paramount importance and healthcare professionals need to support women in these decisions'.

For all practical purposes both sets of guidelines had already pre-empted the changes perceived as necessary, although technically the decision of the House of Lords in *Sidaway* was still a legally binding precedent. The point is now academic as the decision in *Montgomery* (although dealing on the facts with events that occurred in 1999) effectively replaces the old law and the guidelines are subsumed into the new case. Of course they retain their status as 'guidance' and do not have the same force as either primary or secondary legislation. However the court is still entitled to take into account whether or not the treating doctor has in fact followed the powerful and compelling guidance of the profession's governing body.

At §77 the court in *Montgomery* quoted from the 2013 guidelines saying, perhaps a little optimistically, that they are reflected in professional practice:

> 'Work in partnership with patients. Listen to, and respond to, their concerns and preferences. Give patients the information they want or need in a way they can understand. Respect patients' right to reach decisions with you about their treatment and care'.

9.38 In its 2014/2015 report the NHS Litigation Authority summarised the effect of *Montgomery*. The summary includes the following quote:

> 'It is very important to note that a doctor is under a duty to disclose "any material risks", as opposed to those risks which he or she thinks a patient ought to be told about. In other words, this is a recognition that paternalism in the doctor/patient relationship is no longer acceptable'.

This is significant confirmation from a compelling source that such paternalism is 'no longer acceptable'.

9.39 Time will tell, but *Montgomery* is not only persuasive but a decision of considerable authority that is likely to be followed in other common law jurisdictions including Australia, Canada, Namibia, New Zealand, South Africa and others that tend to take their lead from these persuasive courts.

The European Convention States

9.40 That is a very brief summary of the position in common law jurisdictions. But all 47 States that are signatories to the European Convention on Human Rights, with a combined population of over 800 million, have agreed to apply Article 8, the right to privacy and family life. Although there may be minor variations in the actual words used, this has been held by the European Court in a number of cases [141] to include the basic concepts of patient autonomy and the right to bodily integrity in line with the common law.

The judgment in *Montgomery* addresses the Human Rights aspects in §80.

The result now is that a large swathe of the northern hemisphere from Vancouver to Vladivostok has upheld the right of patient autonomy and decision making and adopted patient informed choice over medical paternalism.

Conclusions

9.41 What probably interests doctors, patients and clinical negligence lawyers is the practical effect the decision in *Montgomery* has had; is having; and how it is likely to affect future claims.

First and foremost it seems that little weight will henceforth be attached to the standard NHS Consent Form which will inevitably need revising. All involved know of cases where the form has just been placed in front of the patient with instructions to sign it, often unread and that has been done by a junior nurse or even a ward clerk; frequently just before the patient is taken down to Theatre; and often after administration of pre-medication.

9.42 A case[142] from 2014 in the Supreme Court of Namibia (a well-respected common law jurisdiction carrying considerable weight) involved the sterilisation by tubal ligation of HIV positive expectant mothers at the time of delivery by caesarean section. It was a government sponsored programme trying to minimise transmission of HIV to new-born, a major problem in parts of Africa. There was a carefully structured procedure for advance counselling precisely to ensure fully informed consent to sterilisation and that such counselling and consent was properly documented and certified **before** caesarean delivery and ligation. But in a country of limited resources almost

---

141 Notably *Moscow Community of Jehovah's Witnesses v Russia* ECtHR App No. 302/02

142 LM & Ors v Government of Namibia

inevitably corners were cut; much of the consultation was perfunctory or in many cases non-existent; and documentation (if made at all) reduced to a mere formality. Many young mothers had second thoughts after sterilisation and, with legal advice, brought claims. It was no real surprise when the expert evidence at trial confirmed the obvious: that consent after pre-medication or at an advanced stage of labour, when there was already much pain from uterine contractions, was in reality not informed consent at all and could not be relied on. The government was held liable for non-consensual sterilisation with quite substantial awards of damages.

9.43 Although in the UK the written consent form will still have its place as representing the culmination of the 'dialogue' and thus the final signed recognition and documentation of the patient's wishes, what will really matter is the oral discussion that preceded it. In future it is likely to record the outcome of consultation resulting in consent rather than the process.

Anecdotal evidence suggests that there is already a significant change in both the pre-operative consultation and more especially in note taking and record keeping. For fairly obvious reasons those taking the lead are predominantly senior clinicians in private practice simply because they have more time, better resources including secretarial back-up and probably better legal advice.

9.44 Firstly, much more time has to be allowed for the consultation at which the risks and benefits and also any practicable, especially less invasive, alternatives are explained to the patient. In private practice that time can be found even if it has to be paid for by the patient or insurers. But in the hard-pressed NHS experience suggests that consultation time is still restricted in the interests not merely of costs but of maintaining statistically the required through-put of patients and keeping the managers off the backs of clinicians. So it seems likely that corners will continue to be cut even here. Potentially another '*mid-Staffs'* fiasco is brewing.

9.45 Secondly, record keeping. In future claims based on inadequate or non-disclosure, what was actually said at the consultation (the 'dialogue' referred to in the *Montgomery* judgment and given some prominence) both by the doctor in giving advice on risks and alternatives and by the patient in expressing comprehension and exercise of informed choice, will be critical. The fallibility of human memory, especially of those working under pressure and with a huge work load, is well known and that most cases, coming to court often years after the events in issue, actually turn on what is recorded contemporaneously and proper note keeping. Many a defence fails on inadequate note keeping and faulty memory.

9.46 The result has been that some of the advanced practitioners, especially in private practice, have moved to contemporaneous digital recording of the whole consultation. In some cases they may not necessarily have the recording transcribed but keep it in a memory bank 'just in case'. One consequence is that there is no 'document' in existence to disclose.

That contemporaneous recording is what claimants and their lawyers will want to be produced in disclosure of medical records, whether under the pre-Action Protocol before proceedings or in the course of them. The NHS Litigation Authority may be vulnerable, for some time to come, on non-disclosure or inadequate disclosure of risk invalidating consent until perhaps successive significant awards by the courts force the NHS into changing their practice.

The NHS will in all probability be slow to make the necessary changes simply because firstly it is under resourced. But more especially it suffers from the general inertia, political involvement, and Treasury reluctance to provide extra funds to such a massive organisation in recognising the need for change; responding to it; and allocating the necessary resources.

Common sense suggests that priority ought to be given to obstetrics and to neurosurgery, the two classes of case presenting the highest risk.

9.47 The reverberations of the decision in Montgomery have been of almost seismic proportions as, in addition to the NHS and the Treasury, the medical and surgical professions seek to adjust to the changes. The Royal College of Surgeons of England has been one of those principally affected and they have drafted new guidelines[143] to take account of the changes in law and medical practice. The process has inevitably involved consultation with a wide range of bodies and individuals and that has taken time.

Although the judgment in *Montgomery* was given in March 2015 it has taken until November 2016 to finalise and publish the Guide. To some that seems an almost elephantine period of gestation but it does perhaps give an indication of the size of the task faced by those responsible for the drafting and approval

[143] *Consent: Supported Decision Making–A Guide to Good Practice.* Royal College of Surgeons Nov 2016

processes. The Guide runs to some 44 pages with two Appendices and is available online from the College. Most of the points in the judgment are covered in the above review in this chapter. But there seems to be one significant omission from the new Guide.

9.48 The Supreme Court set out the need for the 'dialogue' between patient and advising clinician and for there to be a record in detail of the substance of the discussion, especially the diagnosis, the proposed procedure, risks, benefits and alternatives. Yet no, or no sufficient, thought seems to have been given as to how this is to be achieved. The Guide contains express references to the acknowledged extra workload on the clinician and the additional time that will have to be found. And yet, at a time when the NHS is under severe financial pressure, there is no indication of extra resources such as longer consultation time and/or digital recording to enable these not only desirable, but legally required, objectives to be achieved.

9.49 In addition to these comprehensive new guidelines the opportunity has been taken by the College to update the guidance on treating those patients who choose not to have allogeneic blood. The new guidance '*Caring for patients who refuse blood: A guide to good practice for the surgical management of Jehovah's Witnesses and other patients who decline blood transfusion*' is believed to have been finalised and available in November 2016.

Both sets of guidelines should be required reading for all those involved in blood transfusion from donor selection through the point of collection, to storage and delivery, right up to the point of completion of transfusion.

9.50 But remember the wise words of H G Wells:

> 'In England we have come to rely on a comfortable time-lag of fifty years or a century intervening between the perception that something ought to be done and a serious attempt to do it.'

Until the NHS wakes up to the enormity of the task it faces and takes the necessary remedial action, there is certainly a strong argument that a purported consent, vitiated by inadequate information and/or non-disclosure of material facts or risk, will continue to represent a happy hunting ground for clinical negligence lawyers.

Chapter Ten

Capacity and Communicating the Patient's Choice

Advance Directives/Decisions at Common Law

10.1 In the context of the judicial re-assertion of the pre-eminence of patient choice the next problem is communicating that choice, especially when the patient is incapable, whether by injury, stroke, anaesthesia or other incapacity from expressing it personally. Hospitals were familiar with written forms of consent to treatment but case specific in elective procedures. However these self-evidently could not provide for the emergency situation. The answer was the written Advance Directive, largely pioneered by Jehovah's Witnesses.

10.2 The first real legal test of the validity and enforceability of such directives was a case in Ontario, Canada. The patient, Mrs Malette, was in a serious car accident in which her husband was killed and she sustained severe facial and other injuries. Upon arrival at hospital for emergency treatment the Advance Directive she carried was immediately brought to the attention of the treating team that was led by Dr Shulman. Shortly thereafter the patient's daughter arrived at the hospital and confirmed to that doctor that the signature on the Advance Directive card was her mother's and requested that he respect her wishes as thereby expressed. Although on express notice of the patient's wishes for non-blood management and the prohibition on using blood, Dr Shulman administered allogeneic blood.

10.3 Mrs Malette, represented by the formidable advocate Glen How QC (mentioned in the Acknowledgments), sued in assault and battery and won. In the leading judgment on appeal upholding the patient's claim the court ruled:[144]

> 'The question to be decided in this appeal is whether a doctor is liable in law for administering blood transfusion to an unconscious patient in a potentially life threatening situation when the patient is carrying a card stating that she is a

[144] *Malette v Shulman and others*—Supreme Court of Ontario, (Court of Appeal), [1990] 67 DLR (4th) 321; [1991] 2 Med LR 162

> Jehovah's Witness and, as a matter of religious belief, rejects blood transfusions under any circumstances. {p. 1}
>
> A competent adult is generally entitled to reject a specific treatment or all treatment, or to select an alternate form of treatment, even if the decision may entail risks as serious as death and may appear mistaken in the eyes of the medical profession or of the community. Regardless of the doctor's opinion, it is the patient who has the final say on whether to undergo the treatment. The patient is free to decide, for instance, not to be operated on or not to undergo therapy or, by the same token, not to have a blood transfusion. If a doctor were to proceed in the face of a decision to reject the treatment, he would be civilly liable for his unauthorised conduct notwithstanding his justifiable belief that what he did was necessary to preserve the patient's life or health. {p.13}
>
> Accordingly, I am of the view that the card had the effect of validly restricting the treatment that could be provided to Mrs Malette and constituted the doctor's administration of the transfusions a battery'.

The appeal against findings of assault and battery and the consequent award of $CAN20,000 and costs was dismissed. The judgment at first instance was upheld both on liability and quantum.

10.4 The Canadian case of *Malette v Shulman* fell to be considered in the British courts a mere 2 years later. One of the interesting features of the English Common Law is the way in which major precedent decisions setting the law for whole generations can be based on the flimsiest of facts. Perhaps the best known example is the House of Lords decision in *Donoghue (or M'Alister) v Stevenson.*[145] This Scots case is the *locus classicus* of negligence ('delict' in Scots law) laying down in common law jurisdictions worldwide what, for more than a century, has founded the fundamental test of negligence, namely duty of care, breach, damage and foreseeability. Although the law is erudite the facts are mundane and, more importantly, questionable. The simple allegation was that the plaintiff had purchased a bottle of ginger beer which she had partly drunk before realising that there was a decomposing snail in the bottle. Although the case went all the way to the House of Lords, there remains a considerable body of opinion that doubts the very existence of the allegedly offending snail upon which the whole edifice of the law of negligence has been constructed.

---

[145] *Donoghue (Mc'Alister) v Stevenson* [1932] AC 562

10.5 A similar question mark over the facts applies to *re T*. As the headnote shows, T's mother was one of Jehovah's Witnesses. Her husband had been uncompromisingly opposed to her beliefs and the marriage had ultimately foundered in divorce when the daughter was only 3-years-old. *T* had been brought up largely by her mother and taught the tenets and beliefs of the Witnesses for the next 11 years but had never progressed to the point of committing herself to that faith by dedication and baptism.

Aged 14 she left her mother's home and went to live with her paternal grandmother. She later formed a relationship with a (non-Witness) boyfriend *C* with whom she went to live and by whom she became pregnant. Thereafter she resumed a close relationship with her father, who was still bitterly estranged from her mother. At 34 weeks pregnancy she was involved in a road traffic accident and admitted to hospital. There her condition worsened. Pneumonia was diagnosed and antibiotics, oxygen and analgesics, including the narcotic drug pethidine, were administered. Her mother was very properly notified of her hospitalisation and condition and visited. During the afternoon, when only her mother had been with her, the patient stated spontaneously to a nurse that she did not want a blood transfusion, that she had been one of Jehovah's Witnesses and retained some beliefs.

10.6 Later that evening she went into labour and was transferred by ambulance a short distance from the general ward, where she had been treated for the post-accident condition, to the maternity unit where she was to give birth. Her mother travelled with her in the ambulance and was for that short time alone with her. And it was those two brief incidents with her mother that laid the groundwork for the erroneous inference of 'facts' upon which a major part of the decision then turned.

Shortly after the arrival at the maternity unit, the patient went into labour and required a caesarean section. The patient again said that she did not want a blood transfusion and was reassured by a junior doctor that blood transfusions were not necessary after a caesarean section. She then signed an elective procedure consent form specifically excluding the use of blood.

Sadly, but perhaps attributable to the effects of the road accident, the baby was stillborn. The patient's condition then deteriorated and she lapsed into unconsciousness. At that point the consultant anaesthetist felt it clinically appropriate to administer blood but was inhibited from so doing by the express terms of the limited consent form that the patient had signed.

Confronted with this dilemma, the father and the boyfriend decided to apply to the court for an order that would enable the unconscious patient to receive the recommended blood transfusion.

10.7 The full history of the emergency *ex parte* hearing late evening and then the main hearing before Ward J. is set out in detail in the judgment of the Court of Appeal and is recommended reading for the serious reader who wants the full facts. Suffice it to say that the judge did not hear from the mother by affidavit or otherwise. She had been served late at night by a process server with a large bundle of papers that meant little or nothing to her. She had no access to a lawyer and, being informed of a court hearing at 10 a.m. the next morning that she might but was not obligated to attend, she might as well have been told she was to appear on the moon. Her daughter was no longer living with her and, as she was fully entitled to do, had made her own decisions on her lifestyle and beliefs. Although the mother still loved her as her daughter, she did not feel that she had anything to contribute to the court hearing, by which time blood had in fact already been administered under the terms of the *ex parte* order.

The mother had no idea that it was going to be suggested that it was she who had raised the idea of refusal of blood and that she had exercised undue influence. She was never heard by the court, and hence never gave evidence that she visited her daughter at the hospital simply out of natural maternal concern for her. At no time did she, the mother, raise the issue of faith or blood transfusion and indeed it came as a complete surprise when her daughter told the nurse that she was a former Witness, still retained some beliefs and did not want a blood transfusion. The mother is adamant that her daughter volunteered this 'out of the blue' wholly unprompted by her.[146]

10.8 Consequently, the judge at first instance, in the absence of hearing anything from the mother, drew the not unreasonable inference that it must have been the mother who prompted the refusal of blood. Given the shallowness, or absence, of the usual strong conviction of a practising Jehovah's Witness and the other factors; *e.g.* her extra-marital relationship and

[146] Personal communication to the author

pregnancy inconsistent with the scriptural beliefs, her condition, the combined effects of the accident, still-birth and medication etc., the judge found that the decision to refuse was not safe to be relied upon in a life threatening situation and thus made the Declaration sought by the father and boyfriend that her signed refusal form should be overruled as inapplicable in the circumstances which had arisen.

And so it came about that one of the most important cases on consent to treatment in English law is founded substantially on an assumption of undue influence by the mother that, like the snail in the ginger beer bottle, is open to serious question.

An order permitting blood was made at first instance and the Official Solicitor on behalf of the patient appealed. The appeal came before a powerful Court of Appeal presided over by the then Master of the Rolls, Lord Donaldson, with two senior Lords Justices, Dame Elizabeth Butler-Sloss, (later President of the Family Division) and Staughton LJ.

10.9 The judgments contain some trenchant observations on patient choice.[147]

Additionally, Staughton LJ. said:

> '... The surgeon will be liable in damages if he operates when there is a valid refusal of consent... In Malette v. Shulman [1990] 67 DLR (4th) 321 a Canadian Court upheld an award of $20,000 to a patient who had been given a blood transfusion in order to save her life but against her known wishes. I doubt if an English court would have awarded such a sum; but the liability would exist'.

10.10 The issue of perceived or possible undue influence has not gone away. The Mental Capacity Act 2005 and its Code of Practice was intended to place on a statutory footing the power of the court to intervene and provide a safety mechanism to safeguard those who lack mental capacity in decision-making including as to medical treatment. However there seems to have been a *lacuna* in providing protection for those adults who do not meet the fairly strict criteria to demonstrate 'lack of capacity' as statutorily defined. The court has moved to fill the loophole by retaining the power to invoke the inherent jurisdiction. Two

---

[147] *re T Adult: Refusal of Medical Treatment* [1992] 3 WLR 782 at 786 D, G, H; 787 B, D; 796 A; 797 H—per Donaldson MR.

leading cases[148] highlight the difficulties and delineate the scope of the protection that the inherent jurisdiction can afford to vulnerable adults. The first related to protection against overbearing parental influence in arranging a marriage. The more recent case ironically reflects the court's concern to protect elderly parents from undue influence from an overbearing son.[149] But in the course of argument, and indeed in the judgment of the Court of Appeal, there are a number of references to *re T* which are all based on the questionable premise of improper influence exercised by the mother in conjunction with religious beliefs.

10.11 However, Staughton J.'s prognosis in *re T* on Quantum of damages has not been fulfilled. As a case in 2002 demonstrated, damages are not so limited.[150] An emotionally vulnerable patient was transfused against her wishes allegedly by mistake but in the face of a valid and applicable signed Advance Directive. The patient, on learning of the secret and unauthorised transfusion, suffered a catastrophic psychiatric breakdown. She sued for assault and damages for Post-Traumatic Stress Disorder and judgment was entered by consent on liability for assault with damages to be assessed if not agreed. The special damages were significant as her daughter had to give up work to care for her mother. The defendant NHS Trust paid into court £100,000 which was accepted with costs in addition. The case never went to trial because the payment into court was accepted but experienced counsel for the patient valued the aggravated damages at not less than £10,000.

10.12 A decision in 1994 demonstrated just how far the concepts of patient competence and autonomy in medical treatment had progressed.[151] *C* was a psychiatric patient detained for the protection of himself and the public in Broadmoor secure hospital. Despite the severity of his psychiatric disorder, he did have lucid moments when he had expressed very specific wishes on medical treatment, especially a profound repugnance and objection to the amputation of any limb. When he developed what was diagnosed as a life threatening gangrene of a lower limb, he stood firm in his rejection of the advised amputation. When the treating team made clear their intention to

---

[148] *re SA (Vulnerable adult with capacity: marriage)* [2005] EWHC 2942 (Fam)

[149] *DL and A Local Authority and others* [2012] EWCA (Civ) 253 (28 March 2012)

[150] *B v University Hospitals Birmingham NHS Trust* Leicester County Court reported in Journal of APIL, Vol. 11:6, December 2001

[151] *re C (Refusal of Medical Treatment)* [1994] 1 Family Law Reports 31 Thorpe J.

proceed to surgery, mental health social workers on his behalf sought and were granted injunctive relief preventing the amputation from proceeding. A very experienced judge of the Family Division ruled:

> '(1) When considering the capacity that entitled an individual to refuse treatment, the question to be decided was whether it had been established that that the patient's capacity was so reduced by his chronic mental illness that he did not understand the nature, purpose and effects of the proposed treatment.
>
> (2) The decision-making process could be analysed in three stages: (i) comprehending and retaining treatment information; (ii) believing it; and (iii) weighing it in the balance to arrive at a choice.
>
> (4) The High Court, exercising its inherent jurisdiction, could rule by way of injunction or declaration that an individual was capable of refusing or consenting to medical treatment and could determine the effect of a purported advance direction as to future treatment. Accordingly injunctive or declaratory relief could extend beyond present to future circumstances'.

What followed was perhaps a salutary lesson that not every prognosis of a fatal outcome is right. Denied by the court order the opportunity of surgery, the treating team had no option but to treat the gangrene conservatively. The felicitous outcome was that the patient recovered with his limb intact.

10.13 Just how far the principle of necessary consent has been further extended was demonstrated by a case of professional misconduct.[152] A female patient underwent anaesthesia for extraction of 4 teeth for which she gave specific consent. A well-meaning anaesthetist decided to administer relief for post-operative pain by diclofenac suppository. He appears to have fumbled the search for the fundamental orifice for insertion of the suppository, straying into the vaginal area, and when the patient emerged from the anaesthesia with her underclothes in some disarray and experiencing some unexpected sensation in her vaginal area, she formed the understandable (but erroneous) belief that she had been the victim of some improper sexual interference whilst under the anaesthetic. She complained to the Professional Conduct Committee of the General Medical Council who, whilst rightly on the evidence rejecting any sexual impropriety, upheld her complaint of failure to obtain informed consent and assault. In a ruling that impacted upon the profession, the anaesthetist (of consultant status) was found guilty of serious professional misconduct and

[152] 'A fundamental problem of consent' Editorial *BMJ,* 7 January 1995; 310:43-8

admonished. The Editor of the *BMJ*, apparently not lacking a sense of humour, wrote the article with the heading including the *double entendre* cited.

10.14 Given the plethora of legal authority and authoritative guidelines both from the Department of Health and from professional bodies, it seemed to many practitioners that the law was beyond dispute. However, in 2002 an NHS Trust refused to accept the wishes of a terminally ill patient (Miss *B*) to discontinue life-supporting treatment or (perhaps even more surprisingly) to transfer her to another unit where doctors were prepared to respect her choice of management options. And this was despite two consultant psychiatrists confirming to them that the patient was, in their professional opinion, competent. Left with no other option, she brought a case which was heard by Dame Butler-Sloss, President of the Family Division,[153] the same judge who had been concerned in the case of *re T* in the Court of Appeal already referred to.

With unerring precision the President put her finger on the fallacy exposed in the arguments advanced on behalf of the NHS Trust. This was to confuse 'patient's best interests', which was a matter of professional and ethical judgment of the treating doctors, with 'competence', which was the legal right of the patient to choose what treatment she would or would not accept.

10.15 In her cogent and compelling judgment the judge stated the following:

> 'It is ... important to recognise that this ... is not about the best interests of the patient but about her mental capacity. {¶ 12}
>
> There is a presumption that a patient has the mental capacity to make decisions whether to consent to or refuse medical or surgical treatment offered to him/her. {¶ 100 (i)}
>
> If mental capacity is not in issue and the patient, having been given the relevant information and offered the available options, chooses to refuse the treatment, that decision has to be respected by the doctors. Considerations that the best interests of the patient would indicate that the decision should be to consent to treatment are irrelevant. {¶ 100 (ii)}
>
> If there is no disagreement about competence but the doctors are for any reason unable to carry out the wishes of the patient, their duty is to find other doctors who will do so. {¶ 100 (viii)}

153 *B and an NHS Trust* [2002] EWHC 429 (Fam)

The treating clinicians and the hospital should always have in mind that a seriously physically disabled patient who is mentally competent has the same right to personal autonomy as any other person with mental capacity'. {¶ 100 (x)}

Risks/Benefit Assessment and the duty to warn

10.16 A key issue is the obligation to assess risks and benefits raised in a case in the Canadian Supreme Court at the end of June 2009, *A.C. v Manitoba,* a blood transfusion case involving a mature minor. The author submits that in the English jurisdiction the *Birch*[154] principle is similarly engaged. By this, in addition to best practice, the treating team were, as a matter of law, obliged to raise and to discuss with the competent adult, mature minor or the parents the risks and benefits of other treatment options. The *Birch* case put a special onus on the treating clinician to inform the patient of alternative (especially less invasive) treatment options and their associated risks and benefits.

10.17 It was a neurology case involving diagnostic choice. The patient was aged 55 with a history of diabetes, not well controlled. She awoke to an extremely severe headache, blurred vision and with her right eye inclined inwards towards her nose. Admitted as an emergency to her local district hospital, she was fortunate to be seen by an eminent professor of neurology who happened to be visiting as an honorary consultant. His view was that she was likely to have a painful condition known as 'pupil sparing right third nerve palsy'. In his experience the most likely cause of this condition in a patient with long-standing diabetes was occlusion of a small blood vessel supplying the third nerve, usually referred to as 'vascular third nerve palsy'. In his professional experience other possibilities (but less likely) were:

a) Posterior communicating artery aneurism which in this context was a bulge in the wall of a blood vessel behind the right eye, leading to the third nerve palsy. The grave risk of such a condition is that the aneurysm, or bulge, may suddenly rupture leading to bleeding into the skull and, in all probability, death.
b) Cavernous sinus pathology, a condition which affects one of the two sinuses on either side of the sphenoid bone. This is the bone forming the base of the cranium behind the eyes and through which the third nerve passes. The problem can be in the form of a tumour, thrombosis

[154] *Birch v University College Hospital NHS Trust* [2008] EWHC 2237 (QB)—Cranston J. *supra*

or infection which, if left untreated can deteriorate to the point of brain damage or death.

10.18 The treatment options in respect of each possible diagnosis were:

- posterior communicating artery aneurism—diagnose as a matter of urgency and, unless excluded, perform emergency surgery within no more than 24 hours;
- cavernous sinus pathology—treat as appropriate but with far less urgency; and
- pupil sparing right third nerve palsy—treat conservatively, the condition typically resolving in six weeks.

The key therefore was urgent confirmation of the CT scan upon which was based the provisional diagnosis and expressly to exclude the potentially life-threatening aneurysm. The professor wrote her up for an urgent MRI scan but unfortunately this was overridden by the consultant radiologist at the district hospital on the basis that, in the light of the CT scan, it was not urgent and there were no slots for MRI available there or at the two associated hospitals that had the facility. Regrettably this was a resource problem far from unknown in the NHS.

10.19 The patient was transferred to the prestigious National Hospital for Neurology and Neurosurgery, part of University College Hospital and known colloquially as 'Queen Square'. This is a tertiary referral centre of excellence with outstanding clinicians and staff. The decision as to which diagnostic tool to use then fell to be considered by those at that unit. Cerebral catheter angiogram was at that time the clinician's preferred invasive option with a known inherent risk in that specialist unit put at 1%. The non-invasive alternative was an MRI scan but, as subsequently emerged, the patient was never offered that option of MRI and so the relevant risks and benefits were never discussed.

Catheter angiogram involved inserting a catheter into the femoral artery and feeding it right up to the aortic branch and the wire onwards into one of the carotid arteries and then the vertebral arteries. It is inevitably a specialist procedure requiring a high level of expertise but it was acknowledged by all experts that it was carried out with proper skill and in accordance with the

Bolam/Bolitho[155] standards so no allegation of negligence was sustainable in respect of the procedure itself. The small but known risk materialised; a clot was dislodged in the procedure and the patient sustained a stroke.

The consequences to her were catastrophic and all the experts involved were later to confirm that it was caused by the catheter angiogram procedure. The trial judge described the consequences thus:

> 'As described in her own words, it has "changed my whole life". She is now classified as disabled, has a weakness down the left side of her body, lacks function in her left arm and hand, cannot carry, has difficulty with her personal care and dressing, and cannot do housework. She was a passionate gardener before the stroke; she has had to abandon that hobby. She played sport and danced, but this is no longer possible. She could not return to her secretarial job although fortunately she can still sit as a magistrate'.

Quantum of damages was agreed at £621,000 but the case went to trial on the issue of liability.

10.20 The claimant claimed in lack of consent amounting to negligent breach of duty in failure to offer and discuss the risks and benefits of the less invasive alternative treatment (the MRI scan) and she succeeded:

> 'Where the Queen Square fell down was in failing to discuss with Mrs Birch, as their own leading neuro-surgeon Mr Kitchen put it, the imaging methods and the comparative risks. For that reason the defendant is liable to her for breach of duty'.—*per* Cranston J. at § 82 of the judgment.

10.21 The author submits that, as a matter of law, the same principle applies to the issue of blood transfusion being the invasive procedure and alternative treatment being the less invasive option. The issue has not yet come to trial in respect of an adult, but in a children's case in which it was raised by the author, counsel for CAFCASS supported the submission in these terms:

> 'It is submitted that the parents correctly raise the issues set out in the case of Birch v University College London NHS Trust [2008] EWHC 2237. While distinguishable on its facts, it is the guardian's position that for the purpose of this application and the purposes of future treatment the Trust is under a duty to keep the parents informed of the benefits and risks of ongoing treatment options. It is also the guardian's position that the use of donor blood for the purposes of renal

[155] *Bolitho v City and Hackney Health Authority* [1998] AC 232 *supra*

> transplant should only be used by the Trust as a last resort and once all other non-blood options have been tried and/or considered'.

In the event on the facts of that case the judge in that case was not called upon to rule definitively on this issue.

10.22 To summarise, there is overwhelming authority that the common law in many jurisdictions throughout the world supports the right of the competent adult to choose treatment options even in a life-threatening situation, and to make a decision binding upon the treating clinicians 'for reasons which are rational, irrational or for no reason.'[156] And the spouse or next of kin has no legal authority to intervene in the implementation of the patient's decision.

10.23 The test of competence laid down by Thorpe J. in the case of *re C,* cited above, was transposed almost verbatim into s.3 of the Mental Capacity Act 2005. For a more detailed consideration of the statutory provisions and the practical application of the law in court proceedings the reader is referred to the seminal work on this topic *Medical Treatment: Decisions and the Law*.[157]

10.24 As a further observation, the problem is not with the law, which is clear, but with its implementation. The Safety of Blood, Tissues and Organs Advisory Committee (SaBTO) issued a consultation paper on 'Patient Consent for Blood Transfusion' that includes the following:

> 'The issue of consent for blood transfusion has been discussed on several occasions by SaBTO. The major concerns are that;
>
>> Patients are not being given information on risks, benefits and alternatives to transfusion or the right to refuse a transfusion;
>>
>> Patients may not be aware they have received a transfusion;
>>
>> Patients who receive blood may go on to donate blood without realising that they should not [Those who have received a transfusion since 1980 are excluded from blood donation];
>>
>> There is inconsistent practice across the UK'.

10.25 On 11 October 2011 the committee held a public meeting under the theme 'Patient consent for blood transfusion' at which a number of eminent

156 *Sidaway v Bethlem Royal Hospital Governors* [1985] AC 871(HL) per Lord Templeman at 904F; repeated by Lord Donaldson MR in *re T, supra*

157 *Medical Treatment: Decisions and the Law* 2nd Edition 2010, Edited by Christopher Johnston, 3 Serjeants' Inn, published by Bloomsbury Professional

speakers presented papers on the outcome of the consultation process and the action plan to implement the various recommendations. In the ensuing discussion strong emphasis was laid on the requirement of patient consent.

In the same month SaBTO published a document 'Patient Consent for Blood Transfusion' prepared by a distinguished working group. It made a number of very sensible recommendations but in so doing raised some serious questions about current practice and especially the extent to which patient consent in sought and obtained *prior* to transfusion. The recommendations on process and governance seem to be largely restatements of the existing position. However, it is those on the next 3 headings that cause some concern.

10.26 Patient Information:

> 'Patients who have received a blood transfusion *and who were not able to give valid consent prior to the transfusion* should be provided with information retrospectively'.

Patient and Public Education:

> 'The UK Blood Services have a key role in helping to educate patients and the public about the risks, benefits and alternatives to blood transfusion'.

Professional Education:

> 'There is a need to support healthcare professionals to improve their knowledge of consent and its relevance and importance in blood transfusion'.

10.27 These 3 recommendations do not sit easily together, especially for the patient who chooses non-blood management. Whilst the second acknowledges the need to help educate patients and the public about 'the risks, benefits and alternatives to blood transfusion', it fails adequately to address the need to help to provide the same education to clinicians and all involved in treatment. It notably fails to make any reference to the *Birch* principle that, where there is a less invasive option, the relevant risks and benefits must, as a matter of law, be discussed and offered as an option upon which it is the patient who makes the final decision.

10.28 But it is the first point that raises disquiet. The whole concept of consent to treatment is that the patient, after being provided with the relevant information about treatment options, then takes the decision *before* treatment. Unless a patient lacks capacity, it is unacceptable and probably illegal for doctors to go ahead with what **they** think is best and only after the event tell the patient what has been done to them.

There seems to be a case for SaBTO and all those involved in clinical governance give these matters a higher priority in implementation.

Chapter Eleven

Ethical Issues and Non-Consensual Treatment

Part A: Confidentiality and Information sharing

Information sharing: the Caldicott principles

11.1 In 1996–97 Professor Caldicott chaired a government inquiry that produced the then appropriate guidelines for those concerned in health and social welfare. The issue was re-visited by a further inquiry, chaired by the same Professor, and the report entitled '*Information: to share or not to share? The Information Governance Review*' was published in March 2013.

11.2 The Chairman's Foreword includes the following:

> 'Our overarching aim has been to ensure that there is an appropriate balance between the protection of the patient or user's information, and the use and sharing of such information to improve care'.

11.3 Chapter One of the Executive Summary starts with the following:

> 'People using health and social care services are entitled to expect that their personal information will remain confidential. They must feel able to discuss sensitive matters with a doctor, nurse or social worker without fear that the information may be improperly disclosed. These services cannot work effectively without trust **and trust depends on confidentiality'.** [Emphasis added]

11.4 The author suggests that a spiritual advisor, concerned with physical, emotional and spiritual health, is *sui generis* with the health and social welfare professionals mentioned. Accordingly the same principles of trust and confidentiality also apply to the disclosure of information that often relates to most intimate personal or family details and are only disclosed in the expectation that they will indeed be treated in strict confidence.

11.5 The original Caldicott Principles as slightly refined by the 2013 Report quoted are as follows:

> '1. Justify the purpose(s)
> Every proposed use or transfer of personal confidential data within or from an organisation should be clearly defined, scrutinised and documented with continuing uses regularly reviewed by an appropriate guardian.

2. Don't use personal confidential data unless it is absolutely necessary
   Personal confidential data items should not be included unless it is essential for the specified purposes of that flow. The need for patients to be identified should be considered at each stage of satisfying the purpose(s).

3. Use the minimum necessary personal confidential data
   Where use of confidential data is considered to be essential, the inclusion of each individual item of data should be considered and justified so that the minimum amount of personal information data is transferred or accessible as is necessary for a given function to be carried out.

4. Access to personal confidential data should be on a strict need to know basis
   Only those individuals who need access to personal confidential data should have access to it, and they should only have access to the data items that they need to see. This may mean introducing controls or splitting data flows where one data flow is used for several purposes.

5. Everyone with access to personal confidential data should be aware of their responsibilities
   Action should be taken to ensure that those handling personal confidential information, both clinical and non-clinical staff, are made fully aware of their responsibilities and obligations to respect patient confidentiality.

6. Comply with the law
   Every use of personal data must be lawful. Someone in each organisation handling personal confidential data should be responsible for ensuring that the organisation complies with legal requirements.

7. The duty to share information can be as important as the duty to protect patient confidentiality
   Health and social care professionals should have the confidence to share information in the best interests of their patients within the framework set by these principles. They should be supported by the policies of their employers, regulators and professional bodies.

These principles should underpin information governance across the health and social care services'.

Part B: Non-Consensual Treatment

11.6 The logical starting point, on this topic of transfusion, for any discussion of medical ethics would seem to be the International Society of Blood Transfusion (ISBT). With the technical support of the World Health Organisation (WHO) which later adopted the Code, in 2000 they published a

Code of Ethics for Blood Donation and Transfusion, later updated in 2006. Further reviews of the Code are believed to be ongoing.

Its objective is described as 'to define the ethical principles and rules to be observed in the field of Transfusion medicine.'

11.7 Under the sub-heading 'Hospitals: patients' it states:

> '12. Patients should be informed of the known risks and benefits of blood transfusion and/or alternative therapies and have the right to accept or refuse the procedure. Any valid advance directive should be observed…
>
> 15. Genuine clinical need should be the only basis for transfusion therapy.
>
> 16. There should be no financial incentive to prescribe a blood transfusion.
>
> 17. As far as possible the patient should receive only those particular components (cells, plasma, or plasma derivatives) that are clinically appropriate and afford optimal safety.
>
> 18. Blood transfusion practices established by national or international health bodies and other agencies competent and authorised to do so should be in compliance with this code of ethics'.

11.8 A number of issues immediately arise from the Code. Firstly, it applies to patients without any qualification as to age. Secondly, it does not differentiate between those having competence and capacity and those lacking these characteristics. Thirdly it makes no provision for the use of force to administer blood to those who chose not to have it or even those cases in which a court may have given authorisation for its use. These 3 points alone give rise to some interesting situations and comparison with the law and practice in differing common law countries is instructive.

England and Wales

The use of forcible restraint to administer non-consensual treatment

11.9 It is submitted that the use of force to overpower any patient, simply to ensure compliance with treatment that the doctor recommends but which the competent patient finds repugnant and resists, is wholly alien to the common law. Professor Len Doyal (referred to later) addresses the ethical objections to such a course. But the British Medical Association in two relevant publications gives guidance as to the position of the treating doctor.

In August 2009 in the guidance[158] for 'custodial settings' the BMA identified some basic principles concerning 'the medical role in restraint and control' intended to be applicable to those held in custody but the principles of which it is submitted should extend to those who object to and indeed may physically resist this particular treatment so that they become subject to restraint and control. The guidance includes:

> 'Restraint should only ever be used as an act of care and control, not as a punishment or a convenience. The use of restraint can result in psychological morbidity, demoralisation and feelings of humiliation. In terms of chemical interventions to control patients, the Metropolitan Police has issued guidance specifically relating to rapid tranquillisation that other practitioners might find useful. It states that rapid tranquillisation should only be performed where equipment for cardiopulmonary resuscitation is present and there are trained staff to use it...
>
> A record should be kept of every use of restraint or force against prisoners.
>
> Prisoners who have been subjected to force should be examined, and if necessary treated by, a doctor as soon as possible.'

11.10 In 2010 the BMA issued specific guidelines[159] for treatment of young people in which there are 15 'Cards' under different topics.

Card 2 'Assessing Competence' raises 4 questions:

> **'Can competence ever be presumed?**
>
> Yes. All people aged 16 and over are presumed in law to be competent to give their consent to medical treatment...
>
> **Can a young person be competent under the age of 16?**
>
> Yes, but this needs to be assessed in each case on a continual basis. Doctors should aim to involve all children and young people in decisions relating to their medical treatment. It is important to recognise when a young person is able to make a valid choice about a proposed medical intervention ...and is therefore competent to make a personal decision. **Doctors should not judge the ability of a particular child or young person solely on the basis of his or her age.** [Emphasis added]

158 *'The medical role in restraint and control: custodial settings'*. Guidance from the British Medical Association August 2009

159 *Children and young people tool kit*—British Medical Association Dec 2010

For a young person under the age of 16 to be competent, s/he should have:

the ability to understand that there is a choice and that choices have consequences;

the ability to weigh the information and arrive at a decision;

a willingness to make a choice (including the choice that someone else should make the decision);

an understanding of the nature and purpose of the proposed intervention;

an understanding of the proposed intervention's risks and side effects;

an understanding of the alternatives to the proposed intervention and of the risks attached to them;

freedom from undue pressure.

Who should assess competence?

GP's who have known the young patient for a long time are well placed to assess the development and maturity but, because these change, it is unwise to rely on any assessment that is is not contemporaneous. Health professionals who assess competence need to be skilled and experienced in interviewing young patients and eliciting their views without distortion. The treating doctor may be the most appropriate person, but other members of the health care team who have a close rapport with the patient may also have a valuable contribution to make.

How can competence be promoted?

When assessing a child's competence it is important to explain these issues in a way that is suitable for their age. A young patient may be competent to make some but not all decisions and clinical staff should promote an environment in which young patients are enabled to engage in decisions as much as they are able. The child or young person's ability to play a full part in decision making can be enhanced by allowing time for discussion'.

Card 4 deals with Consent and Refusal. Notably it includes a paragraph on treatment against a child or young person's wishes:

'Can doctors provide treatment against a child's or young person's wishes?

If a child or young person refuses treatment, just because consent from a parent, or from a court, makes providing treatment lawful does not mean that it inevitably has to be given. Doctors must look at whether harms associated with imposing treatment on a patient who refuses, whether competently or not, should play a part in the decision about proceeding. How critical the treatment is, whether less invasive treatments are available, and whether it is possible to allow time for further discussion with the patient are all factors to be weighed. As much time as is practicable should be taken for the discussion and treatment delayed if that is possible without jeopardising its likely success (see Card 7 on the use of restraint). Doctors must be careful not to apply undue pressure…'.

Card 7 'Use of restraint to provide treatment':

'What factors should be taken into account when considering the use of restraint?

Doctors should consider if imposing treatment could damage the young person's current and future relationships with health care providers and undermine trust in the medical profession…

The following points are relevant to any action taken:

restraint should be used only when it is necessary to give essential treatment or to prevent a child from significantly injuring himself or herself or others;

the effect should be to provide an overall benefit to the child and in some cases the harms associated with the use of restraints may outweigh the benefits expected from treatment;

restraint is an act of care and control, not punishment, and should be administered with due respect;

unless life prolonging or other crucial treatment is immediately necessary, legal advice should be sought when treatment involves restraint or detention to override the views of a competent young person, even if the law allows doctors to proceed on the basis of parental consent;

all steps should be taken to anticipate the need for restraint and to prepare the child, his nor her family, and staff;

wherever possible the members of the health care team involved should have an established relationship with the child and should explain what is being done and why;

treatment plans should include safeguards to ensure that restraint is the minimum necessary, that it is for the minimum period necessary to achieve the clinical aim, and that both the child and the parents have been informed what will happen and why restraint is necessary;

restraint should usually be used only in the presence of other staff who can act as assistants and witnesses;

any use of restraint should be recorded in the medical records. These issues are an appropriate subject for clinical audit;

Who is responsible for the decision to use restraint?

Members of the health team should be given the opportunity to express their views and to participate in the decision-making, although ultimate responsibility rests with the clinician in charge of care. All staff require support, **and must not be asked to be involved in restraining a child without proper training**'.

11.11 The totality of the effect of these guidelines is that, notwithstanding parental consent or even a court order declaring that the proposed treatment would be lawful; the clinical team must pause and weigh very carefully the risk/benefit of physical restraint on the overall welfare of the child. They must have especial regard to the statement:

> 'Doctors must look at whether harms associated with imposing treatment on a patient who refuses, whether competently or not, should play a part in the decision about proceeding'.

The potential for total breakdown of trust and the doctor/patient relationship should not be underestimated.

11.12 In this context there are relevant dicta of Hale LJ. in a leading case[160] involving a psychiatric patient compulsorily detained in Broadmoor Special Hospital:

> 'Whatever the position before the Human Rights Act 1998, the decision to impose treatment **without consent on a protesting patient** is a potential invasion of the rights under Article 3 or Article 8. Super-Wednesbury is not enough. The claimant is entitled to a proper hearing on the merits of whether the **statutory grounds** for imposing this treatment upon him against his will are made out i.e. whether it is treatment for the mental disorder from which he is suffering and whether it should be given to him without his consent "having regard to the likelihood of its alleviating or preventing a deterioration of his [psychiatric] condition"'. [Emphasis added]

This suggests that there are serious limitations to the power to coerce the patient and enforce medical treatment by physical restraint. The reference to Articles 3 and 8 reinforces the submissions under the Human Rights Act 1998.

160 *R (on the application of Wilkinson) v RMO, Broadmoor Hospital Authority* [2001] EWCA Civ 545; [2002] 1 WLR 419; 65 BMLR 15

11.13 However most of this guidance is in the context of a patient under 16. It is submitted that in the case of a competent mature minor patient over the age of 16 the cases should be very rare indeed (if at all) in which force and coercion should be deployed to force treatment that the patient finds wholly repugnant and refuses.

Professor Len Doyal: *Can medicine be torture: the case of children.*[161]

11.14 Professor Len Doyal, an eminent expert in medical law and ethics now retired,[162] has addressed the issue of treatment being forced on children without their consent or against their wishes. Under the potentially provocative title '*Can medicine be torture? The case of children*' he picks up and develops this theme of non-consensual treatment. The entire article is supported by 53 references mainly from peer-reviewed mainstream material. It is dealt with in more detail in chapter 13.

11.15 The Professor notably confirms the best practice referred to above as to the need for the patient's competence to be confirmed by 'a senior paediatrician and child psychiatrist ***who are not involved with the child's treatment'*** [emphasis added]. Experience of court proceedings initiated by NHS Trust lawyers casts considerable doubt on whether this cogent and compelling guidance has ever been read, let alone followed.

The Human Rights Act 1998

11.16 The Act incorporates, albeit to a limited extent, the European Convention on Human Rights.[163] Three articles are primarily engaged on this issue, namely Articles 8 & 9 in conjunction with Article 14.

> 'Article 8:
>
> *Right to respect for private and family life*
>
> 1. Everyone has the right to respect for his private and family life, his home and his correspondence.
>
> There shall be no interference by a public authority with the exercise of this right except such as is in accordance with the law and is necessary in a

---

161 '*Childhood abused: Protecting children against torture, cruel, inhuman and degrading treatment and Punishment:* published by Ashgate Dartmouth

162 Former Professor of Medical Ethics, St Bartholomew's and The Royal London Hospitals School of Medicine and Dentistry

163 Convention for the Protection of Human Rights and Fundamental Freedoms: Rome 1950

democratic society in the interests of national security, public safety or the economic well-being of the country, for the prevention of disorder or crime, for the protection of health or morals, or for the protection of rights and freedoms of others.

Article 9:

1. Everyone has the right to freedom of thought, conscience and religion; this right includes freedom to change his religion or belief and freedom, either alone or in community with others and in public or private, to manifest his religion or belief, in worship, teaching, practice and observance.

2. Freedom to manifest one's religion or beliefs shall be subject only to such limitations as are prescribed by law and are necessary in a democratic society in the interests of public safety, for the protection of public order, health or morals, or for the protection of the rights and freedoms of others.

Article 14:

The enjoyment of the rights and freedoms set forth in [the] Convention shall be secured without discrimination on any ground such as sex, race, colour, language, religion, political or other opinion, national or social origin, association with a national minority, property, birth or other status'.

11.17 The European Court of Human Rights (ECtHR) has held that the right to choose options in medical treatment, including blood or non-blood, is protected[164] and that enforced treatment without consent violates the Convention.

11.18 Attempts to bring an otherwise competent patient artificially within the statutory mental health provisions to enforce treatment have been judicially deprecated and even marked with an award of damages for unlawful detention and assault. In her seminal and peer-reviewed article 'The Right to Refuse Medical Treatment under the European Convention on Human Rights', Elizabeth Wicks wrote:[165]

'The UK courts have also been keen to declare that a "decision to refuse medical treatment by a patient capable of making the decision does not have to be sensible, rational or well-considered". This impressive statement is, however, of little

164 X v Austria, No.828/78; Acmanne v Belgium, No.10435/83; YF v Turkey, No.24209/94; Moscow Community of Jehovah's Witnesses v Russia, No.302/02

165 The Right to Refuse Medical Treatment under the European Convention on Human Rights, Medical Law Review 2001 Volume 9 (17) I March 2001

protection to patients' rights unless it is applied in practice in the most difficult of cases, namely when an acceptance of the patient's decision will result in his death. In these circumstances the UK courts have shown a regrettable tendency to resort to the approach feared by Kennedy—i.e. that a refusal to consent to recommended treatment is evidence of mental incapacity'.

11.19 Further authority is contained in a judgment[166] of the ECtHR given on 23 March 2010, reported by *The Times* of London under the heading 'Medical intervention without consent', in an application against the UK. A paediatrician formed a suspicion of abuse of a girl aged 9 years on incomplete evidence when an available report of a colleague dermatologist provided an innocent explanation for suspect marks. The paediatrician nevertheless arranged for the taking of blood samples and intimate photographs of the girl in the absence of the parents and without their consent. The ECtHR found violations of Article 8 and (on the particular facts) a violation of Article 13 in the failure of the State to provide an effective remedy.

11.20 In summary, the constant theme of these European cases and writings is that the right of choice rests solely with the competent patient. It is not constrained by any requirement such as prior advice from a spiritual, legal or medical adviser. Choice may be based on religious grounds or simply on the particular, even idiosyncratic or irrational, wishes of the competent patient, whether adult or mature minor.

11.21 In the case of minor children who lack maturity to rank as mature minors, the decision-making rests with the parents. It remains with them unless and until, by due process of Convention-compliant law especially Article 6, a court of competent jurisdiction has overruled that choice of medical treatment after hearing proper evidence that conforms to the *Birch* principle of evaluating the risks and benefits of a less invasive option.

11.22 The World Medical Association in its authoritative Declaration of Lisbon on the Rights of the Patient sets out a range of rights accorded to the patient. It unreservedly upholds in Principle 2 the Right to Freedom of Choice and in Principle 3 the Right to self-determination.

Notably in Principle 5 it asserts that a minor 'must be involved in the decision making to the fullest extent allowed by his/her capacity'. Principle 6 governs

[166] *MAK & RK v United Kingdom*, ECtHR Nos. 45901/05 & 40146/06

procedures 'against the patient's will can be carried out only in exceptional circumstances if specifically permitted by law **and** conforming to the principles of medical ethics. [Emphasis added]

The original Declaration was made in 1981 and amended in 1995. Presumably it has to be read in the light of the current law and ethical practice.

Canada

11.23 The general consensus is that Canada is the front runner in according rights of choice to mature minors.

They have taken a hard look at aged based distinctions and whether they unreasonably discriminate against others. It is accepted that such distinctions are a common and necessary way of ordering society. They are by definition arbitrary but within acceptable legal limits 'provided that the age chosen is reasonably relative to the legislative goal' see Gosselin v Quebec.[167]

Eminent author P W Hogg[168] has summarised it thus:

> 'Our laws are replete with provisions in which age is employed as the qualification for pursuits that require skill or judgment. Consider the laws regulating voting, drinking, marrying, contracting, will-making, leaving school, being employed etc. In regulating these matters, all jurisdictions impose disabilities on young people, employing age as a proxy for ability. Such stereotyping is inevitably inaccurate, because individuals mature at different rates.
>
> In principle, the use of age could be eliminated, because each individual could be tested for performance of each function. Age is used as a qualification for no other reason than to avoid or reduce the administrative burden of individualised testing'.

11.24 The Law Commission of Manitoba very sensibly addressed the issue of arbitrary age limits in their report *Minor's Consent to Healthcare* as far back as 1985 and came down firmly against a rigidly fixed limit. The ensuing legislation[169] provided what is in reality a three-tier structure. The practical working of these provisions and the arbitrariness of the different approaches to the over and under 16 year olds was in 2009 tested all the way up to the

[167] *Gosselin v Quebec (Attorney General)* [2002] 4 SCR 429 per McLachlin CJ
[168] *Constitutional Law of Canada* (Carswell, 5th Edition 2007) Vol 2 at p. 668
[169] Child and Family Services Act CCSM C80—assented to 11 July 1985

Supreme Court of Canada in a case [170] involving a patient aged at the relevant time 14 years and 10 months.

It culminated in a judgment that is a masterly piece of judicial writing that ranges widely over the topic, including reviewing especially the extensive materials on maturing adolescents.

11.25 Paragraph 31 of the leading judgment of Abella J (on behalf of four other justices) contains an interesting summary of the lower levels of age that are addressed in the provincial legislation.

> '...a child of 12 years of age or more is entitled to be advised of the proceedings and of their possible implications for the child and shall be given the opportunity to make his or her views and preferences known to the decision maker...Children under 12 can also have their views taken into account if a judge is satisfied that they are 'able to understand the nature of the proceedings' and the judge 'is of the opinion that it would not be harmful to the child'.

Later at paras 46 to 79 there is a review of the common law principles relating to mature minors in not only Canada but other relevant jurisdictions, starting with the general statement:

> '[46] ...However the common law has more recently abandoned the assumption that all minors lack decisional capacity and replaced it with a general recognition that children are entitled to a degree of decision-making that is reflective of their evolving intelligence and understanding'.

The judge goes on to cite Lord Scarman in *Gillick:*[171]

> '...I would hold that as a matter of law the parental right to determine whether or not their minor child below the age of 16 will have medical treatment terminates if and when the child achieves a sufficient understanding and intelligence to enable him or her to understand fully what is proposed'.

The judge went on to review the English cases, notably re R[172]and re W[173] cited in more detail in chapter 14, although there is a compelling argument advanced by experienced medico-legal writers that these cases do not represent an orderly development of the law on mature minors and need to be reconsidered by the Supreme Court.

---

170 *AC v Manitoba* [2009] SCC 30
171 *Gillick v West Norfolk Area Health Authority* [1985] 3 All E R 402
172 *re R* [1991] 4 All E R 177
173 *re W (a minor) (medical treatment)* [1992] 4 All E R 627

11.26 Simply as one example, Margaret Brazier and Caroline Bridge[174] propose the following as a model for autonomous choices:

> '...fully autonomous choice is largely an ideal...The best we can manage is a maximally autonomous choice. In determining whether a particular individual choice demands respect we should look to see whether that choice is undermined by any irremediable defect in the autonomy of the choice in question'.

The argument reaches its most compelling in para [87] of the judgment:

> 'The more a court is satisfied that a child is capable of making a mature, independent decision on his or her own behalf, the greater the weight that will be given to his or her views when a court is exercising its [statutory] discretion. In some cases, courts will inevitably be so convinced of a child's maturity that the principles of welfare and autonomy will collapse altogether and the child's wishes will become the controlling factor. If, after a careful and sophisticated analysis of the young person's ability to exercise mature, independent judgment, the court is persuaded that the necessary level of maturity exists, it seems to me necessarily to follow that the adolescent's views ought to be respected. Such an approach clarifies that in the context of medical treatment, young people under 16 should be permitted to demonstrate that their views about a particular medical treatment decision reflect a sufficient degree of independence of thought and maturity'.

Later at [96] the judge summarised the position by listing eight factors that bear on the issue for determination. This is a carefully considered and mature judicial formulation of principle that commands respect.

The judgment should be required reading for all involved both in formulating policy and indeed its implementation in these cases of mature minors including clinicians, risk managers, hospital lawyers, judges, parents and indeed the mature minors themselves.

Australia

11.27 This jurisdiction of course has its own statutory rules both at Federal level and, albeit with some variation, at State level. Indeed Western Australia is held up as a world leader in government-provided hospital care that has embraced the concept and implemented in practice blood conservation and non-blood management. But on the common law it is almost a mirror image of that

[174] *Children, Medicine and the Law* at p.468

in the UK, especially on this issue of age of competence and capacity to make choices of medical treatment.

11.28 In an important case in March 2013 the court in NSW reviewed the *parens patriae* jurisdiction and its use to force treatment on a refusing mature minor. The patient, a committed Jehovah's Witness supported by his family, had originally been admitted for treatment for Hodgkin's disease. He had accepted conventional chemotherapy but without blood support. Following a relapse the treating oncologist wanted to use much higher doses of different cytotoxic chemotherapy agents which caused, as a side effect, suppression of the bone marrow for which blood support was needed. After a further relapse, even with best available therapy his likely cure rate was only put at '40 to 50 per cent' according to the then current medical literature.

11.29 Re-admitted to hospital in Sydney with pancytopenia and fever, his Hb dropped to 3.5gd/l and chemotherapy was suspended. Given the patient's condition and his adamant stand on non-blood, the hospital went to court for an order that would allow them to administer blood support and thereby re-start the chemotherapy. The patient was then aged 17 years and 2 months, old enough to drive a car; join the military to kill or be killed; and marry and father a child. Perhaps more importantly he was described as 'highly intelligent'. The judge found as a fact that he had researched his own condition. He said he wanted to be responsible for what went into his own body. He explored non-blood treatment on the internet. The treating Professor described him as 'the leader of the team, of he and his parents'. And then the judge declared 'He is clearly a mature minor'.

11.30 Having reached that conclusion and accepted the medical opinion that his chances were at best, with full treatment, only 40-50%, one is entitled to ask what more is a mature minor expected to do to be allowed to take his own decision. Yet under the doctrine of *parens patriae* his decision could be overridden. That is why this decision[175] in Sydney involving a patient only a few months short of his 18th birthday is of special significance.

11.31 In summary, an initially co-operative clinician, aware that the patient was for all practical purposes an adult and should be allowed to choose his

[175] *The Sydney Children's Hospital Network v X*, Supreme Court of NSWL Equity Division Gzell J. 28 March 2013

treatment options despite a court order authorising allogeneic blood if appropriate, modified the treatment to exclude blood. Later when the condition deteriorated, decisions were taken by the hospital authorities that the court order was to be enforced. The patient, by this time only 3 months short of majority at age 18 years, was not merely uncooperative but resistant. The response of the hospital was to call up 3 burly, medically untrained and unqualified security guards who, by sheer brute force, overpowered the patient to enable a sedative to be administered and thence the blood transfusion.

11.32 What is not clear is whether, or to what extent, any consideration was given to the ethical considerations. To the layman, to overpower a competent patient by sheer force in order to administer treatment to which he profoundly objects is totally unacceptable. It was repugnant to a patient with such deeply held religious beliefs. Many would consider it to be a major step down the slippery slope at the bottom of which lies the infamous Dr Mengele and his forced medical experiments on victims in the notorious Auschwitz concentration camp.

Namibia

11.33 The above case in Australia is in marked contrast to a recent case in Namibia recounted in more detail in chapter 21. [176]

Part C: Some Problems in Bioethics and Genetic Testing

11.34 The impact of genetic testing and especially DNA analysis has been dramatic but has, as a side effect, also thrown up some entirely new legal and ethical problems on confidentiality, disclosure and patient rights to information.

The author was invited to make a presentation on this topic to a major Bioethics Conference at the Commonwealth Centre in London. In the course of researching the subject, he came across an item in a medical publication that raised (but did not really satisfactorily answer) a specific problem of the conflicting duties of the treating doctor.

11.35 A husband and wife had a child that was diagnosed with a specific condition, namely spinal muscular atrophy, which was known to be transmitted genetically. They were planning a second child but wanted to be informed, and hopefully re-assured, that the percentage of risk that this second child might too

[176] *ES v AC:* Supreme Court of Namibia SA/2012

inherit the same condition was acceptably low. So the mother and father, with the child, attended a joint consultation with a specialist at which the adults answered questions and all 3 provided the appropriate and necessary blood samples, a demonstrably invasive procedure requiring consent of each adult and of the parents for the child.

When the test results, by genotyping using DNA markers linked to the SMN gene, came back some time later, the specialist called the mother alone back in for a confidential consultation to discuss the test results. The result showed incontrovertibly that there was zero risk of transmission to a prospective second child of the genetic condition inherited by the first. But the unexpected reason was that the tests showed conclusively that the husband could not be the biological father of the first child. It appeared that 'Daddy' was not 'Daddy' after all. Unknown to the husband the mother had, it seems, engaged in some extra-curricular activity outside the marriage by which she had become pregnant. The husband had had no reason to doubt that the child was his and had in good faith accepted her as his daughter.

11.36 The ethical problems raised by the case resulted in some spirited discussion by delegates which showed a wide divergence of views. A specialist doctor in this field, of consultant status, was adamant that the mother **alone** was his patient to whom he owed a duty of confidentiality and therefore not to disclose the non-paternity of the husband. That, however conveniently and perhaps simplistically, overlooked the legal realities:

a) that the husband had been present at a ***joint*** medical consultation with the specialist at which he, together with the wife and child, had provided the requisite samples by invasive procedure for which consent was required and was therefore, on that basis alone, arguably also his patient to whom he owed a duty to tell the truth and provide him with accurate information; and
b) that realistically the husband would inevitably want to know the result of the genetic testing for which he had voluntarily contributed the necessary samples and that result would have somehow to be disclosed. The doctor could not lie to him.

11.37 Quite apart from the family and emotional trauma, the potential financial consequences were significant and long term. One possibility was that they were a fairly wealthy family in which the child could reasonably be expected to live in a nice expensive house; be educated privately; enjoy a life-style that was likely to include ponies, tennis, summer holidays abroad and skiing at Christmas and things of that kind and probably later attend a good quality university fully funded by the 'father'. That represented a contingent liability on him over 21 years of probably not less than half a million pounds sterling. If, on learning of his non-paternity of the child, the husband chose to reject the child and all responsibility for her and to divorce the mother, the financial loss to the child and mother would be potentially enormous. But that all turned on true disclosure of the facts being made to the husband and it was that course that the mother vigorously resisted. And what about the separate interests of the child?

The discussion between medical practitioners, lawyers, laymen and women became quite animated with only one matter upon which there was full agreement: ask the MDU for an authoritative opinion!

Understandably, given the very sensitive nature of the facts, there does not seem to have been published any report of the final outcome.

11.38 But a very similar issue has now been before the High Court in a case decided in May 2015 and publicly reported, albeit with provisions for anonymity of the family.[177]

The facts were described by Nicol J. as tragic and indeed they were. The father had shot and killed the mother. He was convicted of manslaughter (rather than murder) on the grounds of diminished responsibility and ordered to be detained in a secure unit under the appropriate provisions of the Mental Health legislation and where he would receive the necessary treatment. The diagnosis was that he suffered from Huntingdon's Disease which was considered treatable or at least manageable to the extent that he was being prepared for supervised release. His married daughter was a participant in the family and social work therapy that involved joint discussions with those medical practitioners of varying disciplines treating the father.

The treating team had to consider the ethical position of disclosing to the daughter the diagnosis of her father which carried with it the likelihood that she too had inherited the condition of Huntingdon's. In the current state of medical

[177] *ABC v St George's Healthcare NHS Trust* [2015] EWHC 1394 (QB)

knowledge it was not capable of diagnosis during childhood but only on attaining maturity.

11.39 The problems of information sharing under the *Caldicott* principles during treatment came to the fore. The treating team had to consider disclosure to the daughter of the possibility of transmission to her of her father's condition of Huntingdon's disease which she might then herself pass on to any children that she might have. That team doubtless took careful advice from both an ethics committee and probably from top-flight medical lawyers. The conclusion was that they owed their duty of confidentiality to the father and, as he refused them permission to disclose to his daughter even though he had (illogically) disclosed the facts to his brother, they were bound by that duty of confidentiality.

Having thus been kept in the dark, the daughter became pregnant unknowing of the potential transmission of Huntingdon's to the baby. At that stage one of the team of medical specialists, seemingly unaware of the team decision and duty to respect the father's confidentiality, inadvertently disclosed the fact to the daughter, but at a stage in the pregnancy too late for a termination.

11.40 She immediately commenced proceedings against the 3 NHS Trusts responsible for the respective specialists who had been engaged in the joint therapy sessions. Basically her claim was that, by that series of events, there had come into existence between them the relationship of doctor and patient, thus triggering a duty to tell her of the risk to the unborn baby of inherited Huntingdon's and to have done so early enough for the daughter to take an informed decision on whether or not to terminate the pregnancy. She claimed substantial damages, mainly on behalf of the child, but also for herself for the unwanted pregnancy that she was adamant that she would have had terminated had she been told the truth.

The case was duly pleaded in a detailed claim but the NHS Trusts applied for summary strike out on the basis that there was no reasonable prospect of the claimant establishing, on the facts, the existence of a relationship of doctor and patient. Absent such relationship in law, there could not have been a legal duty to disclose.

11.41 The strike out application came before Nicol J. who, after hearing extensive argument from a couple of top Silks and in a careful and well-reasoned judgment, held that, despite the daughter having been present at therapy sessions that had been primarily for the benefit of the father, there had not come into existence the claimed professional relationship of treating doctor and patient **with the daughter.** Absent such proven relationship, there was in law no cause of action alleging duty of care, negligent non-disclosure and foreseeability that had any reasonable prospect of success. The claim was accordingly struck out with costs.

11.42 The case highlights the importance of establishing whether the mere presence of a member of the family at treatment sessions directed to the mental health of the 'patient' father was sufficient to prove the relationship of doctor and patient with such member and thus the usual duty of care that would normally flow from that relationship.

It will doubtless also provide fruitful ground for claimant and NHS lawyers to generate still further litigation on the difficult question of when there does, or does not, exist in law the relationship of doctor and patient with the accompanying consequences of duty of care, breach of that duty and foreseeability of damage.

11.43 The Court of Appeal in late November 2015 gave leave to appeal. Their decision will be awaited with interest as will that of the Supreme Court where the case will probably go. And as Article 8 of the Convention is engaged the case may yet end up in the ECtHR in Strasbourg.

It may even require consideration by Parliament and possibly amending legislation to try and ensure that such a tragedy does not occur again.

Chapter Twelve

The Cost/Benefit Analysis

12.1 There is an erroneous perception that, because blood donors in the UK are volunteers and unpaid, blood is cheap compared with the non-blood alternatives, especially those that emanate from supposedly rapacious pharmaceutical companies. The facts are somewhat different.

12.2 Very little regard was had over several decades to the true cost of blood. The UK government through the National Blood Transfusion Service (NBTS) assumed central responsibility and the method of accounting was fragmented so that, however unintentionally, the true overall costs of both capital and running costs were far from clear.

12.3 The nearest illustration would be to compare the cost per unit as calculated by a commercial undertaking. Suppose that raw materials were available by donation at no cost to the company but that there were costs in collecting, grading, testing for quality, separating components, packaging and distribution, collectively described as 'processing'. Into that calculation is then factored the loss of usable product in the processing and also in expired shelf life, in the case of blood put at 7%. These costs are fairly readily ascertainable and if the number of net units processed and used is divided into the total cost, then a cost per unit can be ascertained fairly simply.

But as those responsible for running any commercial business know only too well, there are major overhead costs attributable to such operations that have additionally to be brought into account. Three major items are readily identifiable namely:

- capital costs and depreciation;
- transport; and
- the now ever pressing issue of final salary pension funding.

Capital costs and depreciation

12.4 To facilitate the harvesting, collection and processing of donor blood, the State provided at a capital cost, not included in any unit cost calculation or the accounts of NTBS, major Processing Centres such as that at Elstree in

Hertfordshire. The recent sale of Plasma Resources UK has highlighted the under-funding of that centre as the sale includes an undertaking from the US purchaser, Bain Capital, to invest £50 million to bring its facilities up to standard. A newer unit at Filton near Bristol is reported to have cost £40 million. No building or plant remains forever and so the commercial accounting practice is to amortise, or write down annually, the original capital cost and thereby arrive at an annual figure to be brought into account on unit cost. Even assuming a fairly generous life expectancy for the sophisticated laboratory equipment needed for fractionating of 15 years and the building of 20 years, the annual amortisation figure for that specialist facility alone should be something of the order of £40 million divided by, say, a middle figure of 17 years which amounts to £2,350,000 per annum. Even taking the more generous figure of a 20 year life, it is still £2 million per annum to be added to the overall unit costs and that is for one facility alone.

Transport

12.5 This is a major cost in terms of:

- expensive specialist and purpose-built mobile blood donor units for collection points;
- refrigerated transport vehicles to meet the strict requirements of transport to processing centres;
- further transport for onward routine daily deliveries to hospitals; and
- emergency 'blue light' distribution to hospitals in special need.

It is a fairly major transport fleet operation in itself in addition to being staff intensive yet neither the running costs nor capital purchase or depreciation on vehicles seem to have been included.

Pension

12.6 No cost for funding 'final salary' pensions for all those involved was included. As the recent financial crisis has highlighted, this can be a very substantial item, even creating a black hole in the capital account in a commercial organisation. Thus when all 3 factors were brought into account, the actual unit cost rose dramatically.

12.7 It was only comparatively recently that unit costs started to become an issue. The NBTS provided blood to NHS Trusts at a cost that seems to have varied from Trust to Trust but which is known to have been of the order of £135 per unit. This represents a heavily subsidised unit cost, probably as great as at least two thirds even if the 3 items outlined above were excluded.

12.8 The situation of costs first came to serious attention in 1998 when an article entitled 'The annual costs of blood transfusions in the UK'[178] was published by Guest et al but published in a professional journal of somewhat limited circulation. The topic was revisited in 2003 when a study was commissioned to be carried out by outside professional experts in medical financing. Catalyst Health Economics Consultants is a professional firm including medically qualified experts, notably Drs Varney and Guest, but outwith and independent of the NHS; commercially astute and with their feet on the ground. They carried out an in-depth study and their report (which received surprisingly little publicity outside the esoteric world of haematologists and blood transfusion specialists) was published in the professionally recognised journal 'Transfusion Medicine'.[179] It is a masterly review of the true costs of donor blood and should be required reading for all those with a serious interest in this topic including the Treasury and, not least, the long-suffering tax-payer who in the end is funding it all.

12.9 For the lay reader some issues are highlighted. Firstly the authors correctly identified the 'costs exclusions' broadly referred to above. But more importantly they broadened the scope to identify and, where possible, cost the following items, a list that is not all inclusive but represents the main heads of cost:

- indirect costs to society, namely the actual costs to the public/employers of donor time off from work (lost productivity/job covering for absence) and/or their leisure time plus travelling costs associated with attending the donor centre, whether fixed or mobile;
- increased demand on hospital resources, notably increased length of bed stay conservatively averaged out at 1 day per transfusion;
- blood transfusion related complications;

178 *Clinical and Laboratory Haematology*. 20. 111-118

179 S.J.Varney and J.F.Guest, Catalyst Health Economics Consultants. *Transfusion Medicine*, 2003, 13. 205-218

- costs of consultants and other senior staff at Hospital Blood Transfusion Committee meetings as required for compliance with monitoring and reporting to SHOT;
- the appointment in each acute unit of a full time and salaried transfusion practitioner;
- capital charges;
- audit fees;
- board member remuneration;
- loss on sale of fixed assets; and
- additional costs of processing due to additional tests required and leucodepletion to reduce transfer of viral and other infections, especially the variant Creutzfeldt-Jakob Disease prion.

Costs exclusions

12.10 First and foremost there is a 7% stock loss from blood donor sessions to ultimate disposal due to processing and quality control or because of expiration of shelf life. Any commercial organisation would, as a matter of urgency, be addressing that as an unacceptable percentage biting into their profit margin.

There are then several costs exclusions identified which in total came to a formidable £919.01 million. That was the figure for 2003, the year of the study, and if the normal annual inflation rate (based conventionally on the RPI) is calculated then it becomes £1,316 million.

Apportionment of costs

12.11 The approximate apportionment between products is red cells 69% (of which 30% is used in cancer patients); 14% in paediatrics; platelets 9%; FFP 6%; and cryoprecipitate 1%.

These costs were all in relation to the 2001 figures that provided the base for the study published in 2003. The author checked with the consultancy firm[180] and was told that no further official up to date study had been carried out. However there was no disagreement with the suggestion that, as a common sense layman's approach, the application of the standard Retail Price Index (RPI) was an appropriate way of broadly assessing the impact of inflation on

[180] Personal communication

those 2003 costs. That leads to the result that the costs per transfusion with inflation added in line with the official RPI, are now cryoprecipitate £1,245; RBC £917; RBC plus FCP £1,463 and RBC plus platelet £1,419.

12.12 As to cost, on the same day in another written answer the minister stated:

> 'Our current estimate, based on information supplied by manufacturers and NHS blood and transplant, is that the cost **per annum** of introducing prion filtration for all United Kingdom blood donations is approximately **£200,000,000'**. [Emphasis added].

This phenomenal sum of public funds that seems to have attracted little publicity would now have to be added to the overall cost per unit pushing it to the point where any commercial provider would inevitably be looking seriously at investing in alternatives.

12.13 Some readers may find the actual figures quite startling. Far from the cost of £135 at which units are supplied to NHS Trusts as a central resource, the actual cost can in some cases be increased by a factor of nearly 10 to well over £1,000 per unit as the figures show and that is excluding the new prion filtration. This is where a comparison with the costs of the major alternative products becomes interesting.

12.14 An important element is the actual effectiveness of EPO. In the world of sport (notably endurance cycling) it has a dirty name and is a banned substance. This is precisely because it is so effective in increasing the level of the oxygen carrying Hb that, particularly in sports in which endurance is predominant, it gives those cheating in this way a serious advantage. The downside for the athlete is the danger of increased thickening of the blood unless the athlete is effectively hydrated to compensate for lost fluid. But in clinical terms where an increase in the Hb is sought without resort to donor blood, it is proved to be effective.

As one case history in chapter 15 shows, it is quite feasible to raise the Hb by 1 gramme per week in advance of planned surgery with a combination of EPO and Iron given as *Venofer*®. This is not mere speculation or theory but proven fact. That must be a factor to be taken into account in conjunction with actual monetary cost. And it eliminates the risk of increased hospital bed stay and all the other known risks associated with blood.

The cost of non-blood alternatives

12.15 The leading authority on costs for practitioners continues to be the British National Formulary (BNF) published jointly by the BMA and the Royal Pharmaceutical Society. From the original handy pocket size carried as standard by most junior doctors on the wards, it has grown to 1,366 pages and now represents a substantial book. An additional change is that it is published to cover a period of 6 months, the current edition running from September 2015 to March 2016.

12.16 The principal item in the context of non-blood management is ferric carboxymaltose branded as *Ferinject*®; marketed by Vifor Pharma and listed at pages 831 and 832. Its indications are 'Iron deficiency anaemia' and it is marketed in vials ready for use and the costings shown are £154.23 for a single vial or £405.88 for 5.

12.17 The highly controversial Eptacog alfa (activated), branded as *Novoseven*® and marketed by Novo Nordisk Ltd, when first available was priced at around $US 5,000 per dose largely for commercial reasons to recover the significant research and development costs. Listed on page 97, it has now come down to a more realistic £525.30 per pre-filled syringe and is for hospitals only. As a potential life-saver in extreme cases of haemorrhage it still represents value for money compared to the cost per unit of allogeneic blood and even more so when multiple units of blood have to be given.

12.18 Despite the (usually uninformed) complaints about comparative costs of non-blood alternatives, these prices have to be seen in the context not of the subsidised price at which allogeneic blood is supplied to the NHS but the actual cost to the taxpayer which, all inclusive, is in excess of £1,000 per unit. At worst non-blood alternatives are cost-neutral and in reality, when skilfully deployed, are often actually cheaper.

12.19 In addition to these pharmaceutical products, there are other techniques available. One is cell salvage. The cost of Cell Savers started high to recoup development costs but have now come down through £8,000 to something of the order of £4,000. Their usage is increasing across a range of conditions and experience suggests that they are indeed cost effective.

Secondly is the *CardioQ*® Oesophageal Doppler Monitor described in more detail in Chapter 4.

12.20 This is just a brief overview of the basics but NHS Trusts and units that have embraced the philosophy of blood conservation and non-blood management have confirmed that in the majority of cases they are certainly cheaper than allogeneic blood and give greater benefit to the patient by minimising known risks and shortening hospital stay.

A comparable study reported from the US in July 2015 was headed 'Costs and outcomes after cardiac surgery in patients refusing transfusion compared with those who do not; a case-matched study'.[181] This is an historic cohort study that aimed to compare costs and outcomes after cardiac surgery in patients who, being Jehovah's Witnesses, refuse blood transfusion with a group of matched patients accepting transfusion. The conclusion states:

> 'Utilising applicable blood conservation measures, cardiac surgery may be performed with similar outcomes and cost from day of surgery to discharge compared to controls in select patients without blood transfusion'.

12.21 The reader will decide for himself or herself but there is strong support for the proposition that, on a simple cost basis alone, most of the non-blood products are cheaper than and at least as effective as allogeneic blood. And given the exclusion of risks and complications; reduced hospital bed stay and the known benefits, there is a compelling argument that non-blood management is indeed cost effective.

12.22 As the history of progression in blood usage demonstrates, those responsible for blood safety have faced major challenges over the years, notably sexually transmitted diseases such as syphilis; hepatitis both B and C; cytomegalovirus; and then the HIV. Each new challenge has been demanding in scientific terms in attempting to devise a fail-safe test to ensure that infected blood does not reach the chain of distribution. This has come in stages and at significant cost. For example, the earliest tests for HIV were based on identifying sero-conversion. However as mentioned above it later emerged that there was a latent period of what became known as 'silent infection' when those infected were either delaying or failing to sero-convert so not showing up on the test. During that period it is accepted that donors capable of transmitting HIV were still being accepted and their blood harvested and distributed.

---

[181] *Transfusion*, Early View (online version of record published before inclusion in an issue). Article first published online; 16 July 2015

12.23 One of the more recent challenges is vCJD. The technology for prion filtration represents another major scientific challenge. Estimates of the prevalence of pre-clinical vCJD or the carrier state in the donor population are largely just that: estimates. But in March 2008 in a written Parliamentary Answer,[182] Dawn Primarolo on behalf of the then Secretary of State for Health referred to one study based on 12,674 tested. She stated:

> 'This suggests a prevalence of about 1 in 4,000 though with very wide ranges of uncertainty and a statistical confidence interval of between 1 in 1,400 and 1 in 20,000'.

12.24 The most recent problem is the Zika virus. According to the report of WHO dated 30 January 2016 it was first identified in Uganda in 1947. The first human case was detected in Nigeria in 1954; it then spread to Pakistan, Malaysia and Indonesia in 1977-78; to Yap in Micronesia in 2007 and thence to French Polynesia in 2013. From there it crossed to Brazil where it appears to have been first reported in May 2015. It has since spread rapidly northwards through the South American continent, the Caribbean, Central America and at the time of writing to Mexico.

The US National Institutes of Health has said, 'Its current, explosive, pandemic re-emergence is, therefore, truly remarkable'.

12.25 Significantly it is spread by *aedes* mosquitos which are the same insects that spread dengue and chikungunya virus found throughout the Americas except for Canada and Chile where it is too cold for them to survive. Unlike the mosquitos that spread malaria they are mostly active during the day and so bed nets only offer limited protection. Having drunk the blood of an infected person they can then infect people they subsequently bite. The WHO also reports that the virus has been isolated in human semen but they say sexual transmission person to person is as yet unconfirmed. It would seem to be almost inevitable. The conclusion is that the route of transmission can be through blood and products originating from allogeneic blood for which there is at present no available test. It logically follows from that that no person living in an area affected by the Zika virus should be a blood donor.

12.26 The WHO expects Zika to spread throughout the Americas but other scientists have warned that countries in Asia could also face large outbreaks.

---

[182] House of Commons: Hansard Written Answers for 11 March 2008 255W and 256W

On 4 February 2016 the health editor of The Times of London reported that '...the NHS banned travellers from giving blood for a month after they returned from a Zika-hit country in an effort to prevent the virus being passed on through transfusions'. A spokeswoman for NHS Blood and Transplant said '...that the precautionary measure was unlikely to significantly affect supplies as most such countries are already covered by six-month bans because of malaria'.

How soon before the virus spreads worldwide? The informed patient may justifiably ask just how safe that makes any blood product, even in the UK which is probably as safe as any in the world.

Clinical Negligence and the NHS Litigation Authority–£28 billion in potential claims

12.27 As with nearly all professions, doctors have for years carried professional negligence insurance to indemnify them against any claims that might be brought. Initially the premiums were reimbursed by the employing NHS even though the insurance providers were private bodies, notably the Medical Defence Union and the Medical Protection Society. But later as the number of employees reached over 1 million (now 1.7m) it was thought more practical for the NHS to take over the risk and more economical to self-fund indemnity insurance.

12.28 The logical extension was the NHS Litigation Authority (NHSLA) to handle the claims, an unquantified proportion of which arise out of the use of allogeneic blood or are due to lack of valid consent under the *Birch* principle. The majority of claims are settled without legal proceedings. In others proceedings are started but, after investigation and pleadings, settled without a trial. A number of cases, especially where there is a serious and/or novel dispute on liability, go all the way to trial. The authority appoints some 12 firms of solicitors throughout the country as specialists in medical claims work to handle these cases.

12.29 The sums involved are substantial. As medical and surgical procedures become more complex, both the number and quantum of claims seem to rise inexorably. Damaged birth claims tend to command the greatest damages, largely due to the need for specially adapted premises and equipment, full time nursing and for lifetime care. But the injury or death of a high earner can also result in a substantial award for loss of earnings. Major advances in, for example, cardiac surgery and intensive care have resulted in prolonged life expectancy for many who, even 30 or 40 years ago, would have been unlikely to have survived.

12.30 The general consensus is that the present system is unsustainable financially and sooner rather than later the government will, however reluctantly, have forced upon it a change to some system of no fault compensation. The overall result may be lower individual awards of damages but at least the injured claimant will be spared the often traumatic experience of long drawn out litigation made worse by the uncertainty of the outcome. The 2015 Supreme Court case of *Montgomery*, involving the mismanagement of delivery of a baby with shoulder dystocia, took 16 years to be resolved.

And the more than 'one third' currently paid to claimant solicitors in costs will at least be available as compensation for injured patients.

12.31 A similar no fault scheme has for more than 30 years been in operation in New Zealand which is often held up as the model to follow. A number of European countries with a state system of health care, including Denmark, Finland, France, Norway and Sweden have similar schemes. They have no fault compensation for what is variously described as a 'treatment injury', 'medical negligence' or 'medical mishap' where payment, although less generous, goes principally to patients or their relatives rather than to lawyers and expert witnesses. Settlements are also far quicker–usually no more than 9 months.

12.32 In the accounting year to 2014 for clinical negligence alone the NHSLA had 11,945 claims (up on the preceding year). For the first time the authority received more than 1,000 claims per month in 6 successive months of the year. It had potential liabilities then of £22.951 billion. Official figures for the accounting year to 31 March 2014 showed that in London alone the NHSLA paid out £470,000 each day in damages–excluding legal costs. The annual operating costs alone of the authority were £4.4 billion.

12.33 The latest figures for the NHSLA are for the year 2014/15 and reflect little change of significance over the years. In the previous year they paid out £1.1 billion in compensation to patients and their legal costs. In the coming year it will be around £1.4 billion. These figures are for clinical negligence only and do not include, for instance, injuries on duty, slipping on wet floors or potholes in car parks.

Perhaps more alarmingly the chairman in his report says:

> '...with accumulated provisions in our balance sheet of over £28 ***billion*** further significant increases are in the pipeline. Currently over a third of what we spend each year is received by the legal profession and, as later pages explain, most of this is paid to claimants' lawyers.
>
> One of our priorities for the year ahead is therefore to work with policy makers, other NHS bodies, clinicians and our scheme members to inform the debate on what might be done to reduce the financial burden on the NHS and increase the availability of scarce resources to the NHS and its patients'.

12.34 The 2014/2015 Report gives the usual breakdown of clinical negligence claims both by number and value. Significantly claims for obstetrics represent only 10% by number but 41% by value. Legal costs continue to assume even greater importance. There was a marked disparity between defence costs at £109.9 million as against claimant's costs of over £326 million.

One particularly disturbing feature is the citation of cases showing costs claimed massively disproportionate to the damages. One claim for £2,000 was settled within 4 months of the letter of claim but the claimant's solicitors presented a bill for £53,529. This on detailed assessment was reduced to £12,146. In a second even more exorbitant claim an offer of £5,000 was accepted. The claimants submitted a bill totalling £121,701 based on an hourly rate of £400 per hour with 100% success fee increasing it to £800 per hour. This was despite the bulk of the work being conducted by unqualified staff. On detailed assessment a number of discreditable matters emerged and the claimant's solicitors, when pressed, refused to disclose any further details in relation to their retainer. The not surprising outcome was that the costs judge ruled that he had 'No confidence in the claimant's retainer' and accordingly the entire claim for costs was struck out. These 2 cases alone seem to raise serious questions about the whole structure of claimant's costs in clinical negligence claims.

12.35 Meanwhile the long-overdue redevelopment of many major and deserving hospitals, such as the Royal National Orthopaedic Hospital at Stanmore in North London, are on hold or delayed for the lack of capital funding of a mere £90 million or so, a figure that is almost insignificant when set against the scale of payouts to claimants and lawyers for clinical negligence. The pressure for change is unlikely to abate.

12.36 A brief postscript on the NHS and its commercial relationship with some pharmaceutical companies. An article in *The Times* of London dated 17 February 2016 carried the headline 'Drugs companies paying hundreds of NHS officials'. It claimed:

> '...through hundreds of freedom of information requests and material from whistle-blowers, it was revealed that the practice of officials taking roles prescribing drugs and in "medicines management" while acting as consultants to pharmaceutical firms is systemic within the NHS. Pharmaceutical companies are spending £30 million a year employing officials and doctors as consultants in addition to £10 million sponsoring their attendance at events, the investigation found. In some cases, senior officials attend more than 20 paid advisory boards a year and earn up to £1,250 a day advising drugs companies on how to sell products to the NHS'.

12.37 If substantiated, the report seems to disclose an alarming conflict of interest very similar to that of the discredited Dr Garetta in France described in more detail in [1.31]. That case occurred more than 30 years ago and yet we still do not seem adequately to have learned obvious lessons from it.

12.38 Most readers will be incredulous that the NHS and/or their legal advisors appear not to have taken the most basic, indeed rudimentary, steps to have tied down contractually those involved in recommending and purchasing drugs on its behalf, precisely to exclude such a demonstrable conflict of interest. The almost inevitable commercial and political repercussions are likely to be on a seismic scale and are awaited with interest.

Chapter Thirteen

Children's Cases and the Legal Progression

13.1 It is one of the strange loopholes in our medico-legal system that there is no mechanism for central recording of those cases where the jurisdiction of the court has been invoked to over-ride the choice of medical treatment of minors. There is no separate database or other method for checking court records in the Royal Courts of Justice (let alone outside London) other than obtaining judicial consent and then laboriously ploughing through literally thousands of cases per year in the family division archives. Those cases that have made the law reports have been at random with no underlying system, criteria or index. But there is no central record in the NHS of such cases, or indeed of outcomes whether good or bad, or significantly, whether blood was actually transfused or not.

13.2 Right up to the 1980's there was an ill-defined legal process for children's cases where the parents were not consenting to the recommended blood transfusion. The benevolent paternalism of the treating clinicians came to the fore and they usually went ahead and transfused anyway, effectively challenging the parents to sue them but secure in the knowledge that they would be supported by the medical defence organisations and judges. The lack of any clear legal process led to some strange results.

13.3 In one bizarre case in which the author was belatedly instructed, an Inspector of the Metropolitan Police had stood in the casualty department of Guys Hospital and solemnly pronounced a Place of Safety Order for the baby to remain precisely where he had earlier been brought by the concerned parents anxious to secure the best available treatment. There was no suggestion that the parents might remove the child and it is difficult to imagine a safer place for the child to be or what practical purpose such an order might have served. This was the then statutory power, the forerunner of section 46 of the Children Act 1989. It was intended to be used for the protection of children, often runaways from home, who were found in circumstances amounting to immediate danger to the child such as, for example, a teenage girl found in a brothel or a young boy in the amusement arcades of Piccadilly Circus that were the notorious haunt of predators looking for 'rent boys'. The law gave the police the power to take the child immediately ***from*** such danger to a place of safety. It was never intended for cases involving serious issues relating to disputed alternatives in medical treatment when the child was ***already*** in a place of safety, and the mere purported making of an order did not in any way confer legal rights that overrode the requirement for parental consent or a proper court order overriding their choice of medical treatment options.

13.4 The legal progression of cases involving medical treatment of children where parental consent is withheld starts with the watershed case of *Baby B* in 1981. Both the parents and very senior and experienced treating consultant paediatrician were agreed that a very seriously impaired Downs Syndrome newborn should not be subjected to major invasive treatment but managed with palliative care until what was expected to be an early death. The local authority took a different view and, to by-pass such combined parental and clinical decision-making, instituted Wardship. That is believed to be the first time that Wardship is recorded as having been invoked in a medical treatment case. Until then it was historically the procedure whereby the property of a minor was protected by the Court of Chancery.

13.5 Over time it had developed into a general protective power over the assets of minors and thus over their person but until this case it had not been extended to medical treatment. Many lawyers and clinicians were troubled at the time by several factors. These included the overriding not only of the parents but of the considered professional decision of the hands-on treating team led by a senior and respected consultant paediatrician. Also the unseemly speed and therefore lack of serious case citation and consideration of legal principle in the proceedings. A judge of the Family Division at first instance sat in the morning, heard inevitably abbreviated evidence and legal submissions with truncated citation of legal authority and gave an *ex tempore* judgment dismissing the application. The Court of Appeal sat in the afternoon in an equally brief hearing and upheld the application to Ward the child and authorise the treatment.

13.6 Many professionals, both medical and legal, were concerned that that is scarcely the way for judges to make new law in such a very sensitive and important area that belonged (if at all) to Parliament. Indeed no less an authority than the then Professor Glanville Williams QC, well-respected Professor of Criminal Law at Cambridge University, wrote a letter that was published in *The Times* of London[183] under the heading 'Life of a child'. It makes compelling reading. One apposite quotation from his concluding paragraph may suffice:

> 'There is a strong argument for keeping the law out of these cases, although it can be kept out only by specific legislation or by a considerable shift of attitude on the part of the judges. When a question is so much a matter of opinion as this one is, the criminal law should stay its hand. It follows from this that the judges should not use the Wardship procedure to supplant the parents'.

13.7 Despite this powerful warning, once the precedent was set local authorities used this procedure as the legal mechanism of choice in medical treatment cases and thereby *inter alia* to override the election of non-blood management made by parents. What made the process so unfair to parents was that the local authorities consistently used the *ex parte* procedure (often late on a Friday afternoon) even when parents were at the bedside and readily available to be given notice (or served with legal papers) and thus involved and have input into the litigation. Acting on the *ex parte* order the hospital often proceeded to transfuse with donor blood, presenting the parents at the *inter partes* hearing on the Monday morning, or later, with an irreversible *fait accompli*. The unfairness was compounded by the un-necessarily authoritarian attitude of many clinicians and especially hospital administrators and/or their lawyers. In one case in which the author was involved the treating team told the parents:

> 'We have a Wardship Order—it's not legally your baby anymore and we will take all the decisions. We do not have to ask your consent for anything'.

That expression of opinion completely overlooked the fact that, despite the blood issue, there were often continuing treatment options where parental input was needed and indeed decision-making should properly have remained with the parents. It was, incidentally, bad in abstract law, as serious decision-making for Wards of Court is reserved to the judge, not the clinician.

13.8 In another extreme case an oncologist, now long retired and not greatly missed, whilst asserting the supremacy of the consultant's decision actually

183 'Life of a child' *The Times* of London 13 August 1981

said to the parents on the ward when they were trying to explain their conscientious stand and seek co-operation in non-blood management:

> 'He's God up there and I'm God down here!'

13.9 One of the problems in the early 1980's was the overall attitude to blood. It was still regarded as the gold standard lifesaving treatment and the view existed that only grossly irresponsible or fanatical parents would refuse it for their child. Secondly the 'Rule of Ten' prevailed so that the conventional transfusion threshold was 10g/dl of haemoglobin. This was based on no scientific criteria (see Chapter 1) but more on agreed defensive medicine to meet the *Bolam* test of 'whether the defendants, acting in the way that they did, were acting in accordance with a practice of competent respected professional opinion'.

The philosophy was that if the clinician transfused at 10 g/dl and there was still an adverse outcome, he would be immune from criticism from his peers, risk managers, judges or coroners and supported by his professional indemnity insurers. If he acceded to the wishes of the parents, he might lay himself open potentially to serious consequences in the event of an adverse outcome. And so he transfused.

Prince v Massachusetts

13.10 For many years attempts by parents to argue relative risks in transfusion practice were dismissed as cranky or even delusional. Sadly the deeply held conscientious beliefs based solidly on Holy Scripture were often treated with contempt and even ridicule. The wholly inappropriate and inapplicable comments in *Prince v Massachusetts*[184] were frequently cited as if conclusive:

> 'Parents may be free to become martyrs themselves but it does not follow that they are free in identical circumstances to make martyrs of their children before they have reached the age of full and legal discretion when they can make the choices for themselves'.

13.11 This demonstrates the dangers of citing a case out of context and it raises the serious question of how many of the commentators have actually read the judgment. Firstly *Prince* was a case that had nothing whatever to do with

[184] *Prince v Massachusetts* 321 U.S. 158 (1944)

medical treatment or blood transfusion. The defendant was the aunt and guardian of her 9-year-old niece. In the evening, out of school hours and at the express request of the niece who was a baptised member of the faith, she had taken her into the small and comparatively risk-free town where they lived.

13.12 There in the public street they together engaged in the evangelising ministry for which Jehovah's Witnesses have been well known for over a century and they were each offering Bible based literature to passers-by for a modest contribution. By chance along came the school attendance officer who (from a reading of the judgment) was already demonstrably hostile to the family and indeed was waiting for an opportunity to act against them. He challenged the aunt, quite wrongly in the view of many experienced lawyers, for breaching the child labour laws on the basis that the niece was 'working and engaged in unlawful selling', and a prosecution was brought on that basis. This was, and remains, legislation aimed at protecting children from exploitation by commercial employers and harks back to the child chimney sweeps of Dickens' era; children down coalmines and the sweatshops that so disfigure some of the Third World countries even today.

13.13 It is highly unlikely that any such prosecution would have been mounted in peacetime but this was 1943/4 and wartime. The US was still reeling from the outrages of U-boats sinking civilian passenger liners with many US citizens, including women and children, amongst those lost and also the surprise attack on Pearl Harbour. Furthermore their troops were engaged in a vicious war with Japan in the Pacific with a very high rate of casualties and in Europe were massing under General Eisenhower for the invasion of Normandy.

Because of the firm stand on neutrality and conscientious refusal to serve in the armed forces, Jehovah's Witnesses were an unpopular minority, whose preaching work was, even in democratic America, subject to intermittent local restrictions, outright ban and harassment that frequently escalated to brutal physical violence. That included their being tarred and feathered and even castrated. Indeed they were the only religious group persecuted even-handedly in Nazi concentration camps; in the Soviet *gulags*; in Japanese prisons as well as in prisons throughout the Allies including the UK, the then Dominions and Colonies, and the USA.

13.14 A detailed reading of the judgment (rather than a mere extract selected out of context) shows a hostile, prejudiced Bench giving a populist judgment against an unpopular minority at a time of war fever. It has no correlation or relevance to medical treatment in the 21st century. The defence submitted that 'the child's presence on the street, with her guardian, distributing or offering to distribute the magazines... was in no way harmful to her nor, in any event, more so than the presence of many other children at the same time and place, engaged in shopping and other activities not prohibited.' Such a logical submission was easily brushed aside by the court as if this child had been mingling with the prostitutes on Times Square or 42nd Street late on a Saturday night.

13.15 What is often omitted from academic writings is the strong dissenting judgment of Murphy J. who seems to have had his feet more firmly on the ground than the majority when he asserted:

> 'It is claimed however that such activity was likely to affect adversely the health, morals and welfare of the child. Reference is made in the majority opinion to "the crippling effects of child employment, more especially in public places, and the possible harms arising from other activities subject to all the diverse influences of the street." To the extent that they flow from participation in ordinary commercial activities, these harms are irrelevant to this case. And the bare possibility that such harms might emanate from distribution of religious literature is not, standing alone, sufficient justification for restricting freedom of conscience and religion. Nor can parents or guardians be subjected to criminal liability because of vague possibilities that their religious teachings might cause injury to the child. The evils must be grave, immediate, substantial. cf. Bridges v California 314 U.S. 252, 314 U.S. 262.
>
> Yet there is not the slightest indication in this record, or in sources subject to judicial notice, that children engaged in distributing literature pursuant to their religious beliefs have been or are likely to be subject to any of the harmful "diverse influences of the street". Indeed, if probabilities are to be indulged in, the likelihood is that children engaged in serious religious endeavour are immune from such influences. Gambling, truancy, irregular eating and sleeping habits, and the more serious vices are not consistent with the high moral character ordinarily displayed by children fulfilling religious obligations. Moreover, Jehovah's Witness children invariably make their distributions in groups subject at all times to adult or parental control, as was done in this case. The dangers are thus exceedingly remote, to say the least. And the fact that the zealous exercise of the right to propagandize the community may result in violent or disorderly situations difficult for children to face is no excuse for prohibiting the exercise of that right.

> No chapter in human history has been so largely written in terms of persecution and intolerance as the one dealing with religious freedom. From ancient times to the present day, the ingenuity of man has known no limits in its ability to forge weapons of oppression for use against those who dare to express or practice unorthodox religious beliefs. And the Jehovah's Witnesses are living proof to the fact that, even in this nation, conceived as it was in the ideals of freedom, the right to practice religion in unconventional ways is still far from secure. Theirs is a militant and unpopular faith, pursued with a fanatical zeal. They have suffered brutal beatings; their property has been destroyed; they have been harassed at every turn by the resurrection and enforcement of little used ordinances and statutes. (See Mulder and Comisky, "Jehovah's Witnesses Mold Constitutional Law" 2 Bill of Rights Review No 4, p. 262.)
>
> To them, along with other present day religious minorities, befalls the burden of testing our devotion to the ideals and constitutional guarantees of religious freedom. We should therefore hesitate before approving the application of a statute that might be used as another instrument of oppression. Religious freedom is too sacred a right to be restricted or prohibited in any degree without convincing proof that a legitimate interest of the state is in grave danger'.

13.16 It took many years and a robust judge to deal comprehensively in the English courts with this concept of martyring. One unwise counsel for a hospital seeking an order for blood transfusion used the quote from *Prince* suggesting forcefully that these parents should not be allowed to martyr the child. The judge's rebuke was swift and robust.[185] He said:

> 'There is no question of these loving and caring parents seeking to martyr this child. They are torn in an agony of conscience between giving the child the best chance of life through the best medical care and at the same time their deeply held religious beliefs. I don't want to hear anything more about "martyring"'.

Counsel backed off and the word seems to have gone round the fairly closed world of medical counsel appearing in these cases. To the writer's knowledge *Prince* has not since been quoted in any of these similar medical cases. Despite that powerful judicial dictum from an authoritative and well-respected judge of the High Court and former Chairman of the Family Bar Association, surprisingly the case is still quoted (inappropriately many might think and selectively without the dissenting judgment) in some well-recognised medical

[185] Johnson J. High Court Family Division—unreported

law textbooks.[186] One of the ironies is that, in giving the case citation of one of the earlier cases where reference was made to it, one learned author makes the wry comment 'where the passage, due to an error by Counsel, is wrongly attributed to Holmes J.'. That in itself raises questions about the diligence of the advocate who cited it but more especially it is a matter of regret that cited selectively, undue weight has been accorded it without the counterbalance of the powerful dissent of Murphy J. quoted above.

13.17 These conscientious beliefs are core values described as such by no less an authority than the Royal College of Surgeons and to breach them would be to compromise Christian beliefs in an unacceptable way.

13.18 It is the same principle as applies to the acknowledgement of any God other than the Supreme Creator. This was the position faced by many early Christians. Whilst they were in subjection to the secular authorities and were thus respectful and obedient to the laws of the Senate and to Caesar as Emperor and secular ruler, they took seriously Jesus' words to: 'Pay back, therefore, Caesar's things to Caesar, but God's things to God'. This brought them into a conflict not of their seeking but simply because they could not worship Caesar *as a god*.

Contemporary historians recount how entire families of Christians, including the very young and the very old, were led into the arena before Caesar and the baying mob. There was an altar with a flame burning and incense provided. They had only to put a pinch of incense on the flame and raise an arm in salute to '*Hail Caesar*' and they and their family could go home. The alternative, which they well knew, was a horrific death such as by being torn to pieces by wild animals, hacked to death by gladiators, or covered with tar and set alight. But because what was required was an act of idolatry in recognising the godship of Caesar, they could not do it. The result was that hundreds or even thousands of Christians died with their families.

13.19 The scale of the persecution is recorded by contemporary historian Pliny the Younger who, while governor of Pontus and Bithynia, corresponded with Emperor Trajan. He reported that the 'contagion' of Christianity

[186] See notably Kennedy & Grubb, *Medical Law* Fourth Edition 2010 at p. 531; Dr Simon Mills BL, *Clinical Practice and the Law;* Christopher Johnston, 3 Serjeants' Inn, *Medical treatment: Decisions and the Law*. Charles Foster: *Choosing Life, Choosing Death: The Tyranny of Autonomy in Medical Law and Ethics:* Heart (2009)

threatened everyone, regardless of gender, age or rank. Pliny gave those accused of being Christians opportunity to deny it or be executed. Any who cursed Christ or recited a prayer to the gods or to Trajan's statue were released. Pliny acknowledged that these were things that 'those who were really Christians cannot be made to do.'

13.17 Some fair minded onlookers (including perhaps a lawyer such as Gamaliel) watching the horrific deaths doubtless thought that at best these Christians were mad not to comply with Caesar's requirements or at least that the parents were totally unfit to bring up their children in a faith that led to such consequences. Had there existed at that time in the Roman culture the legal processes of Wardship and CAFCASS, doubtless the children would have been removed from these Christian homes to be brought up as good pagan worshippers of Caesar. Presumably Caesar's judge would have pronounced on the morality of parents and their rights and responsibilities to their children as did the judge in *Prince.*

13.20 Two thousand years later, many Witnesses perished in the Nazi concentration camps because, for the same principle, they would not say '*Heil Hitler'* (a clear echo of Hail Caesar), or give the infamous raised arm salute, join the Party, wear the Swastika and support the war machine. And what distinguished them from the Jews and others in the camps for whom there was no hope of release was that they had only to give the salute and sign a paper tendered by the Gestapo renouncing their faith as Bible Students and they too could go home.

13.21 Again the issue of their children arose. Reputable historians of the Nazi era record that babies and young ones were seized from their Christian parents and given up to 'good Nazi Aryan parents' for forced adoption. More mature ones were sent to so-called Reform Schools where brutal attempts were made to knock this 'Bible nonsense' out of them. What was so surprising to those who did not know the strength of faith of these Christians was the repeated failure to break the spirit and beliefs of these children.

13.22 The persecution of this small but significant group of Christians was reflected in the comments of the prominent UK jurist, Sir David Maxwell Fyfe QC, who as *rapporteur* had major input into the drafting of what was to become the European Convention on Human Rights. He supported Article 2 of the First Protocol (freedom of education) in these terms:[187]

> '...the object of this Article is to meet what we all know was a terrible aspect of totalitarianism, namely that the youth of the country were brought up so much under the dogmatic teaching of totalitarianism by the agencies or para-agencies of the State that it was impossible for their parents to bring them up in their own religion and philosophical beliefs'.

13.23 It is these underlying principles and core values on the sanctity of life and their higher duty to the Creator that motivate Jehovah's Witnesses when they make their choice of non-blood treatment. It is a moral and conscientious belief based on Scripture.

13.24 Despite the reluctance or refusal of many practitioners to accept this position, there were some progressive clinicians who were beginning to take a harder look at the risk/benefit analysis of blood transfusion as first cytomegalovirus and then hepatitis were followed by HIV transmission, but these practitioners were at that time in a minority. The consequence was that each incident was fought on a case by case basis, slowly pushing back the boundaries of prejudice and ignorance of the benefits of non-blood management.

13.25 Despite the absence of any official records, for over 30 years the author has maintained his own records that clearly demonstrate some important trends. Firstly, only 10 out of 32 orders made (being *permissive* and not mandating treatment) were actually followed through with the administration of blood or blood products peri- or post-operatively and these were mainly cases of blood disorders or prematurity. Furthermore, with the notable exception of a case involving priming of a heart lung machine (subsequently modified by miniaturisation), the author is unaware of any surgical case where the court has given leave and blood been actually administered in the years since 1995.

13.26 That limited percentage of effectiveness immediately raises a pertinent question about public funds and resources in an underfunded NHS. The costs of each application to the Family Division of the High Court (or the Court of Protection) are huge. Simply for an overworked High Court Judge to sit

---

[187] *Religious Liberty and International law in Europe*, Cambridge University Press—Professor Malcolm Evans at p. 274-5

involves a massive support cost in salary, pension, buildings, associate, judge's clerk, recording and transcribing facilities, usher, computers, plus all the administrative staff handling the paperwork in the Family Division. Thus before any legal costs of the applicant NHS Trust, CAFCASS or the parents are brought into account, the court costs to the public purse of a day's hearing in the High Court are unlikely to be less than £8-10,000.

13.27 Because of the gravity of these life and death cases, the preparation will be handled by senior solicitor practitioners with charging rates probably in the region of £300 per hour with all the associated costs of medical records, photocopying and paginating and the multitude of routine costs generated in pleading and filing a High Court application. CAFCASS will have to take an experienced Guardian off other highly skilled and urgent work on children's cases to make full enquiries and prepare a report for the judge. Whilst they are likely to use their own in-house salaried lawyers without charge, these do not come without cost.

13.28 If junior counsel is briefed on behalf of the NHS Trust they will be of significant seniority, perhaps on the brink of Silk, and charging brief fee and refreshers proportionately. In many cases, leading counsel will be instructed. And so to the standing charges of court costs there is likely to be added probably another £10,000 in NHS and CAFCASS legal fees.

13.29 Thirdly are the expert witness costs. Witness statements will be provided from several specialist clinicians and, following Part 35 of the CPR and the Strasbourg case[188] that entitles the parents to have the experts at court for cross-examination, these high-powered experts will take time off from more productive clinical duties to attend court. At the very least, the cover needed for their absence is an additional cost on NHS funds.

13.30 Thus to quote an overall cost ***per case*** of something in the range of £20-£25,000 is by no means fanciful. That sum would fund the capital costs of at least two cell salvage machines[189] plus many courses of treatment with effective recombinant (non-blood) drugs such as the haemostatic agent Factor VIIa *Novoseven*®; r-HuEPO; or products such as *Venofer*® and *Ferinject*®. Yet nowhere is there to be found a cost/benefit evaluation of these court

---

188 *Balsyte-Lideikiene v Lithuania* No: 72596/01, 4 November 2008 p.12 §66

189 e.g *Hemonetics* Cell Saver

applications. On the contrary, each NHS Trust has its own legal budget and most, after a tendering process known euphemistically as a 'beauty parade', will retain solicitors in private practice with all the overheads, profit element and charging rates that implies. The names that recur in these proceedings are the top practitioners in medical law and are usually highly competent. But it might be thought that somebody, somewhere, was keeping an overall eye to see whether these repetitive applications were indeed cost effective to the public purse.

13.31 Once the Children Act 1989 came into force, Wardship gradually fell into disuse and the applications were brought primarily by local authorities under Section 8 for Specific Issue Orders, or orders made under the inherent jurisdiction of the High Court. A notable exception was *re O,*[190] where an over-enthusiastic local authority sought an Emergency Protection Order from Magistrates with late notice to the parents denying them an opportunity to be heard. On appeal to Johnson J., he readily accepted the manifest unfairness to the parents both of the *ex parte* procedure and of the use of the emergency protection procedure.

13.32 Firstly, that is a form of order that merely provides for removal of the child to a place of safety. The child in question was already in hospital to which it had been brought by loving and caring parents seeking the best possible treatment. It is difficult to envisage a safer place. Secondly, this provision does not in fact give to the hospital the right to treat without parental consent. Thirdly, the order is by statute un-appealable for 72 hours, a blatantly unfair provision to parents in medical treatment cases and now possibly a breach of Article 6 of the European Convention which governs fairness of proceedings. Before Johnson J., counsel for the local authority very sensibly did not seek to support either the *ex parte* procedure or the use of the Emergency Protection Order.

13.33 As the judgment shows, the judge set out in terms:

> 'Strenuous efforts must be made to arrange an *inter partes* hearing', and
>
> 'These cases are of such gravity that they should be heard by a High Court judge'.

---

[190] *re O (A Minor) (Medical Treatment)* [1993] 2 FLR 149 Johnson J.

This judgment itself marked a turning point in these cases that was picked up and developed by Booth J. in the case of *re R*[191] that followed only a matter of months after *re O*. In July 2010 Sir Nicholas Wall, then President of the Family Division, had to consider a difficult case of proposed medical treatment (liver transplant) that caring parents resisted as not in the best interests of the child. In the course of his ruling[192] he had to consider whether it was necessary for the law to move on but decided that it did not. He cited and upheld these two cases.

13.34 The third stage of the legal progression came with the reorganisation of the NHS and the creation of largely self-regulating Trusts. This included their acquiring a degree of autonomy and the retainer of their own specialist medical solicitors to act on behalf of the Trust. The result has been that local authorities have effectively dropped out of these blood transfusion cases, NHS Trusts now bring them to the court under the Inherent Jurisdiction of the High Court and the issues are narrowed to that of donor blood only, leaving the major decision-making on treatment options still with the parents. It has been a long haul over some 30 years but the legal status of parental decision-making has made huge strides forward.

13.35 Despite these procedural changes, an analysis of the 32 cases is instructive and reveals some challenging data. Those cases in which blood was actually used fall into three main identifiable categories. These are accepted to be the most problematical areas of medical treatment of minors:

- Haemophilia and the two principal genetic blood disorders, thalassaemia and sickle cell anaemia, where the oxygen carrying red cells are so deficient that, in the present state of medical knowledge and research, only blood support can ensure survival;
- some of the more aggressive childhood leukaemias (notably T-ALL) where it is not practicable to modify the conventional oncology treatment of combination chemotherapy by cytotoxic drugs to exclude blood support and provide feasible non-blood management; and
- low birth weight/premature babies.

13.36 Given the life threatening nature of these 3 categories, most parents will accept, however reluctantly, that there is almost an inevitability in the court

191 *re R (A Minor) (Blood Transfusion)* [1993] 2 FLR 757 Booth J.
192 *LA and SB v AB and MB Medical Treatment* [2010] EWHC (Fam) 1744 and August [2011] Fam Law 789-791

making the order sought. Nine of the cases fall squarely within these categories. One is *sui generis* and highly unlikely to be repeated because it concerned the sole issue of the priming of the heart/lung machine. The priming problems have since been solved by the adaption and miniaturisation of the machine.

13.37 Rhesus conflict is becoming rarer in western medical practice with the use of anti-D post-conception; and the techniques of managing it with multi-lamp ultra-violet phototherapy and other adjunctive therapy have held the bilirubin to acceptable levels, avoided the known risks of kernicterus (damage to the brain) and thereby virtually eliminated the need for exchange transfusion or even blood support.

13.38 That leaves 15 major surgical cases which demonstrate the advances that have been made. The range of surgery now being undertaken successfully without blood includes not simply the fairly routine general surgical procedures but also difficult cardiac repair and complex neurosurgery, often in tiny neonates with blood vessels measured in microns. For those who are interested in knowing not merely ***that*** non-blood management works but ***how*** in practice it works some case histories are set out in more detail in chapter 15.

Ethical Considerations

13.39 The ethos of paediatricians and children's nurses has historically been 'The child first and always'. Thus it is fairly deeply ingrained that parental wishes are only significant if they accord with the treatment being recommended by the clinicians. If the parents take a stand on a particular treatment option, it can at best cause friction with the treating team and at worst lead to undeniably adversarial court proceedings to override the parental wishes. However into this mix also come the wishes of the child.

13.40 Despite the legal concept of *Gillick* competence, it is generally accepted by many practitioners in this field that comparatively young children, especially the long-term chronic sick, often have a genuine insight into and understanding of their condition well beyond their years. For some a huge part of their young lives has been spent in hospital. They are familiar and at ease with the bedside consultation at which, especially in teaching hospitals, medical students and junior doctors are engaged by consultants in very open discussions within the hearing of the child. These child patients quickly learn to 'talk the talk' and can themselves discuss their condition and treatment with sometimes alarming frankness. They not only want but come to expect to be involved in the decision-making process and to have a say in their treatment.

Many specialist children's nurses are familiar with this. They are involved in the day-to-day care, establish a close relationship with the child and as a result the child will often open up and discuss their condition and treatment preferences. It is far from unknown for a child often still under 10-years-of-age to reach a stage where, after frequent and often extremely unpleasant procedures, they say 'enough is enough – I do not want any more'.

13.41 Professor Len Doyal, an eminent expert in medical ethics,[193] has addressed the issue of treatment being forced on children without their consent or against their wishes. Under the potentially provocative title '*Can medicine be torture? The case of children*' he picks up and develops this theme of non-consensual treatment. The entire article, supported as it is by no less than 53 professional references should be required reading for those contemplating overriding consent to treatment by comprehending children. At the risk of the charge of being unreasonably selective, amongst his compelling materials are the following:

> 'Whatever the good intentions of the clinicians, the psychological impact on patients being forced to have painful and sustained medical treatment might well approximate to torture—especially if no legal redress were available for the suffering and indignity they have endured...
>
> Thus a judicial unwillingness to take seriously the right of young people to consent has thrust us back into a situation where persons of designated authority can force medical treatment on them, no matter how competent they may be to decide otherwise. As one noted legal commentator[194] has stated:
>
> > "It seems a strange right which enables a child to say 'yes' but not 'no'..."
>
> There can be no doubt that elective treatments are sometimes forced on children who have verbally and/or physically rejected them...'

13.42 In his conclusion the professor summarises his proposals that:

> '...legal and professional guidelines should be altered where necessary to ensure that:

[193] Former Professor of Medical Ethics, St Bartholomew's/The Royal London Hospitals School of Medicine and Dentistry

[194] Brazier M. *'Medicine, Patients and the Law'*. Harmondsworth, Penguin, 1992:346.

Competence to consent or refuse treatment is decided in the same way for children and adults—the ability to understand, remember, deliberate about and accept the personal implications of proposed specific treatments;

The explicit consent of children should be sought for all elective medical examination and treatment, along with those of parental authority. Their right to refuse should always be respected and their competence to consent should be presumed, unless it has been independently assessed;

When declared incompetent to give consent, children should still be consulted and be given appropriate information and intellectual and emotional preparation for treatment;

When a competent child refuses "necessary" treatment—that which is lifesaving or which prevents permanent and serious disability—this decision should also be respected provided that:

i) it is sustained;
ii) specific reasons are given for it which are consistent with what are known of the child's values; and
iii) competence is confirmed by a senior paediatrician and child psychiatrist who are not involved with the child's treatment.

In emergency situations where there is no time for assessment of competence, children under the age of 16 who refuse necessary treatment can be treated against their wishes. When this occurs and treatment is successful, the young person should be given a detailed written explanation of why the treatment was necessary and why their wishes were ignored;

At the age of 16, all patients should be treated as adults as regards consent to treatment.

[Author's Note: These last two points were written several years before the decision in *AC v Manitoba* and which, for the reasons given, it is submitted should now reflect the law and best practice on Mature Minors].

To the degree that these principles are ignored by both doctors and parents, the medical treatment of children can rightly be said to be cruel and unusual, even when the treatment *per se* is successful and little physical suffering is involved. When there is great suffering and the child's self-respect and trust of adults are permanently and severely damaged, then medicine can indeed be torture'.

Many readers, especially some paediatricians, will find this to be powerful, even provocative, comment, but it is the considered view of an eminent expert in this field that undoubtedly commands respect.

Court intervention or not?

13.43 This is an area in which practice varies widely not merely from NHS Trust to NHS Trust but also between Trust solicitors and even between consultants in the same hospital. The parents of baby *Glass* in many ways did not do other treating teams or parents a favour. The facts were very sad. The baby was seriously impaired and the parents became concerned that the hospital clinicians/risk managers were following a care plan that was likely to lead to a pain free but early death. When the proposed administration of morphine arose, they felt (wrongly on the recorded facts) that the treating team were moving towards accelerating the death of the baby. They remonstrated in robust terms; emotions ran high; tempers flared and it all degenerated into a literal 'punch-up' on the ward, to which hospital security had to be called to restore order.

The ensuing litigation ended up in the European Court of Human Rights, which ruled[195] essentially that parental consent was required to any underage patient lacking competence to decide treatment choices and, absent such consent, a court order must be obtained. As a broad statement of principle few would argue with the reasoning, especially that parental decision-making should only be overruled by due process of law.

13.44 But its practical application has caused many problems. Very few conditions have only one possible treatment. There are usually choices to be made, only some of which involve the issue of donor blood. The treating team may have a preferred option and the parents another. If in every such case the jurisdiction of the court were invoked for a ruling, an already overworked Court of Protection would be swamped with medical cases leaving other often equally urgent work of the court and of CAFCASS and their guardians to grind to a halt. And so, pragmatic solutions continue to apply. The wise dictum of the highly respected former paediatric cardiologist Professor Tynan of Guy's Hospital is the preferred choice of many paediatricians:

> 'Law and medicine don't mix and I would much prefer that this could have been left to be dealt with on the ward between myself and the parents'.

---

[195] *Glass v United Kingdom* [2004] 1 FLR 1019; ECtHR No: 61827/00, 9.3.04

The problems arise when risk managers are involved, followed by Trust solicitors who adhere to a strict interpretation of *Glass*.

13.45 One specific example taken at random demonstrates the problem. A very senior and experienced counsel acting for a specialist hospital with a reputation as a centre of excellence had the non-blood arguments presented together with some compelling professional articles. The Position Statement concluded with this somewhat dismissive paragraph:

> 'It is averred that the potential risks suggested by the parents (at paragraph 6.2 Parents' Position Statement) (i.e. mistake of giving the wrong blood, contaminated blood, transmission of HIV, Hepatitis or CJD, transfusion reaction and immune system suppression) are of such small likelihood that the balance does not weigh against saving B's life with blood products should the same become clinically necessary'.[196]

13.46 This is where the question of trust between clinicians and parents assumes such importance. The Christian community of Jehovah's Witnesses now numbers over 8 million baptised adherents with almost 20 million attending the annual Memorial of Christ's death in 2015. Yet, so far as can be established, there is no recorded case anywhere worldwide of a patient or parents having sued or even filed a complaint of negligence or breach of duty where the choice of non-blood management has been respected, even where there has been a fatal outcome. The only reported litigated cases have arisen where, despite the clear knowledge of the wishes for non-blood treatment, such wishes have been ignored and donor blood has still been given. That was the entire *rationale* that underpinned the leading common law case of *Malette v Shulman* and was followed in the English case.

13.47 In many cases involving children, an understanding is often reached between treating team and parents whereby the clinicians endeavour to honour the parental wishes for non-blood. However the clinicians make it clear that, if they get their backs to the wall and there is a real danger of losing the child, or of grave impairment such as brain damage, they will, albeit as a last resort, use donor blood. The purists will say that this does not comply with *Glass.* It is, however, a pragmatic and workable solution that obviates court proceedings, which are often highly stressful for the parents who have enough to do coping emotionally with the fact of a (by definition) very sick child, and also saves the

---

[196] *re B* Family Division Jul 2004 Holman J. (unreported)

NHS the substantial time and expense of a court application already referred to. It falls neatly into line with the views expressed, albeit informally, by Professor Tynan.

13.48 Thus *Glass* and the legal and ethical realities of paediatric practice sit uncomfortably together and these difficult cases are likely to be resolved on a case by case basis with much turning on the working relationship and degree of trust between clinicians and parents. One important factor is the sheer percentage of cases in which the whole emotionally draining and expensive procedures of a court application are pursued only for the treatment modality at issue never to be employed—what many may regard as an expensive exercise in purely risk management.

13.49 There is now powerful authority, both domestic and at Strasbourg, that Article 8 of the Convention applies not merely to *judicial* but also to *administrative* decision-making. In a lecture by Munby J., as he then was, to the Family Rights Group Conference in 2009[197] he said:

> 'So parents have a right to be fully involved in the planning by public authorities of public authority in the lives of their family and children, before care proceedings have been commenced, while the care proceedings are on foot, as well as after the final care order has been made... Indeed, in principle the procedural safeguards mandated by Article 8 ***apply to all public authorities whose actions may engage someone's Article 8 rights***'. [Emphasis added]

13.50 Perhaps the medical arguments for the non-blood clinical management of children are best summarised in an article in a legal professional journal[198] that demonstrated that there is in fact an increased mortality in critically ill children associated with red blood cell transfusion. But the key legal factor that emerges from the authorities and the practice is that a court order for the use of allogeneic blood and blood products is permissive only. One leading writer summarizes it succinctly:

> 'To avoid confusion or misunderstanding the court should avoid the "authorize and direct" form of order and simply make an order "authorizing" the relevant treatment'.

---

197 Family Rights Group Conference, *Professional Family Advocacy and Safeguarding Children*, 10 June 2009

198 Red blood cell transfusion in critically ill children is independently associated with increased mortality. Kneyber et al. *Intensive Care Med.* 2007; 33: 1414-1422

Thus even after Court intervention the ultimate decision whether to transfuse or not seems to rest with the treating clinician.

Chapter Fourteen

Mature Minors and Consent to Treatment

14.1 The law in England & Wales relating to medical treatment of mature minors and their capacity to give consent to and refusal of specific medical treatments is agreed by many practitioners to be in disarray. Primarily it is governed by a decision of the Court of Appeal[199] made over 20 years ago in which it was held that, whilst s.8 of the Family Law Act 1969 combined with the House of Lords decision in *Gillick* gave a patient under 18-years-of-age in certain circumstances the right to *consent* to medical treatment without parental consent, that did not extend to a right to *refuse*.

14.2 The initial part of the judgment of Nolan LJ. makes it clear that he was dealing with the specific facts of anorexia, the case before him:

> 'I would emphasise that the only aspect of W's welfare with which we are concerned in the present case is her refusal to undergo a particular form of treatment for anorexia. So far in this judgment I have been principally concerned to explain why, as it seems to me, the court has not only the power but the inescapable responsibility of deciding, in that specific context, what is to be done in the interests of her welfare. I am very far from asserting any general rule that the court should prefer its own view as to what is in the best interests of the child to those of the child itself. In considering the welfare of the child, the court must not only recognise but if necessary defend the right of the child, having sufficient understanding to take an informed decision, to make his or her own choice. In most areas of life it would not only be wrong in principle but also futile and counter-productive for the court to adopt any different approach. In the case of medical treatment, however, the court can and sometimes must intervene'.

14.3 It is clear from that passage that the judge is addressing the specific condition of anorexia and its manifestation in that specific patient. It is well known medically that the very nature of the illness of anorexia reduces and in some cases even takes away from the usually teenage patient the capacity to choose whether to take food or not. One medical dictionary puts it thus:

> 'A psychological illness, most common in female adolescents, in which the patients starve themselves or use other techniques such as vomiting or taking

[199] *re W (a minor) (Medical Treatment)* [1992] 4 All ER 627; (1992) 9 BMLR 22 (CA)

> laxatives, to induce weight loss. They are motivated by a false perception of their bodies as fat and/or a phobia of becoming fat'.

Most fair minded people would not disagree with the proposition that, however exceptionally, it is right for the court to intervene in such a case especially where the very illness deprives the patient of real freedom of choice to take in life sustaining nourishment. However the judge went on to broaden the scope of his judgment as follows:

> 'In general terms, however, the present state of the law is that an individual who has reached the age of 18 is free to do with his life what he wishes, but it is the duty of the Court to ensure so far as it can that children survive to that age'.

It is those few words, arguably *obiter dicta*, that have been consistently relied on by lawyers for NHS hospitals when they have sought to invoke the court's inherent jurisdiction and override the mature teenage patient's refusal of treatment.

14.2 Well respected authors have commented negatively on the continuance of this position. The first is the medico-legal writer Professor Margaret Brazier who said:[200]

> 'It seems a strange right that enables a child to say "Yes" but not "No"'.

Also the eminent authors Kennedy & Grubb put it succinctly in their critique[201] of the decisions in *re R* and *re W*:

> 'It is our view that these cases do not properly represent an ordered development in the law and should be considered by the House of Lords when the opportunity arises'.

Attempts to argue a broader right to refuse, in line with the first part of the judgment of Nolan LJ., have consistently been rejected by judges of the High Court (Family Division) who have held themselves to be bound by the second passage under the law of precedent. The author submits that such a position fails to take into consideration the fundamental differences between anorexia (which by its very nature denies the patient free choice) and the choice of non-blood management. Of course there are a few conditions, such as haemophilia, thalassaemia and perhaps T-ALL, where in the current state of medical knowledge the treating team are unable to offer an alternative. But as many of

200 *Medicine, Patients and the Law* - Margaret Brazier
201 *Principles of Medical Law*, Kennedy & Grubb, 3rd Edition at p. 988

the citations in this work demonstrate, with blood loss and anaemia, there are usually alternatives that are both effective and safe.

14.3 This part of the English law on consent to medical treatment, based on an arbitrary and fixed age, seems to be stuck in a time warp at least pre-war (if not Victorian) and enshrined in legislation passed over 40 years ago. The moment of acquiring majority at the age of 18 is supposed to cause what one judge described as a *ευρήκά* moment[202] at which the newly fledged adult mystifyingly acquires instantaneous wisdom, maturity and judgment which he is now free to exercise, even to self-harm and death, provided he does no harm to others. Below that age he is in law deemed to have no such qualities and the benevolent and paternalistic State must have the final say on what medical treatment is in his best interests. This flies in the face of extensive material on maturing adolescents contained in social work, medical, ethical and legal writings and indeed the practical experience of parents, teachers and clinicians treating adolescents daily.

14.4 Whilst Parliament[203] gives a 16-year-old a statutory right to consent to medical treatment, this has been consistently interpreted by the courts as excluding the determinative right to refuse. This age and the right to consent has at common law been extended downwards by the concept of *Gillick* competence[204] yet it still excludes the right to exercise choice where that involves refusal of a treatment option. The anomalies thrown up by the right to consent but not to refuse are legion but two examples may suffice to demonstrate the problem.

14.5 Firstly, a 12-year-old girl, having just attained puberty with all the hormonal and emotional changes that involves, as a result of some unwise and ill-informed sexual experimentation becomes pregnant. She will, in the vast majority of cases, be deemed to have the right and the capacity (including wisdom, judgment and voluntariness) to take the major and irreversible decision to consent to a termination of her pregnancy even though this involves the destruction of a viable foetus and thus the deliberate termination of a life. Arguably, the choice to have the termination must include the refusal of the

---

[202] *A.C. v Manitoba* supra, per Abella J.

[203] Family Law Reform Act, 1969, Section 8

[204] *Gillick v West Norfolk & Wisbech AHA* [1985] 3 All ER 402

alternative treatment option, which is to carry the baby to term, but even at age 12 she is permitted to make the choice.

14.6 At the other end of the spectrum, consider a strapping adolescent male just weeks or even days short of his 18th birthday and in law eligible (*inter alia*) to join the armed forces and kill or be killed on behalf of his country. With a profound conscientious objection to donor blood that he finds repugnant to the scriptural beliefs he has held all his comprehending life, he will have his refusal of blood transfusion overridden by the court in what are deemed to be his best interests. He has not yet had that so-called *eureka* moment and accordingly, in law, lacks the maturity, wisdom and judgment to take his own decision. Procedurally he will have only minimal input into the court's decision and will be highly unlikely to be seen or heard personally by the judge, but will have his views conveyed indirectly via a third party guardian appointed by CAFCASS. The classic dictum of Nolan LJ. cited above, (arguably not an essential part of the judgment that he gave and therefore *obiter dicta*) will be the default position of lawyers for the NHS Trust representing the doctors and CAFCASS representing the interests of the child.

14.7 Johnson J., a wise and kindly judge now retired from the Bench, came very close to allowing a manifestly *Gillick* competent adolescent to decide to refuse donor blood and have the non-blood management of his choice. However, the judge felt himself constrained by the statutory age of majority, as reinforced by the later quoted part of the decision of Nolan LJ., to grant (with manifest reluctance) the order sought by the NHS Trust.[205] The ironic final outcome was that, as in many such cases that have been brought to the court at huge expense to an underfunded NHS, the treating clinicians to their credit did in fact respect the mature minor's deeply held wishes and did not transfuse despite having obtained the leave of the court to do so. Perhaps we in the UK have something to learn from the experience of both Canada and Ireland.

The Canadian approach

14.8 The Law Commission of Manitoba very sensibly addressed the issue of arbitrary age limits in their Report,[206] *Minors' Consent to Health Care* back in 1995, now more than 20 years ago, and came down firmly against any such

---

[205] *re P* [2003] EWHC 2327 (Fam), [2004] 2 FLR 1117, Johnson J.
[206] Minors' Consent to Health Care, 1995

fixed age limit. The ensuing legislation[207] provided what is in reality a three tier structure:

a) at the age of 18 the competent patient has an absolute right of choice of treatment options including the right to refuse what may even be lifesaving treatment in accordance with the principles laid down in *Malette v Shulman,*[208] *Ciarlariello v Schacter*[209] and *re T;*[210]
b) between the ages of 16 and 18, there is a presumption that the minor has capacity both to consent and to refuse so that the patient's decision is ordinarily determinative. It is however capable of being rebutted in a specific case, the burden of proof being on the treating clinicians; and
c) below the age of 16 no such presumption existed.

14.9 The practical workings of these provisions and the arbitrariness of the different approaches to the over and under 16-year-olds was tested all the way up to the Supreme Court of Canada culminating in the judgment dated June 26, 2009. This is a masterly piece of judicial writing that ranges widely over the topic including especially reviewing the extensive materials on maturing adolescents referred to above. It should be required reading for all involved in making and applying the law relating to these cases of mature minors including parliamentarians, clinicians, risk managers, NHS Trust lawyers, judges, parents and indeed the mature minor patients themselves.

A.C. v Manitoba

14.10 The facts:

> 'C was admitted to hospital when she was 14 years, 10 months old, suffering from lower gastrointestinal bleeding caused by Crohn's disease. She is a devout Jehovah's Witness and, some months before, had signed an Advance Medical Directive containing her written instructions not to be given blood under any circumstances. Her doctor believed that internal bleeding created an imminent, serious risk to her health and perhaps her life. She refused to consent to the receipt of blood. A brief psychiatric assessment took place at the hospital on the night after her admission. The Director of Child and Family Services apprehended her as a child in need of protection, and sought a treatment order from the court under

[207] Child and Family Services Act, C.C.S.M. c. C80
[208] *Malette v Shulman* (1987), 63 O.R. (2d) 243 Affirmed (1990), 72 O.R. (2d) 417
[209] *Ciarlariello v Schacter* [1993], 2 S.C.R. 119
[210] *re T (Adult: Refusal of Medical Treatment) (1992)* 4 All ER 649

s. 25(8) of the Manitoba Child and Family Services Act, by which the court may authorize treatment that it considers to be in the child's best interests. Section 25(9) of the Act presumes that the best interests of a child 16 years or over will be most effectively promoted by allowing the child's views to be determinative, unless it can be shown that the child does not understand the decision or appreciate its consequences. Where the child is under 16 years, however, no such presumption exists. The applications judge ordered that C receive blood transfusions, concluding that when a child is under 16 years, there are no legislated restrictions of authority on the court's ability to order medical treatment in the child's "best interests". C and her parents appealed the order arguing that the legislative scheme was unconstitutional because it unjustifiably infringed C's rights under ss. 2(a), 7 and 15 of the Canadian Charter of Rights and Freedoms'.[211]

14.11 There are marked similarities in the law in both jurisdictions in the legal concepts of best interests and the range of protections of the Canadian Charter rights as mirrored in the European Convention on Human Rights.[212] Accordingly, for the purpose of this discussion, whilst the purists may find some minor divergence, they are considered interchangeable.

14.12 Two questions immediately arise. The first is what constitutes the stark difference between adolescents in Manitoba between 16 and 18-years-of-age concerning whom there is a presumption of capacity to take a valid decision on health care and our apparently retarded adolescents in England and Wales who are deemed to lack such capacity?

14.13 Secondly, why can the former have the right, even under the age of 16, to have their choice of treatment options considered by clinicians and advanced personally in evidence before a judge? He may find as a fact that they have the relevant capacity whereas their opposite numbers in England have no such right at all. In an article[213] in a well-known international journal on their right to confidentiality, adolescents were defined as between 10 and 19-years-old. Even in Russia, not known as an outstandingly liberal regime on Human Rights,

---

211 *Canadian Charter of Rights and* Freedoms

212 *Convention for the Protection of Human Rights and Fundamental Freedoms,* Rome 1950

213 Respecting adolescents' confidentiality and reproductive and sexual choices, R.J. Cook and others; *International Journal of Gynaecology & Obstetrics.* Vol 98, Issue 2 pp. 182-187, August 2007

mature minors at 15 years can take their own treatment decisions. In the Netherlands the age of presumption of competence is 12 years.[214]

14.14 The *A.C. v Manitoba* judgment provides some illuminating answers as to a reasonable and balanced approach. The Director of Child Welfare for Manitoba contended for a level of capacity that included 'ethical, emotional maturity—in short wisdom and a sense of judgment' to which he added that the consent must be voluntary and informed. In their decision, set out in a thorough and perceptive judgment, 4 judges of the Supreme Court[215] formulated 7 prime factors, setting them in the following context:

> 'In those most serious of cases, where a refusal of treatment carries a significant risk of death or permanent physical or mental impairment, a careful and comprehensive evaluation of the maturity of the adolescent will necessarily have to be undertaken to determine whether his or her decision is a genuinely independent one, reflecting a real understanding and appreciation of the decision and its potential consequences.
>
> As all of this demonstrates, the evolutionary and contextual character of maturity makes it difficult to define, let alone definitively identify. Yet the right of mature adolescents not to be unfairly deprived of their medical decision-making autonomy means that the assessment must be undertaken with respect and rigour.
>
> The following factors may be of assistance:
>
>> What is the nature, purpose and utility of the recommended medical treatment? What are the risks and benefits?
>>
>> Does the adolescent demonstrate the intellectual capacity and sophistication to understand the information relevant to making the decision and to appreciate the potential consequences?
>>
>> Is there reason to believe that the adolescent's views are stable and a true reflection of his or her core values and beliefs?
>>
>> What is the potential impact of the adolescent's lifestyle, family relationships and broader social affiliations on his or her ability to exercise independent judgment?
>>
>> Are there any existing emotional or psychiatric vulnerabilities?

---

214 Kammerstukken II 1991/1992, 21 561, nr. 11, pp. 33-34

215 *A.C. v Manitoba* supra

> Does the adolescent's illness or condition have an impact on his or her decision-making ability?
>
> Is there any relevant information from adults who know the adolescent, like teachers or doctors?

This list is not intended to represent a formulaic approach. Its objective is to assist courts in assessing the extent to which a child's wishes reflect true, stable and independent choices'.

14.15 Additionally there is cited in the *AC* case the report of an international Consensus Conference on Transfusions and Outcomes that included: [216]

> '...there is little evidence to support a beneficial effect from the greatest number of transfusions currently being given to patients. The vast majority of studies show an association between red blood cell transfusions and higher rates of complications such as heart attack, stroke, lung injury, infection and kidney failure and death'.

As one spokesman put it: 'The results of the conference firmly establish the view that, rather than being a benign procedure, blood transfusion is associated with increased risk of medical complications'.

Discussion

14.16 There is inevitably an element of selectivity in citing from a judgment that extends to some 82 pages but it is submitted that the following represents a fair selection that adequately states the reasoning and the decision in the Canadian case. Binnie J. declared:

> 'Forced medical procedures must be one of the most egregious violations of a person's physical and psychological integrity.... Whether judges, doctors and hospital authorities agree or disagree with C's objection, the decision belongs to her as the Charter is not just about the freedom to make the wise and correct choice; it also gives her the individual autonomy and the religious freedom to refuse forced medical treatment, even where her life or death hangs in the balance, regardless of what the judge thinks is in her best interest'.

14.17 The decision of the judge at first instance, in overruling the choice of a patient aged 14 years and 10 months to refuse donor blood, was held by the Supreme Court to have breached her Charter rights. These are available to all of whatever age, as indeed are European Convention rights in a near mirror image.

[216] 'Blood transfusion and outcomes', *Medical News Today*, 23 April 2009

14.18 There seems to be no reason in logic, social work writings, medical experience or indeed common sense why the law of consent to medical treatment by mature minors in England and Wales should not be brought into line with that of Manitoba or even the Netherlands.

14.19 The prospects of parliamentary time for amending legislation are zero and in any event probably unnecessary. It would seem to rest with the judges that the time has come to re-visit this issue, acknowledge the increasing maturity of adolescents and their rights. Also in the light of very changed conditions, including the Human Rights Act 1998, to recognise the earlier part of Nolan LJ.'s judgment as the effective part (the *ratio decidendi)* and to repudiate the oft cited later dictum as *obiter dicta.*

14.20 Three paragraphs from the Canadian judgment encapsulate their law:

> 'Forced medical procedures must be one of the most egregious violations of a person's physical and psychological integrity against the will of an individual whose refusal is based on a strong religious faith…
>
> If, after a careful analysis of the young person's ability to exercise mature and independent judgment, the court is persuaded that the necessary level of maturity exists, the young person's views ought to be respected'.

Then Binnie J. summarised it this way:

> 'The young person with capacity is entitled to make the treatment decision, not just to have "input" into a judge's consideration of what the judge believes to be the young person's best interest'.

14.21 Although the Canadian judges differed, in the ratio of 6 to 1, as to whether that entitlement is subsumed in the determination of best interests mandated by the legislation under consideration, the author suggests that this decision of 7 eminent Supreme Court judges presents cogent and compelling argument for changing our law on mature minors to give them, subject to capacity, a comparable right both to consent to and to refuse medical treatment.

The progressive criminal law

14.22 The comparative stagnation of the Family Law of England & Wales in respect of the age at which a young person acquires the capacity to choose medical treatment is in marked contrast to the progressive development of the criminal law to adapt to changing conditions. The substantial increase in the incidence of serious cases of child abuse has highlighted the difficulty of successfully prosecuting the offender when the victim is so young. When the author started out in practice in the 1960's it would have been unthinkable for the prosecution to seek to rely on, or for the court to permit, the oral evidence of very young children and certainly not as young as 3-years-old. Additionally at that time in sexual offences the criminal law required corroboration effectively following the 'two witnesses' requirement mandated in the book of Deuteronomy and elsewhere in the Scriptures that the courts had followed for decades. However, the law has moved on significantly not only abandoning the rule requiring a second witness but progressively lowering the age at which a child is considered to have both capacity and competence to give evidence; refining the requirements to make cross-examination more child friendly and comprehensible; and using the now available technology of video links to protect the witness.

14.23 The progression has been most marked over the past 6 years with 5 significant reported cases. The case of *Barker* is perhaps the most instructive. The child was just under 3-years-old when she started to talk about the offences to her foster mother. Her formal interview was recorded when she was 3 years and 3 months and she gave evidence a year later. The Lord Chief Justice ruled that 'delay on its own does not automatically require the court to prevent or stop the evidence of the child from being considered by the jury'.

On the issue of competence, the Court of Appeal said: [217]

> 'Many accreted suspicions and misunderstandings about children and their capacity to understand the nature and purpose of an oath and to give evidence at trial have been swept away'.

The Court went on to apply the statutory test in s.53 of the Youth Justice and Criminal Evidence Act and in holding the child to be competent said:

> 'The question in each case is whether the individual witness, or as in this case the individual child, is competent to give evidence in the particular trial. The question is entirely witness or child specific. There are no presumptions or preconceptions. The witness need not understand the special importance that the truth should be told in court and the witness need not understand every single question or give a readily understood answer to every question'.

[217] *R v Barker* [2010] EWCA Crim. 4

14.24 Little, if any, of these principles or changes in perception of competence of young people seem hitherto to have percolated through to the cases in which a young person chooses non-blood management. And yet it seems that in the criminal law at least, the opinion of those such as Professor Len Doyle, previously cited, about lowering the age of capacity and choice seem to have been substantially vindicated.

The experience of Ireland

14.25 Medical practice in Ireland has for many years been in line with that of the UK but in December 2009 it took a step forward that the UK has been slow to follow. The Law Reform Commission published a Consultation Paper running to over 500 pages, entitled 'Children and the Law: Medical Treatment' which is a comprehensive review of medical treatment with major reforms suggested. Chapter 5 of the Paper is devoted exclusively to the topic 'Refusal of Medical Treatment'. It notes that even the Medical Council states that 'a refusal of treatment against medical advice and parental wishes, is of uncertain legal validity'. There then follows an extensive review of the law of different Canadian Provinces and at §5.51 it deals with the above case of *AC v Manitoba.* The chapter concludes with a series of options for reform which include addressing the issue of refusal of consent. The Law Society of Ireland, representing practising solicitors, has already recommended that minors aged 16 and 17 should have the capacity to consent to and *refuse* medical treatment. In that context the Commission comments:

> 'It would be highly inconsistent and at variance with the principle of autonomy to suggest that a 16 year old who is presumed to have the capacity to make health care decisions can only consent to treatment'.

The Law Commission of Ireland in its later report on 'Children and the Law: Medical treatment' has specifically addressed the issue of refusal of treatment by patients aged 16 and 17. The recommendation now is that they should be presumed to have full capacity to consent to and refuse medical treatment. However they should be subject to a functional test which is 'a case by case test of capacity based on whether the person understands the nature and effect of the specific decision being made'. Significantly however, in the context of a refusal of life-sustaining treatment by a person in this age group, the Commission has recommended that an application may be made to the High Court to determine the validity of the refusal. So even if the law is changed, it seems that decision-making by teenagers is still going to be under the control of the courts.

What the legislature would do to implement the recommendations was awaited with interest. The answer appears to be the Act of 2015 discussed in greater detail in chapter 17.

Chapter Fifteen

Some Children's Case Histories

re C [218]

15.1 *C* was born to parents who came to Britain from Cyprus, where, as in the Punjab, genetic transmission of Thalassaemia is regularly encountered. The newborn survives initially on foetal haemoglobin derived from the mother. As that foetal haemoglobin is eliminated from the system over the ensuing weeks and the baby's new red cells are produced by erythropoiesis (but with inadequate oxygen carrying capacity), breathing distress and cyanosis suggest inadequate oxygenation and the condition is soon diagnosed. As in all these cases, the parents as committed Jehovah's Witnesses wanted the very best care for their baby. They took her immediately to the Royal Free Hospital, a north London centre of excellence. There the tests disclosed the condition and, as the parents were unable for reasons of conscience to consent to the use of donor blood support, an application was made in Wardship following the procedure started in *re B* in 1981. Ewbank J. was a fair but tough judge and his face was granite when confronted by parents withholding consent to, what was then seen as, the gold standard of treatment. The atmosphere in court was initially icy and tense but as the case unfolded and the true nature of the tragic dilemma faced by the parents became apparent, it softened and warmed to an obviously loving and caring mother. The court applied the best interests test and, as the mother was unable to offer any realistic non-blood alternative, and treatment without blood meant an early death, an order was inevitably made and the baby transfused.

re H [219]

15.2 *H* was born at Guys Hospital, discharged home and brought back in by ambulance at 2 weeks as a blue light emergency suffering with breathing difficulties and cyanosis. He was fortunate that he came under the care of Professor Tynan, the senior Consultant Paediatric Cardiologist whose eminent standing in the profession was not merely in the UK but as President of the International Association. He performed with great skill a cardiac catheter-

[218] High Court Family Division 1984 Ewbank J. (unreported)
[219] High Court Family Division 1985 Ewbank J. (unreported)

isation, no mean feat on a tiny baby as it involves inserting a catheter into the femoral artery and feeding it up into the very heart. He effected this without blood and his diagnosis was a serious and life-threatening condition:

- Double outlet right ventricle;
- Ventricular Septal Defect (VSD);
- Interruption of the aortic arch;
- Ductus arteriosus patent; and
- Pulmonary hypertension.

After describing the current treatment, the professor's medical report continued:

> 'The prognosis for this combination of malformation, even with this level of medical treatment is in my opinion extremely poor. It is our opinion that the following surgery is indicated, namely:
>
> Reconstruction of the aorta to establish continuity banding of the pulmonary artery to reduce pulmonary blood flow and to combat hypertension. This surgery is indicated as an emergency.
>
> Although every effort will be made to avoid the use of blood products, with this complex surgery we cannot guarantee that blood or blood products will not be required in order to maintain life'.

The onus then switched to the cardiac surgical team who insisted that, whilst they would do all that they could to meet the parental wishes and to perform the remedial surgery without blood, they would be operating on a baby with a heart about the size of a walnut, performing difficult micro-surgery and, despite all their professional skills, could not eliminate entirely the possibility of a serious bleed. They were only willing to operate with blood available as a fall back, but the parents were unable to consent. An application was made in Wardship and this case too came before Ewbank J.

Whilst waiting to get on before the judge, the professor walked up and down the corridor outside court anxious to reassure both the parents and especially counsel of his position. He said to counsel:

> 'Law and medicine don't mix and I would much prefer that this could have been left to be dealt with on the ward between myself and the parents. However I am only a cardiologist and my surgical team feel they must have the protection of a court order. But I am going to tell the Judge that we are going to do everything

> possible to operate without blood and will only use it as a last resort if we get our backs to the wall and there is a real risk of losing the baby'.

He was as good as his word and went into the witness box to explain in greater detail to the judge precisely that which he had promised counsel. Bearing in mind the climate on blood transfusion in 1985 and that this was a baby a mere 2-weeks-old, even the judge was taken aback but at the end of the professor's evidence in chief said to counsel, with a slightly sardonic smile, 'Well you can't do much better than that!'

The order was duly made and, to the great joy of the parents and the professional sense of achievement of a very skilled team, the complex heart repairs were effected without the use of blood. Sadly the joy was short lived and what happened next serves as a salutary lesson of the need to follow through from operating theatre, through recovery, to intensive care and finally the general ward. Some 72 hours after the surgery, in the course of a ward visit in the early hours of the morning, a night duty junior registrar thought the baby was 'looking a bit peaky' and, without properly checking the Notes in which *No Blood* was clearly recorded, or referring to the professor or his consultant, wrote the patient up for 50mls of blood which the nurse duly gave as instructed.

Everyone involved was devastated when in the morning these facts came out, principally of course the parents. But the professor was outraged that, having given his personal word to the parents, to their counsel, and especially to the judge, blood had been used unnecessarily, without clinical need and especially without reference to him. Despite his seniority and as a mark of the true greatness of the man, he took the trouble to telephone counsel to apologise for what had occurred. He assured both counsel and the parents that rigorous procedures were being put in place to ensure that no such thing could occur again and expressed his deep personal regret and apology that it should have happened at all.

The final twist in the tragedy was that, having made an apparently full and incident free recovery from this major surgery, 5 years later as a seemingly healthy, robust and active child, *H* was struck down with a pneumonic infection of a kind that routinely responds to modern antibiotics. But despite massive input by specialists and the highest quality of intensive care in a high grade hospital, something was seriously wrong with his immune system. He failed to respond to the range of treatments including the most powerful antibiotics available and tragically he died. His parents were too distraught and pre-occupied with the funeral and consoling their extended family to follow through on intensive haematological and pathological tests. But their belief remains that the transfusion of adult donor blood into their 2-week-old baby so suppressed his immune system that, when pneumonic infection occurred, he could not in his weakened state fight the infection despite the intensive treatment given. The case never made the law reports or medical journals and this incident pre-dated SHOT and the reporting system now in place. But there was no other medical explanation offered to explain the death other than suppression of the immune system by the donor blood, or possibly an unidentified infectious agent transmitted by it.

re R [220]

15.3 Soon after birth, *R* was diagnosed with the hereditary condition Transposition of the Great Arteries. In laymen's terms it is the plumbing equivalent of the main inlet and outlet being the wrong way round. There are two possible treatments, each with its own Risks and Benefits. The first is the Switch Procedure. As its name suggests, this involves the disconnection of the great arteries and their re-connection the correct way round thereby restoring the correct blood flow. A major benefit is that, if successful, it is unlikely that further remedial surgery will ever be needed. The risk is that, because of the way that the heart lies, these great arteries are less accessible and the nature of the procedure involves a much greater bleed risk, especially in a tiny neonate.

The Mustard Procedure leaves the great arteries *in situ* but the heart is opened and the flow of blood realigned within the heart. It is a much lower bleed risk but the general belief at that time was that there was a greater likelihood of the need for further invasive remedial surgery, probably in the early to mid-teens. That was a risk the parents felt was acceptable.

This seems to be a classic case for the parents to have the right of decision-making on which procedure was to go ahead. In the light of their commitment to non-blood management, the Mustard procedure had much to commend it. However, they ran up against a very aggressive surgeon who was adamant that ***he*** would make the choice. He also made the wholly unprofessional threat that, if the parents let him have the Wardship Order unopposed, he would try to do

[220] Principal Registry of the Family Division 1985 (unreported)

the surgery without blood but if they opposed him in the Wardship proceedings, he would make sure that he did use blood. Not surprisingly, the professional relationship was at breakdown but even then the surgeon refused a referral to another unit. The local County Council Social Services were contacted by the hospital and Wardship proceedings initiated.

The matter came as a Directions Hearing in Wardship before what was then a Registrar sitting at the Principal Registry in those far off days at Somerset House. Counsel for the parents asked for permission for a referral for a second opinion to Professor Sir Magdi Yacoub who, with his magnificent Paediatric Cardiologist Dr Rosemary Radley-Smith, had agreed to see the child at Harefield. As a team they had already established a track record for pioneering non-blood cardiac surgery. Counsel for the County Council could scarcely resist such a reasonable request for referral to a prestigious unit of world class and leave was granted.

R was duly seen; accepted for the Mustard Procedure and Social Services kept fully informed. *R* was admitted on a pre-planned elective admission and again Social Services, fully informed, did nothing. So the procedure went ahead on the parents' consent; was a success with no blood used and after discharge with reducing reviews from weeks down to months, *R* was finally stood down for annual review. At that stage the parents applied for discharge from Wardship and the balloon went up. A very angry Registrar demanded to know how the court's Ward had undergone major surgery without the consent of the court. The solicitor for the County Council took a real hammering and even counsel for the parents was rebuked, having been unable adequately to conceal a smirk at the manifest discomfiture of the Social Services officials and the original aggressive consultant receiving their come-uppance. However, faced with the *fait accompli* of successful surgery with a full recovery and no further demonstrable need for surgery or court involvement, the Registrar had no realistic option but to order the discharge from Wardship. The parents then applied for and were granted their not insignificant costs against the County Council on the basis that Wardship had been demonstrably of no effect and, had the parents' perfectly reasonable request for a referral been accepted by the first hospital, none of this would have been necessary.

As a post-script, at the time of writing *R* has grown up into a beautiful and healthy young woman now in her late twenties and no remedial procedure has ever been considered necessary. As one holding firmly to and active in the faith of Jehovah's Witnesses she counts herself fortunate to have avoided a blood transfusion.

re G [221]

15.4 *G,* a toddler, sustained third degree burns in a domestic accident. She was admitted to a specialist Burns Unit at Stoke Mandeville where the treating clinicians wanted to use blood products but the parents were unable to give consent. A Wardship Order was made but the child was successfully treated without blood and discharged with uneventful recovery but some minor scarring wholly unrelated to the blood issue.

re S [222]

15.5 *S* was born with spina bifida into a family of Jehovah's Witnesses and in her first eight years of life underwent multiple surgical interventions, all carried out by co-operative clinicians based on parental consent and without donor blood. One of the known complications of this condition concerns kidney and bladder function. The diagnosis was made that, due largely to a defective valve in the drainage into the bladder thereby allowing urinary reflux, one infected kidney was down to less than 10% function. She was referred to a local paediatric urino-genitary specialist consultant who took a very aggressive stance on the use of blood which he said was inevitable. When the parents withheld consent to the use of blood, he consulted with what he claimed was the only other specialist (at a major London teaching hospital) doing this remedial bladder surgery in the country. A Wardship application was filed and at the Directions hearing the consultant told the Registrar in terms that only he and this other consultant were capable of performing the necessary procedure in the UK. Both were adamant that it was impossible and dangerous to the life of the child even to attempt to do the procedure without blood. However the parents had heard, through other parents, of a Paediatric Consultant Urologist who might be prepared to undertake the procedure. So the parents asked for and were granted leave to take the child for a second opinion. The outcome was quite extraordinary. The new consultant expressed amazement at the suggestion that the two named were the only surgeons doing this procedure. He had over

---

[221] High Court Family Division 1986 (unreported)
[222] High Court Family Division 1987 Douglas Brown J. (unreported)

100 Spina Bifida cases on his list at any one time, many of whom needed similar bladder re-construction surgery and he did this procedure regularly. Furthermore he adopted a conservative approach to the use of donor blood with all his patients (irrespective of the parents' religious beliefs or wishes) and the last 30 procedures had all been performed successfully and all without blood. He put this in a robust affidavit that was served on the local authority, who backed down. The case came before Douglas Brown J. and on the parents' application the child was discharged from Wardship, allowing the surgery to proceed on the parents' consent. So far as the author knows, this is the only case in England and Wales where, once court proceedings have been commenced for an order for blood transfusion, a child has actually been discharged from the jurisdiction of the court; the parents left to give the consent to treatment; and for the surgeon to proceed on their consent without court intervention.

In the outcome, the surgeon accepting the referral found that the surgical option proposed by the previous surgeon was in reality the wrong option. The new surgeon performed, without blood, removal of the diseased kidney and repair of the defective valve thereby almost overnight achieving a huge improvement in the general health of the child and her quality of life, especially at school.

One touching feature of the case was when the patient was visited by a little girl, from a family of Jehovah's Witnesses, who had earlier had the same procedure successfully carried out in that unit by the same surgeon without recourse to blood.

S has grown up into a fine young woman and, although inevitably still to some extent impaired by her underlying condition of Spina Bifida that will never leave her, she lives a full and contented life as one of Jehovah's Witnesses and holds down a responsible job in one of the professions.

re E [223]

15.6 As the above list demonstrates, these cases were increasingly coming before the courts but under the protection of anonymity and thus rarely made the Law Reports. In September 1990 *re E* was heard and unreported at the time, but as successive cases raising the same issue followed it through the courts a judicial request was made for it to be reported and so it appeared for the first

[223] *re E (A Minor) (Wardship: Medical Treatment)* [1993] 1 FLR 386 Ward J.

time in 1993. It is a case that has since been extensively reviewed and the subject of comment in a number of leading medico-legal textbooks both nationally and internationally. But even the judgment does not reveal the full extent of this important case and the opportunity is now taken to fill in a number of missing details and set the record straight.

E was a fine young man brought up from birth in a family of Jehovah's Witnesses and learnt those beliefs and core values which he accepted as his personal decision. At age 15 years and 8 months he was a good athlete, standing a full 6 feet tall, big and strong and demonstrating both an enthusiasm for and a prowess at football. In addition he played water polo, a demanding sport that those who know it will acknowledge requires exceptional levels of fitness and endurance. During the early part of the summer holidays of 1990 he started to experience severe abdominal pain and consulted his GP. Unfortunately, he was not referred at that time for specialist review and so several weeks elapsed without a proper diagnosis. Whether or not the delay contributed to the severity of his condition was never established but the golden rule with these conditions is that the earlier they are caught and diagnosed the better the likely outcome. He was finally admitted to hospital on 8 September and 3 days later transferred to a specialist oncology unit recognised worldwide as a centre of excellence. There the diagnosis was made of Acute Lymphocytic Leukaemia (ALL) by then well advanced.

It is a condition in which very immature leukaemia cells accumulate in the bone marrow, destroying and replacing cells that produce normal blood cells. If not caught early, the leukaemia cells are also carried in the bloodstream to the liver, spleen, lymph nodes and ultimately to the brain and testes where they may continue to grow and divide. Unlike Chronic Lymphocytic Leukaemia, its onset and progression can be rapid, accentuating the need for early diagnosis and treatment.

The standard treatment at that time involved cytotoxic drugs which, as the name suggests, kill cells. Unfortunately 23 years ago the state of pharmaceutical knowledge was such that, whilst certain drugs were capable of selectively targeting the malignant cells being produced in the bone marrow, others in use were not so specific and attacked both malignant and healthy cells indiscriminately. They were used in varying combinations, the treatment being known generally as 'combination chemotherapy'. One of the oldest (and still often used) combinations is known by the shorthand acronym CHOP consisting of:

- Cyclophosphamide;
- Hydroxy doxorubicin;
- Oncovin [*Vincristine*]; and
- Prednisone.

Chemotherapy then involved three defined stages:

- **Induction chemotherapy**, the aim of which is to achieve remission by destroying leukaemic cells so that normal cells can once again grow in the bone marrow;
- **Consolidation chemotherapy**, usually a few weeks after the intensive induction phase, is given to destroy any remaining leukaemic cells; and
- **Maintenance therapy** which usually consists of fewer drugs, sometimes at lower doses, and may continue for 2 to 3 years.

Statistically children between the ages of 3 and 7 have the best prognosis; children younger than 2-years-of-age and older adults fare less well. The white blood cell count and particular chromosome abnormalities in the leukaemia cells also influence outcome. The conventional view is that the first 'hit' is the most important and hopefully the first course of chemotherapy brings the disease under control leading to complete remission. However, relapse frequently occurs and leukaemia cells begin to appear again. The disease has a strong tendency to come back, especially in those under 2 years and in adults and the prognosis on relapse at that time in 1990 was poor. For these patients repeat high dose chemotherapy was required and modern treatment now includes allogeneic stem cell transplantation as the treatment of choice.

A leading children's hospital has prepared a brochure that includes a section on chemotherapy designed and written specifically for child leukaemia patients in terms that they can understand. But it does explain in some comprehensible detail the effects of each of these drugs in attacking the leukaemic cells and the side effects some of which are categorised as unpleasant and a few as serious.

Crucially in the case of *E*, because of the delayed diagnosis and the inability of the then drugs to be sufficiently selective against malignant cells only, blood support was an essential part of the care plan. The patient, for reasons of conscience and the core values that he held, could not consent yet there was no viable alternative that in the then state of medical knowledge the family could put forward.

E was intelligent and understood the explanations given to him of his condition, of the recommended treatment and the likely adverse outcome if blood was not used. He took his own personal stand on not accepting blood and his loving parents supported him in that. The treating team, to their credit, took seriously this expression of choice of a patient who met the criteria of *Gillick* competence. Whilst the standard treatment in their judgment had a chance of full remission put at 80%—possibly even 90%—they modified that standard treatment in not deploying the two less specific drugs. The consequences were in part successful because the leukaemic cells dropped from 80% on admission to 24% by Day 10.

In those days it really was blood support or nothing. There was no Recombinant Erythropoietin to stimulate the body's own production of red cells and iron by mouth long preceded *Venofer*® or *Ferinject*®. The serious down side of the non-availability of donor blood support was that the Hb, already down to 8.5 g/dl on admission, was progressively deteriorating through 6.6; 6.1; and 5.6 g/dl. At that level with the prospects of further deterioration to a life-threatening level the hospital sought Wardship to bring the matter before the court. The case was listed for an urgent hearing on Friday 21 September 1990 and came before Ward J. with eminent leading counsel, James Munby QC as he then was (now Munby LJ.) appearing for the *guardian ad litem* Official Solicitor. It was a case that went into the annals of the Court Service, through the Report of the Master of the Rolls[224] as an example of just how fast the court can move in an emergency.

The preceding case, part heard before Ward J., was bumped out of the list and the judge started to hear this case shortly before midday, knowing that the latest Hb reading that morning was now down to a potentially life threatening 4.6g/dl. After some 6 hours of evidence and legal submissions, (the significant parts of which are recounted in the judgment including the Canadian case of *re LDK*)[225] at about 6 p.m. the court rose and the judge went by taxi to the hospital to see the patient personally and alone. It was well after 9 p.m. when he returned to

224 *The Times* Sept 1990— per Lord Donaldson MR.
225 *re LDK; CAS v K* 48 Reports of Family Law (Ontario) (2d) 172

court and, having regard to the extreme urgency of the case, delivered, some 10 hours after starting the hearing, an *ex tempore* judgment as remarkable for its humanity as for the medical precision and legal content on such difficult issues. In the meantime the Associate of the Court of Appeal had been in court and confirmed that arrangements were on stand-by for the Court of Appeal to convene on the Saturday morning to hear an appeal if one were to be brought.

The judge had clearly been impressed by the calm but firm conviction expressed by a young man not yet 16-years-of-age. Late in the judgment he expressed it thus:

> 'There is compelling and overwhelming force in the submission of the Official Solicitor that this court, exercising its prerogative of protection, should be very slow to allow an infant to martyr himself.
>
> In my Judgment [E] has by the stand he has taken thus far already been and become a martyr for his faith. One has to admire—indeed one is almost baffled by—the courage of the conviction that he expresses. He is, he says, prepared to die for his faith. That makes him a martyr by itself. But I regret that I find it essential for his well-being to protect him from himself and his parents and so I override his and his parent's decision. In this judgment—which has been truly anxious—I have endeavoured to pay every respect and give great weight to the religious principles which underlie the family's decision and also to the fundamental human right to decide things for oneself. That notwithstanding, the welfare of [E], when viewed objectively, compels me to only one conclusion, and that is that the hospital should be at liberty to treat him with the administration of those further drugs and consequently with the administration of blood and blood products'.

The final outcome was that *E* was, for the next 2 years and 3 months, treated with the full regime of the four drugs in combination chemotherapy to which the administration of donor blood and blood products was the inevitable support. But at 18-years-of-age the Wardship Order lapsed as a matter of law and he then became entitled as a competent adult to make his own choice of treatment. He stood firm on his conscientious decision not to accept donor blood and, although he accepted modified treatment and survived another 3 years, he died aged 21. The judge in *re P* (*infra* at [15.17]) saw fit to mention this ultimate outcome in the reported judgment in that case.

re C

15.7 Although these were court proceedings in respect of a 2-year-old suffering from acute leukaemia, they are memorable more for the flagrant (and arguably unlawful under a statute of 1913) violation of patient confidentiality by UK newspapers that probably did but certainly should have known better. C's parents lived in a European country where the standard of care was (at least at that time) not of the highest calibre. When their daughter was diagnosed with acute leukaemia, they wanted the very best of care for her but without allogeneic blood. They brought her to the UK to a hospital of international repute but then found that they were only offered treatment that involved donor blood. They then chose not to accept the offer of treatment on those terms, openly discharged the child with full knowledge of the hospital and took her home quite normally by commercial airline. The reaction was almost unbelievable. The UK authorities alerted those in her home country, the police were involved, a court order obtained and a transfusion administered. Unable to pass up a populist photo opportunity, the then President visited (? without lawful consent) and told the parents and the assembled press 'he had personally intervened to impose the treatment'.

Photographs were taken at the bedside with the self-evidently anxious mother and showing the named child, clearly recognisable full face and manifestly distressed whilst recovering from the transfusion. These were then published, with full names, in at least two national newspapers in the UK with an emotive report that elevated the decision by the parents to decline the offered treatment to:

> 'S was last week snatched from a London hospital by her parents, secretly flown back...police issued arrest warrants and watched ports and airports to stop her parents taking her away again'.

A separate photo of the President also featured. As with some of the adult cases recounted elsewhere, it seems that journalist and editorial standards were at a low level. A report was published that was not only inaccurate, inappropriate and intrusive but caused great distress to the family at a time when they were having to come to terms with the serious illness of their young daughter. Moreover it was almost certainly unlawful to identify the child.

re O [226]

15.8 This was a case the judgment in which had a major impact on the conduct of these blood transfusion cases and the fairness of due process to which the parents were entitled if an order was to be made.

O was born prematurely and quickly diagnosed as suffering from neonate respiratory distress syndrome. She was being ventilated but her tiny lungs could not tolerate, without risk, continued pressure of oxygen and the clinicians wanted to give blood. The parents were both with her at the hospital when local Social Services decided, without any warning, to apply to the local magistrates for (of all things) an Emergency Protection Order under s.44 of the Children Act 1989. This was a wholly inappropriate remedy as the baby was already in the safest place it could be: in hospital in intensive care. As previously discussed, such an order did not in any event give to the treating team any authority to override the parental refusal of blood. Furthermore under the statute, no appeal was permitted for 72 hours. When, without having been served or given any formal notice, they learned informally that an application was in the process of being made, the father and a fellow Witness who had been at the hospital supporting the family literally ran to the Magistrates Court but they were not in time. An order had been made *ex parte* on the most limited, indeed flimsy, evidence and without any legal authority being cited.

The parents immediately applied to have the case heard in the High Court and Johnson J. sat in Birmingham as a matter of urgency to deal with it. The judgment is reported and so it would be mere repetition to recount it here. But the following key points were made:

a) an Emergency Protection Order made by lay justices is not an appropriate remedy in these cases;
b) they should be heard by a Judge of the High Court which maintains a rota system for a duty judge to be available, even on the telephone, 24 hours a day 7 days a week; and
c) the *ex parte* procedure can work unfairness and strenuous efforts should be made to arrange a hearing on notice at which the parents have an opportunity to be heard.

---

[226] High Court Family Division, Johnson J. [1993] 2 FLR 149

Although their baby had been transfused, the parents felt an obligation to their fellow believers to challenge the legal process and the way in which their wishes had been overridden without due process and were to that extent successful.

re R

15.9 Not to be confused with the case in paragraph 15.3 above, this case had many similarities. Professor Yacoub again undertook repair of ventricular septal defect at Harefield without blood.

re W [227]

15.10 Congenital cystic adenomatoid malformation of the lung is a nasty condition in a young child. It is a malignant bronchial tumour of epithelial origin. In this case Wardship was granted and an order made permitting blood transfusion. An extremely skilful team at Kings College Hospital, London successfully operated and did not use blood. The child made a full and uneventful recovery.

re P [228]

15.11 A neonate was diagnosed with respiratory distress syndrome. The hospital sought and was granted an order permitting transfusion but the condition of the baby improved without blood, which in the event was never used. This case simply demonstrates that each incident is case specific and some applications to the court are premature.

re M [229]

15.12 *M* was a two week pre-term baby diagnosed with necrotising entero-colitis: an inflammation of the colon and small intestine. It is a serious and life threatening condition in which the abdomen distends; blood and mucous is present in the stools and the high risk is that the bowel may perforate with usually fatal consequences. A highly skilled surgeon from a well-known tertiary referral centre came to court to give evidence in the proceedings for a Specific Issue Order. He spent some time during his evidence in chief explaining to the judge almost apologetically the reasons why he was totally

---

[227] High Court Family Division Waite J. Nov 1991(unreported)
[228] High Court Family Division Ewbank J. Nov 1993 (unreported)
[229] High Court Family Division, Wall J. May 1994 (unreported)

opposed to the use of donor blood if possible. He highlighted in some detail the known risks of donor blood especially to very young neonates and then outlined the proposed procedure. This involved the resection of the affected part of the colon and bringing the bowel out through the abdominal wall to a stoma but in such a way that the procedure would be reversible as the child gained weight and strength, thereby restoring in time normal colon and intestine function. It was major surgery and on a tiny pre-term baby he would be working with blood vessels measured in microns. Despite taking all proper care he had to accept the possibility of nicking a blood vessel and the consequences of a potentially catastrophic bleed. He again apologised for the need to trouble the court but felt that, although the risk was small, he must have blood available as a last resort rather than lose the baby. Not surprisingly, there was no cross-examination—just an expression of thanks on behalf of the parents. The order was duly made and the procedure carried out as promised without blood and with total success. That brilliant surgeon went on to take up a consultant post in a major university teaching hospital where he has continued to teach and practise non-blood management in surgery on tiny infants. He was in the forefront in his speciality with neonates in pushing back the boundaries of bloodless surgery.

re M

15.13 A criminal case in Tallinn, Estonia, involved a mother and foetus with a serious Rhesus incompatibility. Under the old Soviet system there had been poor primary care, no anti-D and the problem had been compounded by the then social convention of using termination as a form of contraception. By the time she became one of Jehovah's Witnesses *M* had already undergone 8 terminations. Her obviously useless contraceptive device failed yet again and she fell pregnant but this time she refused, on grounds of Christian conscience, the termination offered and indeed strongly recommended. The foetus was suffering from advanced symptoms of Rhesus incompatibility to the level of *hydrops foetalis* which carries a very high risk of mortality. To give the baby an outside chance of survival, the mother agreed to her labour being induced early but the baby was born seriously ill and died 48 hours later. During that period she had been asked for consent to blood transfusion but had withheld consent on the grounds of her religious beliefs and conscience. The media got hold of the story and an overzealous prosecutor, seemingly influenced by public opinion, charged her with causing the death of the baby, the equivalent of manslaughter. However at trial at the end of a lengthy cross-examination the chief prosecution witness, the senior and vastly experienced clinician in charge of the tertiary intensive care unit, agreed that the baby was born a 'non-survivor', with or without blood. Despite this clear evidence from his star witness disproving causation (an essential ingredient of the prosecution's case) the prosecutor ploughed on, but the mother (contrary to all experience of conviction in a legal system deeply ingrained with the Soviet mentality) was acquitted.

However, whilst on bail awaiting trial her contraception had failed yet again and she had fallen pregnant. This time the aggressive prosecutor said he would ensure that this baby was given blood. A very fair judge had then allowed her to leave the jurisdiction to have her baby in a unit in Sweden where they had experience of non-blood management in even severe cases of Rhesus incompatibility. Immediately after birth the treating team implemented an aggressive course of therapy including multi-lamp ultra-violet phototherapy. Adjunctive therapies included oral charcoal, which has been found to help bind the bilirubin and speed up its excretion. This highly experienced team were able to let the bilirubin level rise right up to the line at which conventionally exchange transfusion is undertaken but held off. For a while the bilirubin level hovered at the cut-off point on the graph but then, to the relief and satisfaction of all concerned, fell back. No transfusion was ever given. This was one of the many cases in which the late Nigel Vukovich (see chapter 2) had given advice on diet and the use of natural vitamin and mineral supplements during the pregnancy. The mother remains totally convinced that these made the difference in enabling the treating team to avoid the use of allogeneic blood. The child is growing up healthy and unimpaired and now has no adverse effects of the non-blood management of a difficult condition.

re S [230]

15.14 *S* developed an extremely unpleasant growth known as a lymphangioma on his neck and jaw. It was the size of a large orange and still growing. For an 8-year-old at school it was, quite apart from the pain, grossly disfiguring and a social embarrassment.

One leading text-book describes it thus:

[230] High Court Family Division Mar 2001 Bracewell J. (unreported)

> 'Occurs in both triangles and may reach a massive size necessitating decompression/debulking. The ramifying and multilocated nature of the lymphatic cysts makes extirpative surgery exceedingly difficult and risky'.

An outstanding surgeon was willing to operate without blood but risk managers to his NHS Trust insisted on applying for a court order that was duly granted by a judge of the High Court. Technically demanding surgery, rightly described as 'difficult and risky' was carried out by a cooperative team without blood transfusion and the young patient made a full and uneventful recovery.

re H Wilms Tumour [231]

15.15 Wilms Tumour (otherwise known as nephroblastoma) is a malignant tumour of the kidney found in children. It is rare over the age of 8 years and the most obvious symptom is an abdominal swelling. Treatment is by nephrectomy followed by radiotherapy and cytotoxic drugs. The parents were unable to consent to the recommended blood support and an order was made. The nephrectomy was successfully performed without resort to donor blood and the immediate progress of the further treatment was similarly concluded without blood. The final outcome is currently unknown but is believed to be full remission for more than 5 years which, in oncology terms, rates as recovery.

re O [232]

15.16 *O* was a neonate born with some of the symptoms of Rhesus Conflict outlined above. There was considerable pressure on the parents to consent to blood which they resisted. Because of the experience of the 'Tallinn' and other cases in the effective use of multi-lamp phototherapy with some adjunctive therapies, when an application was made for an order for blood, the parents resisted it, seeking to hold to non-blood management. Johnson J. gave leave to the hospital to use blood but expressly on the limited basis that the hospital would do all that they could to treat the bilirubin level without resort to donor blood. This was, in fact, achieved by the use of triple lamp phototherapy with a bilirubin blanket but there were serious parental concerns about iatrogenic anaemia. This is the expression for anaemia caused by the actions of the treating team, in this case taking multiple samples too frequently and of much too great a volume. In the first 23 days of life the hospital had taken 34 samples

---

[231] High Court Family Division Jul 2002 (unreported)

[232] High Court Family Division 2002 Johnson J and HH Judge Pearlman (unreported)

of blood. Most were of 1 ml, which may not sound a great deal but in reality represented 7.5% of the baby's total circulating volume. After discharge home, the visiting nurse did not bring a micro-sampling kit. So a sample equivalent to that provided by an adult had to be drawn off to provide enough volume to satisfy the lab computer. Then a further sample was taken on a Saturday when there was no laboratory facility open at that (major) hospital. The sample was sent to another hospital 10 miles away and was lost in transit. So yet another sample had to be taken from a tiny baby that was fighting for every drop of Hb and oxygen carrying capacity. Because of the existence of the court order, the not unreasonable protests of the parents went unheeded, even though there is a considerable volume of professional literature on the very risks of iatrogenic anaemia. Fortunately despite the manifestly sub-optimal treatment in drawing off so much blood simply for testing, the baby survived and has made an uneventful recovery without blood being given.

re P [233]

15.17 This case of Hypermobility Syndrome with impacted bowel raised in a serious form the present inadequacy of the law to acknowledge the increasing capacity of mature minors. The NHS Trust sought an order and CAFCASS were joined as the guardian of a patient aged just short of 17 years. They instructed a local solicitor to interview the teenage patient with particular reference to whether he was considered to be *Gillick* competent to consent to his treatment. A senior solicitor, on the Law Society children's panel and with considerable experience of children's cases, formed the very firm view that the patient was indeed competent to choose his treatment options. The solicitor went further and confirmed that, in his professional judgment, the patient was a demonstrably believing and active member of the faith of Jehovah's Witnesses in which he had been brought up from birth; that the patient's personal and deeply held religious beliefs and core values should be respected and he should not be compelled to submit to forced transfusion of donor blood. This did not square with the default position of CAFCASS, which was that no patient under age should be entitled to refuse treatment in accordance with the *Nolan* dictum. See chapter 14.

The solicitor felt so strongly about the case that he instructed separate counsel to represent the patient and indeed, although he practised some distance from

---

[233] *re P* [2003] EWHC 2327 (Fam), [2004] 2 FLR 1117 Johnson J.

London, at some professional inconvenience attended the High Court himself. The court was thus faced with the rather unedifying spectacle of counsel for CAFCASS urging the making of the order and counsel independently instructed for the underage patient resisting it on the basis of *Gillick* competence attested to and supported by a very competent and senior solicitor. The judge in the course of argument came as close as could be to refusing the order. He even indicated that the time might come when he would find a 17-year-old competent to decide. However, he found himself constrained by the 'Nolan' dictum of the Court of Appeal already discussed and made the order.

The final outcome was that the treating clinicians, perhaps heeding the compelling arguments of Professor Len Doyal, belatedly felt that it was not in the best interests of a manifestly competent and comprehending patient to force upon him the treatment that he found repugnant and with which he was not willing to cooperate. Despite the order giving leave, no blood was given. The patient lived beyond 18 years but later sadly died from complications unconnected with the issue of blood or non-blood management of his condition.

15.18 October 2003 saw two cases each involving highly complex neuro surgery.

In the first, ***re W,***[234] the condition was ependymoma of brainstem and fossa craniotomy. In lay terms this meant a malignant growth about the size of a large plum but located in a very difficult place at the brain stem. An extremely skilful and co-operative neuro-surgeon, wanting to accommodate the parental wishes for non-blood surgery, agreed to modify the usual procedure and, on his NHS Trust seeking an order, explained this to the judge. It involved going in and removing two thirds of the growth at the first session; coming out and sewing up and letting the boy recuperate. After several weeks he had him back in theatre and very skilfully, in the most difficult part of the complex procedure, removed the final third of the malignant growth. No blood was used and the boy made a complete and uneventful recovery.

15.19 The second case the same month involved Foramen Magnum decompression.[235] This is high risk neurosurgery because it involves the spinal cord where it passes through a hole in the bony structure of the occipital bone.

[234] High Court Family Division Oct 2003 Bennett J. and Black J. (unreported)
[235] High Court Family Division Oct 2003 Johnson J. (unreported)

As the name suggests, there was compression on the spinal cord that had to be relieved. Another brilliant neuro-surgeon was willing to try without blood and this case came before Johnson J. who by this time was becoming more than familiar with the arguments for non-blood management. At the urging of the NHS Trust the judge, again following the *Nolan* dictum, made the order on the basis of use 'as a last resort' but yet again no blood was used and there was a full and uneventful recovery.

Natalie M [236]

15.20 Natalie was born with severe congenital heart defects:

- right atrial isomerism;
- complete atrioventricular septal defect;
- double inlet right ventricle;
- double outlet right ventricle;
- sub-valvar pulmonary stenosis;
- atrioventricular vale regurgitation;
- dextrocardia; and
- supraventricular tachycardias.

These were complex diagnoses but essentially, for the layman, her heart had only one pumping chamber with multiple complications. Over the years she had Bilateral Glenn shunts and many out-patient consultations at an eminent tertiary unit with major surgery in contemplation. She was under regular monitoring by her GP but even so the system let her down. To try and diminish the pumping load on her defective heart it was prudent to keep her blood thinned and she was on *Warfarin*. At a routine GP visit she was seen by a *locum* with no experience of her or her complex condition who, without reference to the cardiac unit under whose highly specialist care she was, changed her medication to aspirin. Neither she nor her mother were warned of the side effects of internal bleeding well known to be associated with long term aspirin use, or to watch for possible occult blood being passed in her stools. She attended school normally and engaged in the activities of her Christian Congregation including the evangelising ministry. However her mother noticed that she was increasingly tired and would come home from school or meeting and go immediately to bed to sleep for a couple of hours.

[236] High Court Family Division Apr 2004 Kirkwood J. (unreported)

She was recalled to the cardiac unit as an outpatient, largely because a decision needed to be taken as to whether the treating team were going to attempt an extremely difficult repair or put her on the list for a transplant. A prudent consultant asked for an up to date blood test, especially Hb, and it came back at a mere 7.4g/dl. As that level of anaemia was well below the then recommended transfusion threshold of 10g/dl there was very serious concern and request to the mother for consent to start donor blood transfusion immediately. As she had consistently done for the 14 years of Natalie's life, the mother could not on grounds of conscience consent and indeed Natalie herself, arguably *Gillick* competent, was adamant that she did not want blood. The consultant surgeon wanted Natalie in theatre with an Hb of 15g/dl to allow for the expected blood loss of such major heart surgery.

As an impasse was reached, an application to the court was filed. Ivor Cavill, an expert in iron supplementation, was consulted by the mother's lawyers about the use of r-HuEPO (*NeoRecormon*®) in conjunction with *Venofer*® iron supplementation. He gave a very firm opinion that it would be possible to increase Natalie's Hb level by up to 1 gramme of per week. Armed with that evidence the mother argued before the judge to be allowed to try that regime as there was no urgency for the surgery itself and the judge, in the face of the cogent and compelling evidence from Mr Cavill, granted leave. Ironically the paediatric haematologists at the cardiac unit involved had no experience of this combination of r-HuEPO and *Venofer*® and so had to be gently led through the procedures. As promised by Mr Cavill, the Hb did indeed rise at the predicted rate and in fact reached a remarkable level of 16 g/dl in just 9 weeks. All of this was off-licence but it demonstrated beyond contradiction that this regime is capable of achieving such an increase.

Despite the achievement in reaching the Hb level required for surgery, for clinical reasons wholly unconnected with the issue of blood or the period of treatment with the non-blood regime outlined, Natalie's condition deteriorated significantly; the window of opportunity for the transplant closed and tragically she died before it could be effected.

This case, suitably anonymised, was discussed at the NATA Seminar in Prague.

re B [237]

15.21 *B* was a neonate with Transposition of the Great Arteries. However, there were additional complications of ventricular septal defect (VSD) with abnormal coronary anatomy. In contrast to the earlier case of *re R* above [15.3] the Mustard procedure was not an option and it had to be the Switch procedure. The cardiac surgeon was willing to try non-blood techniques but in that unit they did not have available at that time the miniaturised Heart/Lung bypass equipment that could be primed with non-blood. The parents wanted their baby to be treated by that surgeon and unit and so were in no position to dispute the inevitable order that was made on the application of the NHS Trust. However, that case is notable for the fact that, although the parents could not put forward a non-blood alternative, the judge in his formal judgment commented:

> 'The Court must be astute to ensure that non-blood alternatives have been considered before making an Order'.

For those parents who in the 1980's had been used to the almost rubber stamp making of an order as requested by the hospital and the reluctance to listen to the non-blood arguments, this judicial comment marked a major step forward.

re B [238]

15.22 This was a Rhesus conflict case in Ireland involving twins *in utero*. The first treating hospital correctly diagnosed the Rhesus conflict but wanted to give an intra-uterine transfusion to the foetuses. The mother refused consent, as in law she was entitled to do, and indeed discharged herself. She secured a referral to a team at University College Cork, who were willing to treat so far as practicable within the choice of the mother as to non-blood management. The treating team had the difficult task of balancing the need to keep the foetuses in the womb for as long as possible to reduce the risk of anaemia of prematurity and yet induce delivery to deal with the bilirubin level before it reached the point where it presented a serious risk to either or both newborns. They succeeded in reaching 33½ weeks gestation. Immediately after birth they commenced aggressive multi-lamp phototherapy to address the bilirubin and this was successful. One twin was diagnosed with anaemia as moderate and the other as mild. The Health Service Executive (not the hospital) went to court to

[237] High Court Family Division Jul 2004 Holman J. (unreported)
[238] High Court Dublin Jan 2008 Laffoy J. (unreported)

obtain a 'protective' order, which was granted. Both twins were put on a course of erythropoietin and iron, which lasted after discharge from the delivery unit for another 10 weeks. But the treatment was successful without blood transfusion and the twins are now thriving and healthy with no adverse consequences. In March 2011 the mother was interviewed on Cork radio FM. Whilst preserving confidentiality, she gave a graphic account of her experience, compounded by the trauma of the court involvement, but at the same time expressing heartfelt appreciation for the quality of care that she and the baby had received at the hospital.

re C [239]

15.23 This case is considered in more detail in the chapter on Ireland. C was a very premature baby, 24 weeks and 5 day's gestation, which is right on the brink of viability. A High Court judge granted leave for blood 'as a last resort' but a highly skilled unit in the Coombe Hospital in Dublin successfully managed the anaemia of prematurity without blood. To the great joy of his loving parents *C* was discharged home at just over 11 weeks after birth, still scarcely a term baby. He very rapidly put on weight and at the time of writing is thriving to the point he rapidly caught up with all the growth criteria expected of a full term baby and is developing as a normal healthy child.

[239] High Court Dublin Oct/Dec 2009 Birmingham J. (unreported)

Chapter Sixteen

The Expert Witness

16.1 At first reading, this chapter might seem to be not merely superfluous but, in the light of the leading work[240] on this topic, written by no less an authority than Lord Justice Wall, former President of the Family Division of the High Court, possibly even presumptuous. However, experience of these cases in which the High Court is asked to overrule refusal of consent to medical treatment, notably blood transfusion, suggests that NHS lawyers and even CAFCASS seem to treat these cases as in some way *sui generis* and not subject to the provisions of Part 35 of the Civil Procedure Rules (CPR) and the concomitant Protocols and Practice Directions.

16.2 The majority of children's cases requiring expert medical evidence are indeed brought under the Children Act 1989 and much expert evidence is directed to the section 31 'threshold criteria' and the determination of whether the child is suffering or likely to suffer significant harm. However, at his paragraph 3.5 on page 14, Wall LJ. specifically refers to proceedings brought in the High Court under the inherent jurisdiction. This is the usual legal mechanism now deployed by NHS Trusts to bring these matters before the court for a declaration that it will be lawful to over-ride the parental treatment choice and thus to transfuse.

16.3 It would indeed seem difficult to argue that a case that by definition involves two diametrically opposed views on proposed (or at least recommended) medical treatment can do other than involve expert medical evidence. The difficulty arises when, as is often the case, the NHS Trust seeks to rely primarily on the evidence of the treating clinician(s). Wall LJ. at his chapter 33 addresses this under the heading:

> 'What if you are the treating clinician'?

In particular, at Note 3, he highlights and quotes from the report of a working group convened by the Royal College of Pathologists and the Royal College of

[240] *A Handbook for Expert Witnesses in Children Act Cases;* The Rt Hon Lord Justice Wall, Family Law 2nd Edition: Jordan Publishing Ltd

Paediatrics and Child Health entitled, *The Role of the Expert Witness* and published in September 2004:

> '...It is our view that paediatricians involved in the acute management of patients should not be expected to give expert testimony in cases involving those patients. It is a *sine qua non* that doctors treating patients must develop partnerships with them and with the immediate family to ensure the best medical outcome. This will inevitably result in a degree of intimacy and therefore subjectivity when evaluating the case as a whole. This is the opposite of what is required of the expert witness, who should be objective, impartial and detached'.

16.4 Thus the court should be looking for evidence in two categories. Firstly, if (despite the advice of the Working Group) treating clinicians are involved, then they are arguably bound by the *Birch* principle and the duty to advise on the less invasive alternatives together with a comparison of the risks and benefits. Experience suggests that it is very rare for them to address in detail the non-blood alternatives, even though these almost certainly represent the less invasive option. Further, as the treating clinician is most directly involved with the day to day care of the child, such evidence, as the Royal College Guidelines quoted indicates, is highly likely to contain a subjective element. The court, as the substitute decision-maker, is entitled to precisely the same information as the parents should receive, so as to make a properly informed choice, and should accordingly be looking for an objective appraisal. It should also be mindful of the dictum of Holman J. cited in chapter 15 on Children:

> 'The court must be astute to ensure that non-blood alternatives have been considered before making an Order'.

16.5 Secondly, the court will be looking to be assisted by a genuinely independent and objective expert whose approach meets the general test of an expert. The general principles applicable to all experts preparing reports for, or giving evidence to, any court or tribunal were laid down by Creswell J. in *The Ikarian Reefer* in 1993.[241] Not long before, Cazalet J. had given similar guidance for experts in the Family Division.[242]

---

241 *National Justice Cia Naviera SA v Prudential Assurance Co Ltd (The Ikarian Reefer)* [1993] 2 Lloyds Rep 68 at pp. 81-82

242 *re R (A minor) (Experts'* Evidence*)* [1991] 1 FLR 291

16.6 The facts giving rise to the *Ikarian Reefer* judgment were comparatively simple. The Panamanian registered vessel ran aground; fire broke out in the engine room and she was a total loss. The owners claimed on their insurers, who repudiated liability on the basis that the fire was caused deliberately with the connivance of the owners and it was a fraudulent insurance claim. It was a classic case in which expert evidence predominated and Creswell J. took the opportunity to set out what has become accepted as the definitive common law authority governing expert evidence. This has been conveniently summarised as:

- The evidence of an expert witness should be independent, objective and unbiased.
- The evidence of an expert witness should relate to matters within his field of expertise.
- The expert should state the facts and assumptions which form the basis of his expert opinion.
- The expert should consider facts which are capable of detracting from his opinion.
- The expert should clearly indicate when a matter falls outside the ambit of his expertise.
- Where this is so, the expert should indicate that he possessed insufficient information to form more than a provisional opinion.
- Where the expert could not swear that the content of his report was true without adding a qualification, the expert should state the qualification.
- Where this is so, the expert should indicate that, following the exchange of expert's reports, his opinion has changed.
- The expert should provide the other party with photographs, plans, calculations, analyses, measurements, reports, etc. to which his evidence refers.

16.7 From that broad definition of the principles governing the role of the expert there has been a progressive review of the functions and duties of the expert witness in family proceedings that has involved not only Practice Directions from the President but also a number of decided cases. One principal matter of concern is the self-evident difference in role between the treating clinician and the outside expert brought in to report independently. As Thorpe LJ. said so pithily in a case in 2000:

> 'It ought to be elementary for any professional working in the family justice system that the role of the expert to treat is not to be muddled with the role of the expert to report'.

16.8 The whole issue was comprehensively reviewed in a landmark article[243] in the August 2012 issue of *Counsel* by Jo Delahunty QC of 4 Paper Buildings and Kate Purkiss of Coram Chambers, leading and junior counsel respectively, who had appeared for the parents first in a lengthy criminal trial at the Old Bailey alleging the murder of their much loved younger boy. This was followed by a six week fact finding hearing in the Family Division in care proceedings relating to the older sister. The case highlighted precisely the difference in approach between the treating team, who were totally convinced that the injuries were non-accidental, and a range of defence experts who demonstrated clearly that the mother 'had severe vitamin D deficiency that she had passed on to her son *in utero* leading to congenital rickets which became more severe as she continued to pass on the deficiency through her breast milk'. The judge in the criminal trial stopped the case and directed an acquittal. In the family proceedings Mrs Justice Theis refused the local authority's application for a Care Order on the basis that she 'could not be satisfied, on the balance of probabilities that any of the fractures or the traumatised fissure were as a result of inflicted deliberate harm caused to J. The fractures could have been caused by the day to day handling of a young baby due to the particular fragility of J's bones as a result of the severity of his undetected rickets'.

16.9 In her extremely thorough judgment dated 19 April 2012[244] the judge reviewed the law on the proper approach to expert evidence in the family courts. In particular she cited the compelling words of Butler-Sloss P. in a case in 2004 that included the following: [245]

> '(iv) The court must always be on guard against the over dogmatic expert, the expert whose reputation or *amour propre* is at stake or the expert who has developed a scientific prejudice.

[243] *Counsel*: Journal of the General Council of the Bar. August 2012 at pp. 26-29
[244] *LB Islington v Al-Alas and Wray* [2012] EWHC 865 (Fam)
[245] *re U; re B (Serious Injury: Standard of Proof)* [2004] 2 FLR 263 at § 23

(v) The judge in care proceedings must never forget that today's medical certainty may be discarded by the next generation of experts or that scientific research will throw light into corners that are at present dark'.

16.10 The duties of an expert were later incorporated in the relevant Practice Direction issued by the President of the Family Division.[246] Paragraph 3.1 states the 'Overriding Duty' thus:

'An expert in family proceedings relating to children has an overriding duty to the court that takes precedence over any obligation to the person from whom the expert has received instructions or by whom the expert is paid'.

The next paragraph then defines the 'Particular Duties' of the expert and (although not copying them verbatim) sets out in detail the principles alluded to in *The Ikarian Reefer* with very strong emphasis on the independence of the opinion expressed.

16.11 However the whole re-structuring of the family courts system into a unified Family Court has been under review under the Family Justice Modernisation Programme chaired by Ryder J.[247] One specific issue is the evidence of experts which at present not only consumes a great deal of court time but (more importantly in the current financial climate) absorbs what many consider to be a disproportionate amount of financial resources. One of the key factors in the modernisation plan is to shorten the time taken to reach a decision in the interests of the child. Under the heading 'Public law case management' at §47 the proposals state:

'If an expert is required, any expert evidence that is necessary is likely to be provided by a single or single joint expert so that an issues resolution hearing can be listed at about 20 weeks to identify the issues which remain and list the final hearing shortly thereafter'.

16.12 The pressure to reduce the amount of expert evidence is perhaps demonstrated in the Fourth Update Family Modernisation Programme, an extract of which is quoted in the article in *Counsel* cited above:

'...to further reduce the need for expert evidence in both standard and exceptional tracks, we will enlist the help of the Family Justice Council and join with the

[246] Practice Direction: Experts in Family Proceedings Relating to Children. Sir Mark Potter 1 April 2008

[247] Judicial proposals for the modernisation of family justice, Ryder J.

> Government in the publication of peer reviewed research as to evidence-based good practice. Not only will pathway documents be available giving guidance as to the form and content of materials for use in court, but judges will have available to them research materials which are uncontradicted i.e. generally accepted by a reasonable body of professionals. That would not of course prevent a dispute being heard relating to such materials but it will concentrate minds as to the need for the same in many cases'.

Further:

> 'the Care Monitoring System Guidance for Practitioners suggests that a form of order in relation to the decision on the instruction of an expert will include the reason for permission being granted such as *the absence of expert evidence from local authority/CAFCASS or an identified necessity on a relevant issue outside the skill and expertise otherwise available to the court'.*

16.13 Perhaps the most compelling criticism of a proposed change in culture relating to expert evidence is the concluding part of that section in the article in *Counsel*:

> 'We are very concerned that a change in culture which restricts the use of expert evidence where the local authority already has such evidence, and where the interim threshold on very basic terms has been established, may be interpreted restrictively by the family courts: in reality this will impact mainly on Respondent parents in contested care proceedings. The burden of proof rests with the Local Authority in care proceedings. Where it adduces expert evidence, a Respondent should not be denied the opportunity to call expert evidence to challenge that opinion. The suggestion in the Programme is that a library of approved research material may take the place of the experts themselves. In a case such as *Al Alas & Wray,* such restriction would have resulted in catastrophic injustice'.

Those are indeed strong words but when looking at the case overall, the treating teams at UCH and at GOSH were world class experts with strongly held and expressed professional opinions and yet the inescapable fact is that they were wrong. It took independent experts instructed by the coroner and the defence to prove the vitamin D deficiency underlying the (previously undiagnosed) rickets in the deceased child and thereby secure the acquittal of the parents on the grave charge of murder. Even then the local authority persisted, albeit unsuccessfully, in the allegation of non-accidental injury as the basis for care proceedings in respect of the elder sibling.

The two named hospitals are each held in high regard and the evidence of their expert clinicians would in normal circumstances be accepted and acted upon. And yet the warning of Butler-Sloss P. cited above 'against the over dogmatic expert, the expert whose reputation or *amour propre* is at stake or the expert who has developed a scientific prejudice' seems to have been fulfilled.

The very real fear remains that the proposed changes and reliance on 'a library of approved research material' (in effect a *Bolam* library representing the conservative views of the medical profession) could so easily lead to a real and catastrophic injustice unless the parents are allowed to call proper expert evidence in rebuttal.

16.14 An additional difficulty can easily arise in the actual drafting of the expert's report. There is a long recognised practice of the expert(s) conferring with counsel before the final report is perfected and disclosed to the other side. But it is not without risk. The facts of the case of *Whitehouse v Jordan* probably represent the nadir of failure by two experts and counsel to deal properly with the preparation of a joint report.

16.15 Baby Whitehouse suffered catastrophic brain damage at birth. The allegation was that Dr Jordan, the Senior Obstetric Registrar had, in the course of a forceps instrumental delivery, applied too much force and pulled for too long thereby causing the ultimate brain damage. Expert evidence was crucial and two eminent professors of obstetrics were instructed on behalf of the plaintiff. Although the plaintiff won at trial, the Court of Appeal overturned the finding of negligence and this was later upheld in the House of Lords. However both appellate courts in the course of ruling on negligence were scathing about the circumstances of the preparation of the experts' reports.

16.16 In the Court of Appeal Lord Denning said: [248]

> 'In the first place, their joint report suffers to my mind from the way it was prepared. It was the result of long conferences between two professors and counsel in London, and was actually settled by counsel. In short, it wears the colours of special pleading rather than an impartial report. Whenever counsel "settle" documents we know how it goes. "We had better put this in". "We had better leave this out" and so forth. A striking instance is the way in which

[248] *Whitehouse v Jordan* [1980] 1 All ER 65 (CA)

Professor Tizard's was "doctored". The lawyers blocked out a couple of lines in which he agreed with Professor Strang that there was no negligence'.

16.17 Later, in the House of Lords, Lord Wilberforce addressed the same issue: [249]

> 'One final word. I have to say I feel some concern as to the manner in which part of the expert evidence called for the plaintiff came to be organised. The matter was discussed in the Court of Appeal and commented on by Lord Denning. While some degree of consultation between experts and legal advisers is entirely proper, it is necessary that expert evidence to be presented to the court should be, and should be seen to be, the independent product of the expert, uninfluenced as to the form or content by the exigencies of the litigation. To the extent that it is not, the evidence is likely to be not only incorrect but self-defeating'.

Although this case pre-dates the CPR, it is still good law on the principles that should govern the inter-action between experts *inter se* and experts and lawyers at the stage of preparation of the report. For a plaintiff's expert to be talked out of his professional view that there was no negligence really is unacceptable.

16.18 In summary, the author accordingly submits that, whatever the practice hitherto in these blood transfusion cases, there is a compelling argument that Part 35 is engaged with all that that involves.

16.19 That immediately raises questions about the role of the court and the pre-hearing management, the necessity for leave to obtain and adduce expert evidence, and more especially that the expert be wholly professional and objective in fulfilling the overriding duty to assist the court. It especially means that, even though initiated by the NHS Trust on behalf of the treating team with a view to obtaining an order that the parents resist, the proceedings are first and foremost ***non-adversarial.***

16.20 All concerned in these cases could do no better than read Wall LJ.'s succinct instruction intended for the expert witness:

> 'The importance of the non-adversarial principle for you is that you are not there to support one side or the other. You are there to give your objective professional opinion to the judge on the points which are within the area of your expertise in order to assist the judge to reach a conclusion which is in the best interests of the child or children concerned'.

---

[249] *Whitehouse v Jordan* [1981] 1 WLR 246 (HL)

16.21 This leads on to the *Birch* principle discussed in more detail at [10.16] and the duty to advise on the less invasive alternative treatment option. It should be incorporated in the instructions of the NHS lawyers that the medical witnesses (of whatever speciality) address the issue of risks and benefits including conservative and/or non-blood management. They will, of course, have to follow the several Protocols and Practice Directions to include the updated requirements relating to the mandatory certificates to be included. These go further than the earlier procedures and require the witness to certify his awareness of and familiarity with not merely Part 35 of the CPR but the Practice Directions and Protocols. At present this seems to be honoured in the breach in these blood cases, with the witness statements merely including the standard format of Declaration of Truth.

16.22 It also seems highly likely that in the near future expert witnesses will have to address the issue of competence of mature minors aged under 18 years. Following the ruling in the Canadian Supreme Court in the case of *AC v Manitoba* there are compelling arguments that the long-standing decision of the Court of Appeal[250] and the 'Nolan' dictum so frequently relied on (although arguably *obiter dicta*) may no longer be either appropriate at Common Law nor European Convention compliant, namely:

> 'In general terms, however, the present state of the law is that an individual who has reached the age of 18 is free to do with his life what he wishes, but it is the duty of the Court to ensure so far as it can that children survive to that age'.

It is highly probable that the issue will be tested at least by inviting the Court of Appeal to re-visit its own decision, if not taken direct to the Supreme Court under the 'leap-frog' provisions, and expert evidence on the mental capacity and competence of the minor is likely to feature significantly.

16.23 In addition to the law, further consideration will probably have to be given to the cogent reasoning of Professor Len Doyal on the ethical issues raised in overriding the treatment choice of a comprehending minor discussed in chapter 11.

16.24 The role and duties of an expert witness were extensively reviewed by the Supreme Court in a case decided in March 2011.[251] The solicitors acting for

---

[250] *re W (a minor) (Medical Treatment)* (1992) 4 All ER 627 (CA) (1992) 9 BMLR 22 (CA)
[251] *Jones v Kaney* [2011] UKSC 13

the claimant in a personal injury claim arising out a road traffic accident had instructed a consultant clinical psychologist to report on the long-term effects of injuries asserted by the claimant. The defendants instructed a consultant psychiatrist who took a different view, that the gravity was being exaggerated by the claimant. Following usual practice on restricting multiple expert evidence, the district judge ordered the two experts to hold discussions and to prepare a draft joint statement. The claimant's expert on the telephone then changed her opinion and somewhat rashly deferred significantly to the defendant's expert. The upshot was settlement of the personal injury claim on terms less favourable to the claimant. He then went after the expert who claimed immunity from suit but the Supreme Court ruled against her and upheld liability. The court held that there was no good public policy reason for granting the immunity claimed and that liability existed. In future all experts will have to take this into account in compiling their reports and giving evidence. Additionally it would seem to be the course of prudence for them to check that their Professional Indemnity Insurance covers the risks disclosed by this case.

Transparency

16.25 In what many lawyers appearing in family cases regard as a significant shift in policy on confidentiality, the President of the Family Division of the High Court, in a judgment in May 2011, [252] ruled that there was little reason in family proceedings for a refusal to disclose the report of an expert witness. The judge, who had heard care proceedings in respect of the three children, had been highly critical of the report of Dr M., a paediatrician. The Care application had, in the event, been withdrawn by the council and the judge had made an exceptional order that they pay £100,000 costs towards the mother's legal aid costs.

16.26 Given these highly unusual events, an investigative journalist then wanted access to the detail including the report of the expert witness of which the judge had been so critical. The President said that he would like to see a practice develop in which expert reports would be routinely disclosed and the media able to comment both on the report and the use to which it had been put in the proceedings. Each case would need consideration as to whether or not there was an outstanding welfare issue that needed to be addressed by a

[252] *In re X, Y and Z (Children) (Expert witness: Identification)* Family Division May 11 2011

continuing order for anonymity. How this develops in practice will be awaited with interest but hopefully the prospect of more transparency may concentrate the minds of experts before they put pen to paper.

16.27 Over the years there has been so much misinformed, emotive and sometimes outright hostile reporting of these blood cases (see Emma; Maher; and Gilman chapter 7*)* that it is encouraging to see the President reminding the media of the wise dictum of Lord Hobhouse in the House of Lords that: [253]

> 'No public interest is served by publishing or communicating misinformation'.

16.28 One final matter is that the quality of the evidence put before the court in children's cases is increasingly coming under close and professional scrutiny. The government commissioned a report conducted by Professor Jane Ireland, a forensic psychologist at the University of Central Lancashire. She was given unprecedented access to expert witness evidence from 3 courts. In her report published in May 2012 she found that 20% of reports were written by people not qualified for the task; a further 20% were by people writing outside their area of knowledge and qualifications; 65% of the reports were 'poor' or 'very poor' and only 1 in 10 experts were practising in the field in which they were giving advice. Unsurprisingly, Professor Ireland called for an urgent review of the entire system. How much of this translates into the children's blood cases is problematical. However, the wider welfare of the child and family play a major part in the consideration by the court in addition to the technical medical evidence. This research by a distinguished professor will undoubtedly carry weight.

16.29 In summary, there may have to be a reappraisal of how the medical evidence is presented and reported in these contested blood transfusion cases.

---

[253] *Reynolds v Times Newspapers Ltd* [2001] 2 AC 127 at p. 238

Chapter Seventeen

Ireland

17.1 Although having a written Constitution of which it is justifiably proud, Ireland's jurisprudence is still substantially common law based. The law on Consent to Treatment is reviewed in great detail in the leading case of *In re a Ward,*[254] a decision of the Supreme Court that has stood the test of time since 1996. The case was in many ways the mirror image of *Bland*[255] in that, although the origins of the injury causing the condition were different, it came down to an end of life decision.

17.2 These end of life cases are by definition most distressing for the immediate family and they have exercised clinicians and the courts. But in order to arrive at a reasoned judgment as to whether, on the particular facts before it, it was lawful for the clinicians to withdraw life-sustaining treatment, the judges had first to review the law on consent to treatment and the rights of the competent patient to decide treatment options. Only then could it proceed to the law on the court's substituted decision-making process where the patient was no longer competent.

17.3 The extract from the judgment of Denham J. is set out here in the context of the specific law of Ireland.

> '331. The right to life is the pre-eminent personal right. The State has guaranteed in its laws to respect this right. The respect is absolute. This right refers to all lives—all lives are respected for the benefit of the individual and for the common good. The State's respect for the life of the individual encompasses the right of the individual to, for example, refuse a blood transfusion for religious reasons. In the recognition of the individual's autonomy, life is respected'.

17.4 A major blood scandal took place in Ireland between 1976 and 1994. The following account is based on the official report into the issue.[256] In 1961 the Blood Transfusion Service Board (BTSB) had been created as an Executive Agency, known as a 'state sponsored body'. It was a separate legal entity with a

---

254 *In re a Ward of Court (withholding medical treatment)* (No 2)[1996] 2 IR 79

255 *Airedale National Health Service Trust v Bland* [1993] 2 WLR 316

256 *Report of the Expert Group of the BTSB 1995; Report of the Tribunal of Inquiry into the BTSB 1997*

board of management reporting regularly to the Minister for Health who, in political terms, was accountable to the *Dáil* (the Irish Parliament) for the activities of the BTSB.

17.5 BTSB's main functions were to manage the national blood transfusion service and ensure a safe and adequate supply of blood to meet the needs of the population, based on voluntary blood donors. In reality BTSB operated with minimal ministerial oversight. Decision-making remained predominantly with the medical and scientific professionals responsible for managing its day to day activities.

17.6 In the early 1970's, the BTSB had been responsible for the distribution of a blood product anti-D. This is a well-known and scientifically approved blood component used in Western medicine specifically for those pregnant women whose blood grouping was Rhesus Negative. It is recognized that the Rhesus conflict of a pregnancy with a Rhesus Positive father, if left untreated, was likely to lead to increasing foetal problems in subsequent pregnancies. The primary cause is that the pregnant mother has been sensitised to the D antigen. The problems included raised levels of bilirubin in the foetus, potentially leading to jaundice and, in extreme cases, to kernicterus and *hydrops fetalis*, each with the potential to cause fatal brain damage. The nature of the problem is such that with each successive pregnancy the Rhesus problems multiplied causing what came to be known colloquially as 'blue baby syndrome'. This is discussed in considerably greater detail in chapter 8.

17.7 The recommended prophylaxis is to give the mother postpartum (including even ectopic pregnancy or pregnancy terminated by spontaneous miscarriage) a large enough injection of anti-D to prevent her manufacturing anti-D herself. This reduces or eliminates the Rhesus conflict in any subsequent pregnancy. The problem is sufficiently well known that the Royal College of Gynaecologists has issued guidelines for Rh prophylaxis.

17.8 In 1976, it first came to the attention of the BTSB that one of the donors whose blood had contributed to a batch of anti-D had been diagnosed with infective hepatitis. Although aware of this, senior staff continued using the donation in the preparation of subsequent batches of anti-D. In 1977, the BTSB were notified that a number of women who had received anti-D had developed hepatitis but senior staff, without any or any proper investigation, attributed such diagnoses to environmental factors and took no further action.

17.9 By the early 1990's a blood test to establish the presence of Hepatitis C became commercially available. Blood samples from the 1977 incident had been retained and were then submitted for re-testing using the newly available technique and tested positive. When this was drawn to the attention of senior staff they again chose to take no further action to investigate the matter.

17.10 However, in a separate incident another donor's blood tested positive for Hepatitis C and staff chose to ignore that result believing it to be a false positive. The consequence was that the donation went forward for processing and again was ultimately used in multiple batches of anti-D.

17.11 In January 1994 a member of staff at a regional blood bank had completed a study that showed a high incidence of women donors testing positive for Hepatitis C. Further investigation showed that the common denominator was that they had each received anti-D. Upon being informed of this, the Minister decided that it was necessary to inform the wider public and to demonstrate that decisive action was being taken. A screening programme was put in place; all available stocks of anti-D were recalled; and the *Dáil* and the public generally were reassured that the matter was now under control. However the incident became a political scandal later described (with echoes of André Picard and the Krever Commission in Canada) as 'the greatest health scandal in the history of the State'.

17.12 Sadly, the securing of the stable door was long after the horse had bolted. Over 1,000 women were identified as having been infected over the years and they joined together as a group under the banner *Positive Action* to do battle with the government for proper compensation. Those who want to pursue the history of this incident in greater detail should turn to Anne-Marie Farrell's seminal work *Contaminated blood and political scandal in Ireland.* [257]

17.13 The ensuing litigation only served to enhance the public perception of a medical and political cover up. Brigid McCole, a mother of 11 children and who had been infected by contaminated anti-D, brought a High Court case which was supported by *Positive Action* and many journalists and members of the public. In the Spring of 1996 the case was listed for trial that October. In the pre-trial preparation her lawyers accused the BTSB of deliberately withholding documents that showed that the batch of anti-D, which included that given to

[257] *Scandals in past and contemporary politics* by John Garrard and James Newell, Chapter 11 pp.163-173

her in 1977, had come from a donor previously diagnosed with infective hepatitis. Sadly, before the case could come to trial Brigid McCole died from the effects of her Hepatitis C. In the ensuing rancorous publicity the *Cork Examiner* described the political ineptitude as 'the worst crisis of its kind in public administration…in the history of the State.'

The scandal rumbled on with public concern expressed that the incident 'violated the traditional social and religious role accorded in Irish society to women as mothers, now infected by a deadly disease by a state institution to which they had entrusted their well-being'. Further that it showed 'a government more intent on limiting its financial liability than addressing the needs of the victims'.

17.14 It is difficult to assess the full long term impact on the Irish public whose faith in the ability of a previously respected institution BTSB to deliver safe blood products had been devastated. Over the years, laborious efforts have been made to establish safe procedures and products and restore credibility so that there is now a full time Haemovigilance Consultant Haematologist whose primary function is to try and secure safer blood. But understandably some mistrust of donor blood and blood products remains.

17.15 One aspect that cannot be ignored is that, in addition to the hardship to the patients and families of those infected, there has been the massive cost to the Irish taxpayer. The average pay-out in compensation was the Euro equivalent of £750,000 per victim of Hepatitis C and those infected with HIV received £101,000. In 2009 an independent enquiry in the UK chaired by Baron Archer of Sandwell (The Archer Inquiry referred to in chapter 5) had recommended that British victims be compensated on the same level as those in Ireland. These Irish figures were cited in a claim for compensation brought in the UK by a claimant, Andrew March, who was refused payments reflecting parity with the payments in Ireland. The UK Department of Health tried to argue that the Irish blood transfusion service had been at fault but there had been no such facts demonstrating fault in the UK. Holman J., in proceedings for Judicial Review, ruled on 16 April 2010 that the UK government's approach 'has been and remains infected with error'. [258]

[258] *March v Department of Health*, Judicial Review, 16 April 2010 per Holman J.

Non-blood management

17.16 The advance and acceptance in Ireland of non-blood clinical management has been slower than in the UK but steady progress is being made.

17.17 In January 2008 a mother, pregnant with twins, was diagnosed with Rhesus conflict. Because of her inability on grounds of conscience to consent to the use of donor blood, proceedings were instituted in the High Court in Dublin. [259] In that particular Unit, the clinicians had established a track record for successfully using the techniques of non-blood management. The mother wanted treatment in that Unit so, although there was no consent, equally there was no serious opposition to the making of an order. The outcome was that the twins were born with raised bilirubin levels but were successfully treated with ultraviolet multi-lamp and adjunctive therapy. They made an uneventful recovery without any blood being used. This is yet another example of a permissive order being obtained by the State, at considerable cost, but no blood ever being given.

17.18 The further case of *Baby C* demonstrates the advances that have been made in managing without blood the very low birth-weight pre-term neonates. *C* was born at a mere 24 weeks and 5 days, weighing 750 grammes. An exceptionally skilled and committed team at the Coombe Hospital, Dublin treated the baby. Leave was given by Birmingham J. to use blood as a last resort. *Baby C* was gradually weaned off the ventilator and EPO and at 11 weeks after birth was discharged home without blood being used. He continued to thrive and is now a normal child with no apparent residual effects.

Physical Restraint

17.19 Even if court authority for permission to transfuse is obtained, the author submits that there can be no order for physical restraint of the patient outwith the existing Mental Health legislation. Many patients will find repugnant the mere concept that such draconian powers can be sought at all (as they have been, notably in Australia), let alone in secret without the patient or their representatives having any opportunity to argue to the contrary. To many it seems a very slippery slope at the end of which lie the appalling lessons of Dr Mengele and his enforced medical experiments on victims in the Nazi

[259] *re B & W,* High Court, Dublin Chancery Division, Laffoy J. unreported

concentration camps and the more recent Soviet misuse of enforced treatment in psychiatric units of those who merely dissent from the government in power.

17.20 There are relevant dicta of Hale LJ. in a leading UK case involving a psychiatric patient compulsorily detained in Broadmoor Special Hospital:[260]

> 'Whatever the position before the Human Rights Act 1998, the decision to impose treatment without consent on a protesting patient is a potential invasion of the rights under Article 3 or Article 8. Super-Wednesbury is not enough. The claimant is entitled to a proper hearing on the merits of whether the statutory grounds for imposing this treatment upon him against his will are made out i.e. whether it is treatment for the mental disorder from which he is suffering and whether it should be given to him without his consent "having regard to the likelihood of its alleviating or preventing a deterioration of his [psychiatric] condition"'.

17.21 On this issue of the legality of physical restraint the reader may wish to consider also *Irish Mental Health Law* at pp. 300–301.[261] The additional submission is now made that it is not for a judge at first instance, let alone *ex parte*, to make new common law. The court cannot authorise forcible restraint of a patient in hospital outside the relevant provisions of the existing Mental Health legislation that provides for this contingency in very circumscribed terms relating to violent psychiatric patients. If such a change in the law is to be accomplished it is for the *Oireachtas*, after full public debate, and not for the judiciary, especially in an *ex parte* hearing and with no relevant authority cited to the judge.

17.22 Dr Simon Mills BL expressly referred to these procedural safeguards in his leading textbook on *Clinical Practice and the Law in Ireland*.[262] At paragraph [4.40] he writes:

> 'Where it is proposed that a patient will be treated in the face of a refusal and where there is uncertainty about the patient's capacity to refuse, a court may be asked to rule on the lawfulness of treatment in the circumstances. Although there is no considered Irish case law on the issue of applications to the court in respect of doubtfully competent individuals, there is [here citing St George's NHS Trust supra] substantial guidance from the English courts that where it is proposed to

---

[260] *R (on the application of Wilkinson) v RMO, Broadmoor Hospital Authority,* [2001] EWCA (Civ) 545; [2002] 1 WLR 419; 65 BMLR 15

[261] *Irish Mental Health Law*, Anne-Marie O'Neill, February 2005, First Law Limited

[262] *Clinical Practice and the Law*, Dr Simon Mills BL, 2nd Edition, 14 November 2007, Tottel Publishing

> seek a court order declaring the patient's refusal of treatment invalid, then that application should be made on notice to the patient and the patient should, where possible, be represented at the hearing of the action'.

Most patients, especially parents, are likely to feel that these represent the minimum safeguards against over-zealous or coercive medical intervention to which the patient, of whatever age, is not consenting.

17.23 Finally is the proposed change in the law covering the age of consent to treatment. Following a long consultation process by the Law Commission of Ireland and its report 'Children and the Law: Medical Treatment', the recommendation was that mature minors of 16 and 17-years-of-age should be deemed to have capacity both to consent to and to refuse treatment. However this was to be subject to a functional test which is 'a case by case test of capacity based on whether the person understands the nature and effect of the specific decision being made'. Significantly the Commission recommended that an application could be made to the High Court to determine the validity of the refusal. How that would work out in practice remains to be seen.

The Act of 2015

17.24 In the meantime after more than 3 years of deliberation the long awaited Assisted Decision-Making (Capacity) Act 2015 was finally passed into law by the President on 30 December 2015. At the time of this second edition going to print the Act still has no commencement date which is explained by the need for time to draft, publish and bring into effect firstly the Regulations which will have legal effect albeit as secondary legislation. Also the Code of Practice cited in the statute which will be advisory but nevertheless of considerable importance in the fact finding deliberations of any court. The consensus of the distinguished speakers at the National Assisted Decision Making Conference sponsored by the HSE on 22 February 2016 was that this work was unlikely to be finished by the end of 2016. It now seems likely to be well into 2017.

17.25 It is of interest that as a matter of policy the legislature seem to have retained the common law concept of the Advance **Directive** as laid down in the 1990 Canadian case of *Malette v Shulman* as subsequently approved and adopted into UK law by such cases as *re T* and in 2015 in Namibia in *ES v*

AC.[263] This seems to indicate at least some support for the principle of the right of patient choice having priority over medical paternalism and especially that, in the event of disagreement, patient choice is to prevail.

This is in marked contrast to the comparable UK Mental Capacity Act of 2005 that was supposed to replace but incorporate the common law principles but in fact changed the terminology from ***Directives*** to ***Decisions.*** That is more than a mere cosmetic change of title but a significantly retrograde move from binding directives back to medical paternalism as to whether to comply. This new Irish law seems, in that respect at least, to provide more protection to patient choice.

17.26 A number of general matters can usefully be gleaned even from the Act itself at this stage. For instance, the Preamble at page 9 makes a reference to the European Convention of Human Rights as one of the applicable principles even though there does not seem to be any specific reference to the Convention within the lengthy Interpretation Section 2, the Schedule of Statutes or elsewhere in the body of the Act.

17.27 Section 8 sets out what are defined as 'Guiding Principles'. Section 8(7) (b) and (c) are perhaps two of the important principles. If an intervention is made on behalf of a [patient], the intervener <u>shall</u> [note the mandatory ***'shall'***]:

> 'b) give effect so far as is practicable, to the past and present will and preferences of the relevant person [patient] insofar as that will and preferences are reasonably ascertainable; and
>
> c) take into account the beliefs and values of the relevant person…'

This would seem to give express statutory priority and protection to religious beliefs and values as representing the basis of the choice of non-blood management.

17.28 There are then pages of provisions in the Act that would not seem material to this issue although of general application in the context of patients who lose capacity e.g. by injury or dementia. End of life decisions are the subject of special provisions that do not seem relevant in the context of choice of non-blood management.

---

[263] *ES v AC*. Namibia Supreme Court see chapter 21.11

Capacity

17.29 Section 3 deals with a person's capacity and says at the outset that it is to be construed '*functionally*'. Section 3(2) sets out the defining considerations for assessing a person's lack of capacity. It follows almost *verbatim* the 3 stages enunciated by Thorpe J., the well-respected judge of the English Family Division, in the celebrated case of *re C*. set out in more detail in [10.12].

How this provision of '*functionally*' is to be reconciled with the total failure of the Act to provide for Advance Directives for those mature minors who are under 18 years but have functional capacity is a question that may yet have to be answered in the courts.

Part 8

17.30 Part 8 of the Act at page 83, under the heading 'Advance Healthcare Directives', then deals in detail with these relevant matters, starting with a comprehensive definition section.

Section 83(2) is perhaps one of the more important provisions relating to the validity of patient choice:

> 'A relevant person who has attained the age of 18 and who has capacity is entitled to refuse treatment for any reason (including a reason based on his or her religious beliefs) notwithstanding that the refusal:
>
> (a) appears to be an unwise decision;
> (b) appears not to be based on sound medical principals; or
> (c) may result in his or her death'.

17.31 Thus the disagreement of the treating team with the religious or indeed other beliefs or values of the patient is no basis for overriding a valid refusal of treatment. This may assume extra importance when considering the rights of the pregnant woman set out below.

17.32 Section 84 sets out in detail the new provisions that will be mandatory in a new Healthcare Directive. It would seem that there will have to be significant and substantial changes to the drafting of new Directives to make them compliant with the statute and thus valid, registrable and enforceable.

One crucial provision is the mandatory requirement in subsection (6) that, analogous to Wills, **all four persons are present** at the same time and each signs in the presence of the other three. This will need careful consideration and compliance as the Minister has under subsection (9) the power to issue specimen forms and it will be necessary to ensure compliance generally.

Notification

17.33 For the first time there is a power for the Minister to make regulations to require that notice of a Directive be given to him and to maintain a register. How he proposes to make this work with at least 6,000 potential patients in Ireland, each renewing their Directive each year, remains to be seen. The issue of fees payable may become crucial. Many may wonder why they should have to pay for merely indicating their choice of treatment options in an Advance Directive. Is that 'proportionate' or 'necessary' under the Convention? One also immediately suspects a potential resource problem as in Namibia with the HIV infected mothers.

Some Specific Cases for Consideration

17.34 Provided their Directives are compliant with the Act, male persons over the age of 18 seem to have much the same protection as that given by the common law. The same applies to females over 18 but with the exception of those of child bearing age to whom special rules apply as set out below.

The lower age limit is set under the Act at 18 years. This makes no provision for mature minors who actually have capacity as defined in the Act – the principle of 'functionality'. There could be an argument based on the common law e.g. the Canadian Supreme Court case of *AC v Manitoba*. Additionally or in the alternative there may well be room for challenge under the European Convention on the grounds of Article 14 discrimination in conjunction with Article 8 interference with the family. These matters will need careful consideration once the Regulations and Code of Practice have been published.

Pregnant Women

17.35 Section 85(6) deals with this topic. It introduces a legal concept of a possible competing interest of the supposed rights of the unborn child. This is contrary to the UK legal concept, supported by case law, that the foetus has no legal interest until a live birth. The mother retains sole decision making until such a birth. Only then may the court intervene to protect the 'child' as a live person having a separate legal identity.

As a matter for legal argument, there is a manifest discrepancy within the Act especially with section 83(2) above.

17.36 One of the less attractive provisions of section 85 to many who support patient choice is the introduction in subsection (6)(a) of the concept that where 'complying with the refusal of treatment would have a deleterious effect on the unborn, there shall be a presumption that treatment should be provided or continued'.

This begs the question of choice. There are always two choices in proposed medical or surgical treatment: to intervene or not to intervene. Even if the option to intervene is accepted, there are invariably options as to the way in which to intervene. The choice of option A inevitably means the rejection of option B. But does the mere rejection of one option whilst accepting another available and medically accepted option involve 'refusal'?

17.37 Subsection (6)(b) then provides for the referral of the issue to the High Court.

The crucial part of subsection (6)(c) reads:

> 'In determining an application under paragraph (b) the High Court shall have regard to the following:
>
> (i) the potential impact of the refusal of treatment on the unborn;
> (ii) if the treatment that is refused were given to the directive-maker, the invasiveness and duration of the treatment and the risk of harm to the directive-maker'.

This has all the hallmarks of a compromise at the debate stage between the secular humanists who uphold the absolute right of the mother to choose her treatment options without consideration of any supposed rights of the unborn and those who hold that as a matter of law life starts at the point of conception in the womb and that the foetus thus has an independent legal right to protection.

17.38 The real issue is on what legal basis the High Court is supposed to resolve the dilemma. Further, it does not address the possibility of the mother seeking injunctive relief to prevent any intervention on the unborn. The statute merely requires the judge to 'have regard to' these issues. It does not give him any express power to override the choice of the mother that is arguably determinative under both the common law and under Article 8 of the Convention.

With the exception of the wholly irresponsible mother, especially those addicted to alcohol or non-prescribed drugs, the vast majority of pregnant mothers do indeed 'have regard to' the unborn baby they are carrying. Most go to great lengths to protect its welfare.

Similarly GP's, midwives, obstetricians and others giving ante-natal care 'have regard to' the unborn child and most do so in an exemplary fashion – that is why they are in the profession.

17.39 What the Act does not provide is any guidance of the manner in which the judge is to 'have regard to' these issues. Unanswered topics include:

a) patient choice and therefore non-intervention;
b) evidence to be adduced;
c) the burden of proof;
d) the admissibility of independent expert evidence;
e) what criteria is the judge supposed to apply;
f) to what extent (if at all) the judge is entitled under the statute to make any order (presumably Declaratory only);
g) the extent to which the nature and detail of the intervention that the judge seeks to declare will be lawful for the treating team to administer;
h) enforceability and
i) costs including Legal Aid.

These sensitive topics will need extra and very careful consideration and have the potential for causing extensive litigation.

17.40 Article 40.3.3 of the Irish Constitution (as amended in 1983) states:

> 'The State acknowledges the right to life of the unborn and, with due regard to the equal right of the life of the mother, guarantees in its laws to respect, and, as far as practicable, by its laws to defend and vindicate that right'.

In her seminal work '*Medicine, Ethics and the Law*'[264] Professor Deidre Madden at chapter 6 reviews extensively serious problems of interpretation

[264] *Medicine, Ethics and the Law*, 2nd Edition 2007, Deidre Madden, Tottel Publishing Ltd

including the formation of the human embryo and its development to the stage where it becomes capable of a live birth. The new Act introduces still further complications particularly as to the interaction of that Article of the Constitution when considered in the light of the Strasbourg case law.

How the courts will approach and resolve these potential conflicts is difficult to foresee.

17.41 There is an entirely new procedural regime of application to the Court, surprisingly brought down to the jurisdiction of the Circuit Court, save in cases of end of life decisions and also of the unborn foetus both of which are expressly reserved to the High Court.

17.42 The Act further tightens the requirements for validity of the actual document by making express provisions for (*inter alia*) attestation almost analogous to those applicable to the making of a Will. There is also a requirement for deposit and registration of each Directive that seems to suggest an absence of serious thought to the numbers involved. There must be many who, especially in an aging population, for other and personal reasons may wish to sign an advance directive as to what is to happen to them when they lose capacity, for example by the onset of dementia. But there are also many persons within Ireland for whom it is a fundamental tenet of their faith that they will not accept allogeneic blood. Unless adequate resources are provided by the relevant department of government, there must be a serious risk of overload in trying to cope with the level of registrations, most of which will be renewed annually and therefore required to be registered each year.

17.43 A number of other criticisms can justifiably be levelled at the legislation. For example the Act only applies to those over the age of 18. This completely ignores the common law rights of mature minors to choose their treatment options and indeed to do so by advance directive. The clear example set by more progressive countries such as Canada seems to have been completely ignored. And although the preamble to the Act makes specific reference to the European Convention, scant regard seems to have been given in this context to Articles 6, 8 and 14 and the extensive case law at Strasbourg.

17.44 In short, once the procedural formalities have been completed and the Act, Regulations and Code are in place, there would seem to be considerable scope for challenge that may go all the way to Strasbourg. Consideration may even have to be given to the possibility of striking down some provisions as being incompatible with the Convention.

Chapter Eighteen

A Wider Perspective

18.1 It may assist to consider some comparative law that, although it may not be strictly binding, is persuasive and indeed to be taken into account. The common legal bond between most of the countries in Europe is now the European Convention on Human Rights[265] applicable to the 47 States who at the date of writing are High Contracting Parties. However, there are other additional treaty and professional obligations that bear on the topic of patient consent to medical treatment.

18.2 The common law is supported by medical practitioners at an international level. The World Medical Association (WMA), established in 1947, now has a membership of 84 national medical associations and represents some 9,000,000 medical practitioners. The respective medical associations of the UK and Ireland as members of the WMA are both signatories to The Declaration of Lisbon[266] that includes the following:

> 'The following Declaration represents some of the principal rights which the medical profession seeks to provide to patients...
>
> (c) The patient has the right to accept or to refuse treatment after receiving adequate information;
> (e) The patient has the right to die in dignity;
> (f) The patient has the right to receive ... spiritual and moral comfort including the help of a minister of an appropriate religion'.

18.3 A majority of member states of the Council of Europe recognize the right to 'integrity' as applied to medical interventions in a separate Convention:[267]

> 'Article 1:
>
> Parties to this Convention shall protect the dignity and identity of all human beings and guarantee everyone, without discrimination, respect for their

---

265 *Convention for the Protection of Human Rights and Fundamental* Freedoms, Rome 4.11.1950

266 1981 Statement of the World Medical Association (of which the BMA was a founder member)

267 *Convention on Human Rights and Biomedicine* ETS 163

integrity and other rights and fundamental freedoms with regard to the application of biology and medicine.

Article 5—General Rule

An intervention in the health field may only be carried out after the person concerned has given free and informed consent to it.

This person shall beforehand be given appropriate information as to the purpose and nature of the intervention as well as its consequences and risks. The person concerned may freely withdraw consent at any time'.

18.4 One example of how this works in practice is from Spain, where the Constitutional Court has made the following statement:[268]

> 'This court has declared that religious liberty—considered to be a subjective right of a fundamental nature—is based on the recognition of a framework of liberty, and a sphere of free will on the part of the individual. That is, it recognizes the right of citizens to act in this field with complete freedom from coercion by the state or any other social group. And it has also stated in relation to a similar problem to the one under consideration, that coercive medical treatment constitutes a violation of that fundamental right, unless there were a constitutional justification'.

Similar provisions apply in many other Member States and some citations are set out below.

18.5 This leads to a consideration of the European Convention on Human Rights. Firstly, in the preamble, all Contracting States assume a positive obligation in terms that they 'shall secure to everyone within their jurisdiction the rights and freedoms defined'. The use of the imperative 'shall' is significant. Also the Convention applies to all physically present within the jurisdiction irrespective of nationality, immigrant status or any other factors, including migrant workers, temporary visitors or even illegals.

18.6 In defining this positive obligation, the European Court of Human Rights at Strasbourg (ECtHR) has held that any interference in rights defined in the Convention must be subject to an appropriate sanction, even if committed by private parties.[269] The mere existence of a legal system is not sufficient if no action is taken to secure the rights in question.

---

[268] Cassation Appeal Number 3164/94 of 4 November 1996

[269] *X & Y v Netherlands,* (26 March 1985) 8 E.H.R.R. 235

18.7 The principal articles engaged by this issue of Consent to Treatment are Article 8, the right to respect of private life together with Article 14, freedom from discrimination on the grounds of (*inter alia*) religion where this is the motivating force behind the choice of non-blood treatment. In extreme cases, Article 3, the prohibition of torture, inhuman and degrading treatment, and Article 5, the right to liberty and security, may also be engaged.

18.8 The former European Commission of Human Rights (whose functions have been subsumed in, and all applications go to, the Court) held that compulsory medical intervention is an interference with the right to respect for private life under Article 8 of the Convention:[270]

> 'In respect of Article 8 (Art. 8) of the Convention the Commission recalls that a compulsory medical intervention, even if it is of minor importance, must be considered an interference with the right to respect for private life'.

The court has also stated relative to Article 8:[271]

> 'There was no dispute as to the applicability of Article 8 (art. 8): the facts underlying the application to the Commission concern a matter of "private life", a concept which covers the physical and moral integrity of the person …'

18.9 The Commission further stated:

> 'The Commission considers that the taking of a blood sample constitutes an interference with the applicant's right to respect for his private life within the meaning of Article 8'.

If taking an unauthorized blood sample constitutes interference, it would seem impossible to argue against the corollary that forcing of blood transfusions contrary to a competent adult patient's known and recorded decision is an even more egregious interference with the right to respect for private life.

18.10 Non-consensual or coercive medical intervention by forcibly restraining the patient or rendering him powerless to resist by anaesthesia also interferes with the patient's right to liberty and security of person, a right guaranteed under Article 5 of the Convention. Indeed there is a compelling argument that such a violation of patient trust and bodily integrity is in some

---

270 *Peters v The Netherlands,* Application 21132/93 (Comm. Report 6 April 1994) (cf. No. 8239/78, Dec. 4.12.1978, D.R. 16 p. 184; No. 8278/78, Dec. 13.12.1979, D.R. 18 p. 154 and No. 10435/83, Dec. 10.12.1984, D.R. 40 p. 251).

271 *X & Y v Netherlands*, (26 March 1985) 8 E.H.R.R. 235

circumstances capable of amounting to degrading treatment as defined by Article 3.

18.11 The only defence to claims of violations of these various articles could be if the State could discharge the burden of proof and show that the overbearing of the expressed will of the patient:

a) was in accordance with law;
b) had a legitimate aim;
c) was necessary in a democratic society;
d) met a pressing social need; and
e) was proportionate.

18.12 But implicit in this would be a reversion to the benevolent paternalism that the doctor knows better than the patient what is best for the patient. This is the clinical best interests argument so roundly rejected by Dame Elizabeth Butler-Sloss when she upheld the competence test and the right of the competent (though seriously disabled) adult, Miss B, to choose her treatment irrespective of the prognosis of a fatal outcome.

18.13 Attempts to bring an otherwise competent patient artificially within the Mental Health provisions to enforce treatment have been judicially deprecated and even marked with an award of damages for unlawful detention and assault. In her seminal and peer-reviewed article 'The Right to Refuse Medical Treatment under the European Convention on Human Rights', Elizabeth Wicks wrote:[272]

> 'The UK courts have also been keen to declare that a "decision to refuse medical treatment by a patient capable of making the decision does not have to be sensible, rational or well-considered". This impressive statement is, however, of little protection to patients' rights unless it is applied in practice in the most difficult of cases, namely when an acceptance of the patient's decision will result in his death. In these circumstances the UK courts have shown a regrettable tendency to resort to the approach feared by Kennedy—i.e. that a refusal to consent to recommended treatment is evidence of mental incapacity'.

---

[272] *The Right to Refuse Medical treatment under the European Convention on Human Rights*, Medical Law Review 2001 Volume 9 (17) I March 2001

18.14 The author of that article went on to cite Judge LJ. in the English Court of Appeal[273] who said:

> 'When human life is at stake the pressure to provide an affirmative answer authorising unwanted medical intervention is very powerful. Nevertheless, the autonomy of each individual requires continuing protection even, perhaps particularly, when the motive for interfering with it is readily understandable, and indeed to many would appear commendable'.

18.15 Were further authority needed; it is contained in a judgment[274] of the ECtHR given on 23 March 2010, reported by *The Times* under the heading 'Medical intervention without consent', in an application against the UK. A paediatrician formed a suspicion of abuse of a girl aged 9 years on incomplete evidence when an available report of a colleague dermatologist provided an innocent explanation for suspect marks. The paediatrician nevertheless arranged for the taking of blood samples and intimate photographs of the girl in the absence of the parents and without their consent. The ECtHR found violations of Article 8 and (on the particular facts) a violation of Article 13 in the failure of the State to provide an effective remedy.

18.16 In summary, the constant theme of these European cases and writings is that the right of choice rests solely with the competent adult patient. It is not constrained by any requirement such as prior advice from a spiritual, legal or medical adviser. Choice may be based on religious grounds or simply on the particular, even idiosyncratic or irrational, wishes of the competent adult patient. In the case of minor children who lack maturity to rank as 'Mature Minors', the decision-making rests with the parents. It remains with them unless and until, by due process of Convention-compliant law especially Article 6, a court of competent jurisdiction has overruled that choice of medical treatment after hearing proper evidence that conforms to the *Birch* principle of evaluating the risks and benefits of a less invasive option.

Procedural Fairness

18.17 The second relevant aspect of Convention law is procedural fairness. The part of Article 6 that bears on civil procedures states:

---

[273] *St. George's Healthcare NHS Trust v S* [1998] 3 All ER 673 at 688

[274] *MAK & RK v United Kingdom* ECtHR Nos. 45901/05 & 40146/06

> '1. In the determination of his civil rights and obligations or of any criminal charge against him, everyone is entitled to a fair and public hearing within a reasonable time by an independent and impartial tribunal established by law'.

The ECtHR has held that domestic courts must be, and appear to be, impartial.

> 'The Court recalls that the Contracting States are under the obligation to organise their legal systems so as to ensure compliance with the requirements of Article 6 paragraph 1 (art.6-1); ...impartiality is unquestionably one of the foremost of those requirements. The Court's task is to determine whether the Contracting States have achieved the result called for by the Convention, not to indicate the particular means to be utilised'. De Cubber v Belgium, 9186/80 (26 October 1984) A.86 §35, 7 EHRR 236

18.18 This bears on appropriate procedures to safeguard the rights of patient or parents when the court jurisdiction is invoked to override withholding of consent to donor blood. The use of the *ex parte* procedure is disapproved in the common law cases outlined in [13.31], notably by Johnson J. in *re O* and Booth J. in *re R.* Both of these cases precede the Human Rights Act 1998 but remain good law. Thus, to attempt to go behind the back of the patient or parent to secure a court order inevitably violates the concept of fairness.

Pan-European Cooperation

18.19 Two examples may demonstrate the increasing commonality of approach to non-blood management throughout Europe. The first is the organisation Network for the Advancement of Transfusion Alternatives (NATA). Founded in France by a small group of practitioners minded to pursue bloodless surgery, it has now grown into a prestigious and well-respected international force in evaluation of and advancement of the general concepts and, more especially, bringing the ever increasing techniques and products into main stream practice. The regular NATA Conferences attract eminent speakers to present papers and stimulate discussion. The Journal *Transfusion Alternatives in Transfusion Medicine* (TATM) is ranked as one of the most respected, peer-reviewed and authoritative sources on this topic. The Editorial Board is a veritable Who's Who of eminent practitioners in this field throughout Europe and further afield including at least 3 well-recognised experts from the US.

18.20 As further evidence of cooperation, there is a group of experts who have unique experience of managing the multiple victims of major bomb explosions. Although Northern Ireland had at one time the unenviable but principal experience of treating victims of bomb blast and gunshot, terrorist attacks across Europe, including the Madrid train bombing, have now widened the number of clinicians who have had to treat the victims of these major incidents. Spain has formed an organisation *Sociedad Española de Medicina de Catástrofes* (SEMECA)[275] that took the initiative in bringing these experts together at a special conference in Seville in 2004.

18.21 One of the eminent specialists with wide experience is Professor Vitaliy Slepushkin from Russia. He has over 15 years' experience of specific practice in 2 major war zones—Chechnya (including the devastated city of Grozny) and North and South Ossetia, a less well publicised area but with a high rate of attrition in terrorist bombings. He was also the senior clinician treating the survivors of the infamous massacre at the school at Beslan in September 2004. Of the 1,100 hostages taken by a Chechen warlord, 777 were children, but in the rescue operation by Russian security forces, using tanks, thermobaric rockets and other heavy weapons and a series of explosions and subsequent fire, 334 hostages died and severe injuries were sustained by 783 others. By sheer volume of patients, as well as by professional disinclination against donor blood, Professor Slepushkin has had to treat without donor blood; frequently because it simply was not available. In Grozny, for example, the local blood bank had been bombed. He is a respected clinician within Russia and the recipient of a number of national awards including 'The Calling', a special award for medical staff providing assistance to the victims of terrorist attacks.

Professor Slepushkin's detailed presentation at the SEMECA Conference outlining his experience; the techniques of non-blood management and the favourable outcome was well received and made a significant contribution. He is also a man of integrity and courage who is prepared to give professional and objective medical evidence in unpopular causes and before hostile courts.

The harmonisation of medical best practice

18.22 Just as the European Convention and the Declaration of Lisbon have sought to harmonise ethical relationships, so there has been a progressive move

[275] *www.semeca.org*

towards harmonisation of medical best practice in many of the European states. There are many citations in the footnotes to this work that demonstrate a fairly consistent approach to blood conservation strategies in hospitals and universities throughout Europe, along with serious attempts to reduce the incidence of donor blood transfusions. In 2002, a large scale study[276] of 145 intensive care units throughout Europe confirmed that the length of hospital stay and incidence of organic dysfunctions and mortality were significantly higher among the patients who received blood transfusions than among those who chose non-blood management. The study, which also showed that transfusions were associated with immuno-suppression problems, allergic reactions and infectious transmissions, encouraged the use of bloodless medical and surgical techniques. The professional journal in which it appeared is based in the US and it does not seem to have received the public attention, at least in Europe, which the issues raised would seem to justify.

The following, although not intended to be exhaustive, represent an additional selection of quotations from authoritative medical and legal professional sources in 10 different countries as a representative sample of unity of approach.

Austria

18.23 The European Court of Human Rights stated[277] that the Witness parent's choice of medical treatment without the use of blood transfusions should not in any way have impaired her right to custody of her children.

Belgium

18.24 The Juvenile Court in Liege stated[278] that Jehovah's Witnesses are 'well informed of the alternatives to blood transfusions and may engage competent medical services when necessary.'

Professor Dr Karel Dobbelaere, a member of the Belgian Royal Academy acknowledged in a social survey:[279]

---

[276] Jean Louis Vincent at al. Anaemia and Blood Transfusion in Critically Ill Patients, 288 *Jour Amer. Med. Assoc.* 1499-1507 (2002)

[277] *Hoffman v Austria* No. 15/1992/360/434 (ECtHR 1993)

[278] No. RRQJN 66/93 58219 FAM

[279] Authenticated November 12, 1996 by the Apostille of the Belgium Minister of Foreign Affairs

'Jehovah's Witnesses co-operate closely with the medical staff and they love their children. If a blood transfusion is prescribed, they request an alternative treatment out of respect for their convictions. In many large hospitals effective techniques have been developed to accommodate them'.

England & Wales

18.25 A detailed review of the relevant law from the UK is set out in chapter 9 but the following is one of the key citations: [280]

'This appeal is not in truth about the "right to die" ... This appeal is about the "right to choose how to live". This is quite different, even if the choice, when made, may make an early death more likely...

An adult patient who, like Miss T., suffers from no mental incapacity has an absolute right to choose whether to consent to medical treatment, to refuse it or to choose one rather than another of the treatments being offered... This right of choice is not limited to decisions which others might regard as sensible. It exists notwithstanding that the reasons for making the choice are rational, irrational, unknown or even non-existent.

The law requires that an adult patient who is mentally and physically capable of exercising a choice must consent if medical treatment of him is to be lawful ... Treating him without his consent or despite a refusal of consent will constitute the civil wrong of trespass to the person and may constitute a crime...

... the next of kin has no legal right either to consent or to refuse consent...'

France

18.26 The Conseil d'Etat in a case involving the right of a Witness patient to refuse blood transfusions stated: [281]

'..the right of an adult patient to give his consent to a medical treatment, when in a position to express himself, is a fundamental freedom'.

Professor Bernard Hoerni, former President of the French National Order of Physicians (Ordre National des Medicins) said that the position of Jehovah's Witnesses: [282]

'..has incited doctors...to adapt treatment protocols in order to take these personal factors into consideration, just as for each patient other personal, organic or

---

[280] *re T* [1992] 3 W L R 782 per Donaldson MR *supra*
[281] *Valerie and Isabelle Feuillatey* Conseil d'Etat Edict Aug 16 2002
[282] Attestation of Bernard Hoerni Jan 31 2007

physiological factors are taken into consideration. The decision to accept or reject a treatment is, however, always the right of the patient, when he is conscious and lucid, and free of external coercion. I met with individuals with firm and respectable convictions who also understand and respect the position and behaviour of doctors who sometimes find themselves in emergency situations. I have never known of circumstances during which these people have constituted a threat to public order'.

Additionally a survey[283] in France confirmed that 97% of Jehovah's Witnesses in that country have a family doctor and do not hesitate to go to hospital for treatment of serious health problems.

Germany

18.27 The ECtHR ruled:[284]

> 'Even a minor interference with the physical integrity of an individual must be regarded as an interference with the right to respect for private life under Article 8 if it is carried out against the individual's will'.

Ireland

18.28 The Supreme Court has held:[285]

> '§312. Medical treatment may not be given to an adult person of full capacity without his or her consent. There are a few rare exceptions to this e.g., in regard to contagious diseases or in a medical emergency where the patient is unable to communicate. This right arises out of civil, criminal and constitutional law. If medical treatment is given without consent it may be trespass against the person in civil law, a battery in criminal law, and a breach of the individual's constitutional rights. The consent which is given by an adult of full capacity is a matter of choice. It is not necessarily a decision based on medical considerations. Thus, medical treatment may be refused for other than medical reasons, or reasons most citizens would regard as rational, but the person of full age and capacity may make the decision for their own reasons.
>
> §331. The right to life is the pre-eminent personal right. The State has guaranteed in its laws to respect this right. The respect is absolute. This right refers to all lives—all lives are respected for the benefit of the individual and for the common good. The State's respect for the life of the individual encompasses

283 SOFRES, *Survey of Jehovah's Witnesses in France,* October 1998

284 *Storck v Germany* ECtHR No. 61603/00 Judgment 16.09.2005

285 *In re a Ward of Court (withholding medical treatment)* —per Denham J. (No 2) [1996] 2 IR 79

> the right of the individual to, for example, refuse a blood transfusion for religious reasons. In the recognition of the individual's autonomy, life is respected'.

The Assisted Decision Making (Capacity) Act 2015 was passed into law on 30 December 2015. It still awaits a commencement date and drafting of the Regulations and Code.

Italy

18.29 The Council of State has observed[286] that 'the individual's right to free choice of treatment, in the absence of legal provisions that make certain medical treatment obligatory, is guaranteed at constitutional and legislative levels, and therefore any refusal to accept blood transfusions is lawful'.

Russia

18.30 Professor Anatoly P. Zilber, Chairman of the Department of Intensive Care and Anaesthesia, Petrozavodsk University and Republican Hospital of Karelia, Russia has in supporting their stand on non-blood management stated of Jehovah's Witnesses:

> 'They do not abuse alcohol, they do not smoke, they are not money hungry, they do not break their promises, nor give false witness...It is not a mysterious sect, but law abiding citizens... They are respectable, happy people, interested in history, literature, art and life in all its aspects'.

Other aspects of artificial oxygen carriers, especially *Perftoran*® and non-blood management are discussed in chapter 19.

Spain

18.31 One example is the Spanish consensus statement on alternatives to allogeneic transfusions: the 'Seville Document'.[287] This document sets out the composition of the expert panel and the methodology. It then reviews a range of procedures and associated techniques for non-blood management supported by 142 cited references. Its value primarily is that it demonstrates how in yet another European country blood conservation strategies and non-blood management are being co-ordinated countrywide at an official level with government funding for the project.

---

286 Council of State—Italy—First Dept. Section No. 1390/96, Jul 30 1986

287 *Med Clin (Barc)* 2006;127 (Supp 1): 3-20 and *Transfusion alternatives in transfusion medicine* 8, 178–202

Additionally a senior vascular surgeon acknowledged:[288]

> 'This successful surgery program has been made possible thanks to you [Jehovah's Witnesses], who with much effort and determination, have finally convinced us that transfusing blood is not always the best alternative. Thank you on our behalf and on behalf of all those patients you have indirectly benefited'.

Switzerland

18.32 A High Court in Switzerland has ruled[289] that the right of a patient to self-determination is 'an absolute right' and that 'what is decisive for the patient's choice is the expression of his own will and not the opinion of the doctor about what is in the interests of the patient.' Accordingly 'the patient's right to self-determination is extremely broad.'

Summary

These citations are merely selected extracts from a substantial body of professional writings (medical and legal) that uphold the basic right of the adult patient to choose what is, or what is not, done to his own body. The position of minors and the age at which they acquire legal responsibility and capacity for decision-making, inevitably varies considerably between jurisdictions.

Children and Court Intervention

18.33 At [13.43] there is a discussion of the effects of the case of *Glass v United Kingdom*[290] and its impact on paediatric practice when there is a divergence of views between the treating team and the parents. It would be mere repetition to include the same discussion in this chapter but clearly there are issues that, whilst the judgment is in strict law binding only on the United Kingdom, impact throughout the 47 Convention States who are under Treaty obligation to 'take in to account'. The European practitioner may find it helpful to read the full judgment and weigh it against the practical experience of co-operation between clinicians and parents obviating the necessity for highly stressful and expensive court proceedings.

---

288 Dr J.M. Revuelta, Chief of the Cardiovascular Surgery Section of the *Marques de Valdecilla* University Hospital Santander, Spain; Letter to Branch Office of Jehovah's Witnesses, Spain November 23 2007

289 Federal Tribunal, Switzerland

290 *Glass v United Kingdom* [2004] 1 FLR 1019; ECtHR No. 61827/00, 9.3.04

18.34 To round out this consideration of the European perspective, the European Court of Human Rights on 10 June 2010 gave a landmark judgment in a case[291] from Russia. An alliance between the Russian Orthodox Church and an anti-cult body, both virulently hostile to Jehovah's Witnesses, had prevailed upon a sympathetic prosecutor to bring a civil action to liquidate the legal entity that represented that faith in Moscow. The prosecutor, in opening the case, made the remarkable admission that she had no facts upon which to base the claim and that no less than 5 criminal investigations had turned up no evidence of illegal activity. Nevertheless that did not prevent her making wide assertions of conduct supposedly breaching the Charter and justifying the draconian penalty of liquidation, some of which impinged on Jehovah's Witnesses' refusal of donor blood and choice of alternative clinical management. The case proceeded entirely upon an examination of the faith's Scriptural beliefs and literature and degenerated into an old-fashioned heresy trial. After a formidable 116 days in the domestic courts including trial, appeal and retrial, the order was made and so the aggrieved victims took their case to Strasbourg.

18.35 The judgment should be required reading for any involved in Human Rights as the Court went through allegation by allegation refuting each one. In the context of the issue of choice of non-blood management the prosecutor had made the absurd allegation that Jehovah's Witnesses 'incite their members to commit suicide by refusing medical treatment'. The Court dealt with this allegation in robust terms that it would be mere repetition to summarise. The relevant section is at paragraphs 131 to 146 and is felt to be of sufficient importance for it to be set out in full as an Appendix to this work.

18.36 As a matter of Convention law, this judgment is binding on Russia only. But the other 46 High Contracting States have by the Convention entered into treaty obligation 'to take account of' the Court's jurisprudence' so this case is likely to be cited in many cases yet to come. Finally, it is notable that in the context of European Law the European Court has cited with approval both the Canadian case of *Malette v Shulman* and *re T* from the UK.

18.37 As a post script and to show that Europe is very much in line with international thinking and practice, the experience of Australia and China is instructive.

---

[291] *Moscow Community of Jehovah's Witnesses v Russia* No. 302/02

Australia

18.38 As far back as 1957 in Australia a Director of a major Blood Transfusion Service wrote his own warning on blood transfusion:[292]

> 'In Australia the majority of blood transfusions are administered in public hospitals by recent graduates in medicine. On such doctors rests the responsibility for the judicious use of human blood, a task which should not be lightly undertaken.
>
> Resident medical officers soon discover that blood is available for the asking and, perhaps, are inclined to use it without due regard for those who give this blood voluntarily, without proper consideration of the indications for its use and sometimes as a placebo for anxious relatives. Having mastered the satisfying technique of transfusion, it is only natural that some should desire to use the technique as often as possible. These are serious charges, but they are not without foundation. Incompatible and even fatal transfusions have frequently occurred in patients who have not required the transfusions.
>
> The injection of infected blood usually produces profound protein shock followed by septicaemia if death does not occur in the early stages. It is not possible to detect infection from the appearance of the blood. A number of other diseases have allegedly been transmitted by blood transfusions but syphilis and malaria are the only two of importance'.

In Australia the concept of freedom and choice is highly valued and led to the establishment of 'bloodless medicine' at an earlier stage than many other countries. The famous Kaleeya Hospital in Freemantle, Western Australia, has pioneered bloodless surgery for many years. Now the arrangement has been put on a more formal basis with the Government of Western Australia Department of Health becoming, it is claimed, the first in the world to adopt 'bloodless surgery'.

A report[293] in the recognised State newspaper said as follows:

> 'The WA health system will become the first in the world to adopt a "bloodless surgery" policy that could significantly reduce the use of blood transfusions and save the State tens of millions of dollars. The pioneering approach, known as patient blood management, is used at Freemantle Hospital—reducing its use of

[292] Dr R J Walsh, Director of New South Wales Blood Transfusion Service: Sydney University Medical Journal Vol 147, 1957

[293] *The West Australian*, April 2 2011

blood—and will be rolled out across all hospitals. Experts say it is safer for patients and will help avoid a looming shortage of blood as more people have cancer and orthopaedic surgery.

Under the program, patients going into hospital for surgery will have a blood test several weeks before to check if they need therapy such as iron supplements to treat anaemia. Doctors will also be encouraged to use surgical techniques that minimise blood loss.

Chief medical officer Simon Towler there was good evidence the new approach was safer for patients and led to faster recovery and shorter stays in hospital. He said the use of blood products in Australia was a billion dollar industry, with a unit of blood costing about $700.

Transfusions would still be there if needed, but when there was a safer alternative it should be used, Dr Towler said. "We're the first jurisdiction in the world to take this on as a system-wide program and we're going to set a challenge for the world," he said. "We're confident this approach will work, will be better for patients and could save tens of millions of dollars for WA Health."

Dr Towler said the need for blood would rise with the population ageing and the 50 per cent rise in demand for cancer services over the next decade. The biggest users of blood products in hospital were people aged 70 and over and more were having surgery.

"Unless we get better at how we use blood, we could get into supply problems down the track," he said. "We're doing this to make the best use of the blood we have."

The program would encourage GPs referring patients for surgery to check blood counts well ahead of time, he said.

Australian Red Cross Blood Service transfusion medicine specialist Lynn Aston said Australia had one of the safest blood supplies in the world but it was not risk-free, nor was the practice of people using their own pre-collected blood. "We will always need donors but demand keeps increasing and our rationale is that we should be giving blood to people who need it but if there are safer alternatives we should be using them," Dr Aston said'.

18.39 In October 2011 the Alfred Hospital in Melbourne pulled off what was claimed as a remarkable 'first' in non-blood management. A 33-year-old woman involved in a severe car accident sustained major injuries including an almost severed spinal cord, collapsed lungs, fractured skull, fractures to the ribs, cheekbone and elbow and a ruptured spleen. Not surprisingly these extensive injuries had caused major blood loss but as one of Jehovah's Witnesses transfusion of allogeneic blood was not an option. Researchers have for years been working to find a viable synthetic blood. The hospital turned to the US Navy who, with exceptional cooperation from all involved including the manufacturer, border inspection agencies, an ethics committee and the airline carrier flew in 10 units of the synthetic bovine-derived product HBOC-201.

With remarkable generosity the drug manufacturer stood the main costs involved. The infusion almost immediately raised the patient's level of haemoglobin and probably prevented imminent heart failure. Although in a coma for a week after the transfusion of this product she has since made a remarkable recovery.

China/Asia

18.40 China faces similar problems in trying to ensure safe transfusions and non-blood management is rapidly becoming Government policy. A change in the law, effective 1st August 2012, is designed by the Ministry of Health to spell out best practice and to put blood conservation and non-blood management on a legal footing. Hospitals graded AAA and AA will be monitored as they implement patient blood management in accordance with Article 23:[294]

> 'Article 23
>
> Clinical institutions should vigorously develop their blood conservation technique, develop auto transfusion, from pre-operative to post-operative blood conservation management system, apply the suitable measures to patients who satisfy the appropriate techniques and make the practical outcome part of the evaluation criteria for the department'.

18.41 Significant advances have been made in patient blood management.

Dr Shander of the prestigious Englewood Hospital in New Jersey is acknowledged to be one of the world's leading experts. In November 2015 he conducted a lecture tour that took in the Philippines and then China.

The Philippine Society of Anesthesiologists hosted a seminar in Manila attended by about 40 key health-care experts at which Dr Shander gave a

---

294 www.moh.gov.cn

presentation on PBM. A report of the open forum that followed it was of 'a lively discussion that ran for an hour and a half'.

18.42 Dr Shander then moved on to China where he gave a series of presentations in the cities of Beijing, Shanghai and Xiamen. He shone the spotlight on the evidence supporting the management of anaemia without blood but by reducing phlebotomy (iatrogenic anaemia). Also on cell salvage; ESA; iron and other nutrients. His focus was on innovative solutions to the systemic risks of allogeneic blood transfusions.

All major hospitals within the Beijing City radius were notified and urged to send representatives to his presentation at the Beijing Red Cross Blood Center. As a result, the auditorium was filled to seating capacity and with others standing.

18.43 Next was a meeting with anaesthesiologists at Peking Medical College Hospital, one of the country's leading hospitals. During his presentation, a department head commented 'You are fortunate to have been able to gain experience caring for Jehovah's Witnesses'.

The following day he addressed another full auditorium of surgeons and anaesthetists at Fu Wai Hospital, National Center for Cardiovascular Diseases. They have been actively promoting PBM and in the last five years have reduced red cell transfusions by over 50%.

18.44 A successful tie-up between the Clinical Transfusion Committee of the Shanghai Medical Association and Zhongshan Fudan University Hospital ensured a large audience of health experts and local authorities were on hand to hear his presentation 'New Paradigm in Patient Blood Management'. As a keynote speaker at their annual meeting Dr Shander commended over 1,300 health experts at the Chinese Society of Cardiothoracic and Vascular Anaesthesiology for placing PBM at the top of their priority list.

18.45 In summary, in recent years there has been a surge of interest in PBM demonstrated by the establishing of the China Blood Management Association and the ongoing drafting of a national PBM Protocol.

Chapter Nineteen

Artificial Oxygen Carriers—The Experience with Perftoran® /Vidaphor

19.1 An interesting divergence of approach has emerged between the more prosperous West and the cost-restricted Russia. In the West, non-blood products have been directed principally to the 3 stages of treatment namely:

- achieving haemostasis as quickly as possible e.g. *Novoseven*®;
- immediate volume replacement; and
- agents to replace the lost iron and to stimulate naturally erythropoiesis to replace the lost Hb e.g. r-HuEPO and *Venofer*®/*Ferinject*®

Russia, on the other hand, has pursued the development of non-blood oxygen carrying substances.

19.2 The primary factors have undoubtedly been cost driven. The research and development costs of the major pharmaceutical companies worldwide are phenomenal. But they are commercial companies operating in an environment where a patent has only a limited life. Once the patent has expired, then commercial competitors can replicate and market the product at considerable profit but without having incurred the huge initial outlay in R&D that led to the original discovery. In addition to the R&D costs and those of the patenting process, the modern testing and safety procedures to secure approval for the use of the product from the appropriate licensing authority and the necessary Product Licence are themselves onerous and can run to hundreds of thousands of euros or dollars. The original discovering company has to make a commercial return, both to recoup the original investment and to satisfy its shareholders. The almost inevitable consequence is that when a newly patented product first comes to market, the price at which it is made available reflects that urgency to recoup the outlay and maximise profit before the patent protection expires.

19.3 One of the simplest examples is the haemostatic agent Factor VIIa marketed as *Novoseven*®. The original research was directed to treatment for those haemophiliacs who were especially deficient in this vital clotting factor. A Product Licence was issued for this narrow avenue of treatment but as its efficacy was proved, the 'off-licence' applications expanded rapidly. A remarkable case history [4.36] was presented at one of the NATA conferences by the chief trauma surgeon at the major unit in Jerusalem involving an Israeli soldier. The medical community worldwide monitors new developments such as this and it has not taken long for the (still off-licence) use to extend to a wide range of specialities where major blood loss is encountered, including obstetrics and postpartum haemorrhage. Although perhaps not as dramatic as the case of the Israeli soldier, the original uses of r-HuEPO and Iron in renal patients have been similarly extended although the cost of each course of treatment has now come down to a more realistically affordable level.

19.4 Despite their obvious life-saving benefits to patients, none of these products has achieved the ultimate goal of the pharmaceutical industry which is 'artificial blood'. And the cost factor has undoubtedly driven Russia to seek to develop a low-cost alternative approach that will minimise recourse to these Western products that are too expensive for a cash limited state medical service.

19.5 The real starting point for an artificial oxygen carrier came in 1989 with the discovery by the Green Cross Corporation of Osaka, Japan of a perflurocarbon substance patented as *Fluosol*®. It was hailed at the time as a major breakthrough but given a limited FDA licence initially for coronary balloon angioplasty. There was no doubting its oxygen carrying capabilities and indeed the marketing material included a graphic display of a live mouse totally immersed in the liquid and still breathing. The product had the obvious advantages of eliminating certain major problems with donor blood, especially mismatch and transmission of viral and bacterial infections. However as experience of its use in practice extended, some shortcomings became increasingly apparent. One was the half-life *in vivo,* which was in reality down to about a mere 2 hours. This meant that repeat infusions were necessary, pushing the patient potentially into fluid overload. All involved in critical care following major blood loss know that evaluating the actual loss and thus the appropriate amount of volume to replace is an inexact science. The skill is to replace sufficient fluid but not to overload the patient.

19.6 The second risk area was the emergence of a statistically significant risk of (*inter alia*) stroke. Thirdly, the product had a low PFC content (20% volume) and fourthly it involved a labour intensive preparation. In essence, whilst the oxygen carrying capacity of perfluorocarbons was established as a principle, the reality was that *Fluosol*®, the first generation product, was not the complete package and its use was discontinued in 1994. Nonetheless, the research was far from wasted but the development of the process diverged.

The Basics

19.7 To understand just how far Russia has come with the development of *Perftoran*® as a synthetic blood product, it is helpful to understand some of the basics about perfluorocarbon emulsions (PFCE). Due to their inability to remain mixed with aqueous solutions, liquid perfluorocarbons must be prepared as emulsions in water and salt before being used in patients. The PFCE particles are spherical, averaging about 0.2 microns in diameter with a perfluorocarbon core and a thin egg yolk phospholipids surfactant as a coating. The small diameter is a major factor in increased tissue perfusion. In the production, PFCE molecules are mixed with water, salts and the surfactant via high pressure homogenisation, and sterilised with high pressure steam. The entire process takes 12-14 hours with close to 100% yield of product and can be achieved on a large scale at no great cost. By comparison, the generally accepted loss in blood collection, testing, storage and distribution is 7%.

19.8 Some of the advantages are immediately apparent:

- due to the synthetic nature of the product it has a shelf life of 2 years;
- it minimises the risk of infection or immunologic reaction resulting from a transfusion of donor blood (mismatched blood type, mismatched Rh factor, transmission of HIV and hepatitis B);
- oxygen delivery is markedly enhanced. PFCE's dissolve oxygen (unlike haemoglobin which binds the molecule) which allows them to:
    i) load/unload oxygen twice as fast as haemoglobin;
    ii) extract 90% of the transported oxygen; and
    iii) deliver the amount of oxygen of 1-2 units of red blood cells in one unit of PFCE (100-110 ml);
- over about 4-12 hours after infusion, the PCFE particles are removed from the circulation via normal respiration by simple evaporation in the lungs;
- the reduced diameter of the particles at 0.2 microns means that oxygen transport is facilitated into the narrower tissue spaces. The PFCE particles travel in the plasma near the vessel walls and between RBC's. The largest gaps between RBC's exist in the microcirculation

and as a result PFCE's provide the most benefit to smaller vessels. Also, where there are local areas of vasoconstriction or blockages of the vessels, some plasma can still pass through and deliver PFCE's/oxygen to the tissues.

19.9 In summary, *Perftoran*®, registered in 1996, is an improved first generation PFCE building on the experience of *Fluosol*® and taking it to a new level in both oxygen transport and cost efficient large scale production. The result is that it has become the substitute of choice for oxygen carrying in non-blood clinical management in Russia. The practicalities of its progressive use have been amply demonstrated. The serious researcher will find literally scores of citations in professional and peer-reviewed literature in Russia on the excellent *Perftoran*® website www.perftoran.ru (bi-lingual in Russian and English). A key article giving a very good overview '*Perftoran:* Plasma Substitute with Oxygen Transporting Function' was published in a respected medical journal and has been translated into English.[295]

19.10 There have been several catastrophic explosions and fires in coal mines in Kuzbass, South Western Siberia. This is one of the largest coal fields in the world, over 27,000 square miles; 200 miles of underground tunnels and produces more than 30% of Russia's coal. One explosion of methane combined with coal dust caused grave thermal injury with 35 killed; but there were survivors and they were successfully treated with *Perftoran*®. Professor Slepushkin was one of those in the forefront of the treating team. At the Proceedings of the Russian Scientific Conference at St Petersburg in 2004 several papers were presented and subsequently published in the *Collection of Proceedings*. The papers were variously titled but included:

- 'The first results of the use of *Perftoran* in intensive care of miners having a grave combined injury due to explosions in Kuzbass coal mines';
- '*Perftoran* as a new standard for anti-shock treatment of grave combined injuries due to explosions in coal mines'; and
- 'New aspects of intensive care of a grave thermal injury in its acute period'.

---

[295] A.M. Golubev, Translated from Byulleten '*Eksperimental'noi Biologii Meditsiny* Vol 124 No. 5 pp. 484-492, May 1998

19.11 In addition to these specific experiences, on the *Perftoran®* website under the heading 'Clinical Application/Surgery, traumatology' there are numerous published papers demonstrating its application in a wide range of treatments that include:

- acute lung injury syndrome;
- peritonitis;
- burn shock;
- cardiac surgery;
- severe trauma and blood loss;
- traumatic injury of the spinal cord;
- thermotoxic injury;
- cardio resuscitation;
- elderly patients undergoing abdominal operations;
- thermal injury during military operations in Chechen Republic;
- treatment of open fractures;
- grave craniocerebral injury;
- maxillofacial surgery; and
- oncology microsurgery.

19.12 The author recounts one example from his own professional experience in Russia. In 2004 Mrs T.V. Salnikova was an innocent pedestrian when two cars collided very close to her. One bounced off the other and careered off the road, striking her lower body and causing multiple injuries. She carried an Advance Medical Directive accepting all non-blood management but excluding consent to any allogeneic blood or blood products. At the trauma unit, the treating team respected her choice of treatment and she underwent an emergency amputation of a lower limb. Her Hb fell to 3g/dl but with good quality critical care she survived. *Perftoran®* was deployed with r-HuEPO and other adjunctive therapies and slowly her Hb climbed back to 4.8g/dl. However she had also suffered other serious organ damage that, on any conventional statistical view, significantly reduced her chances of survival even had she been prepared to accept donor blood. Infection and sepsis set in, complicating her underlying diabetes, and although she survived for some 22 days in all, she finally succumbed to the combination of multi-organ injury and failure brought about largely by infection.

19.13 A criminal investigation into the 2 drivers, with a view to prosecuting either or both for causing the death by dangerous driving, attributed her death solely to the injuries sustained in the impact with the car that hit her, but there was insufficient evidence to prosecute and the investigation was formally closed. Under Russian law that finding of cause of death was conclusive and it gave rise to an *estoppel* against the prosecutor alleging a different cause of death.

19.14 However, 5 years later a local prosecutor, on instructions from the Prosecutor General, brought proceedings against the Local Registered Organisation (Congregation) of Jehovah's Witnesses in Taganrog of which the deceased had been a member.[296] One amongst many bizarre allegations was that the religious literature (published and accepted worldwide) 'incited' members to commit suicide by refusing medical treatment and that Mrs Salnikova was a victim of such incitement. Professor Slepushkin, having reviewed the clinical notes, gave robust evidence as an expert witness for the defendant LRO.

19.15 His primary conclusion was that the patient had been correctly and skilfully managed without blood. Because of her multi-organ injuries, the prognosis was not good and he cited a recognised professional article that put the probability of mortality as high as 86%.[297] Once sepsis set in, the patient was, for all practical purposes, a non-survivor. However, he went further in his analysis of her condition in that, in his considered professional opinion, blood was actually contra-indicated. An exchange between him and the prosecutor cross examining made his conclusions absolutely clear:

> '**Prosecutor**: So a transfusion would not have saved her in any case?
>
> **Witness V.D. Slepushkin**: No, I think that she would have died sooner if she had had a blood transfusion.' [Cassation Appeal, paragraph 473]

19.16 In addition, the professor dealt with a number of issues bearing on blood transfusion and the benefits of a conservative strategy and non-blood clinical management:

---

296 *Prosecutor of Rostov Region v Taganrog Local Registered Organisation of Jehovah's Witnesses*, Rostov Regional Court and Supreme Court of the Russian Federation Judgment 8 December 2009

297 *Sepsis—Monograph:* V.V. Moroz with co-author. Petrozavodsk: Intel Tek, 2004

- Of the patients who choose medical treatment without blood transfusions, only 11.5% do so for religious reasons.
- In a medical study of 5,000 persons seriously wounded in the Chechen conflict, the mortality rate of those receiving blood transfusion was 34.6% while the mortality rate of those who did not receive blood transfusions was 31.8%. [Cassation Appeal,[298] paragraph 474]
- Alternatives to blood transfusions, including *Perftoran,* are widely available in all hospitals in the Russian Federation.
- In the last 15 years, there has been a sharp decline in the use of blood transfusions by clinicians in the Russian Federation and worldwide.

19.17 The professor further cited a number of additional professional articles supporting non-blood management.[299,300,301,302]

> 'Mortality during multiple organ failure, independent of whether blood components are transfused or not, is up to 70% and that without septic complication; during multi organ failure affecting three or more organs lethality is 96-98%.'

In addition he cited one of his own published papers.[303] Faced with this overwhelming and independent expert evidence the court had no realistic alternative but to acquit.

The Prosecutor's case against the congregation in Taganrog is still ongoing.

19.18 On the wider issue of the right of the patient to choose non-blood management under the Russian system, a conclusion from the Perm Heart Institute, dated July 17, 2009, No. 0105/464 notes:

> 'Concerning representatives of the Religious Organisation Jehovah's Witnesses. According to their religious teachings the internal use (transfusion) of medicines of non-human biological (animal) origin (donor blood and blood products are not allowed. In this case, doctors do not have the right to the final decision, since by

---

298 *Prosecutor of Rostov v Taganrog LRO,* op *cit*

299 Research and Practice Conference Papers V.V.Chalenko, I.V.Andozhskaya, A.A. Redko et al

300 Optimising the delivery of intensive care to wounded and ill civilians in a local military conflict, Doctoral dissertation of D.D. Adayev

301 Intensive care for multi-organ failure among surgical patients, A.P. Geigorenko et al Belgorod State University

302 Sepsis at the beginning of the 21st century: Classification, Clinical-Diagnostic Concept and Treatment—Russian Association of Specialists in Surgical Infections ('RASSI')

303 A comparative study of patients with massive blood loss, Receiving and Not Receiving Hemotransfusion (V.D. Slepushkin, D.P. Doev)

law they are not authorized to decide matters of a religious nature. We find comparable contradictions with representatives of other confessions (Judaism, Islam, and Buddhism regarding organ transplants, etc.). A significant amount of positive experience has been gained at the Perm Heart Institute in bloodless surgery including surgeries performed on representatives of the religious organization of Jehovah's Witnesses'.

The Western development of oxygen carriers

19.19 By contrast, whilst Russia has vigorously promoted research and production of *Perftoran*® as an improved first generation, most pharmaceutical companies in the West have diverged and pursued second generation perflurocarbons. They include *Oxygent*® and *Oxycyte*® both of which are still undergoing the trial processes in the US and the European Agency for the Evaluation of Medical Products but the author is not aware of any comparison evaluations with *Perftoran*®. However for further scientific reading, the excellent *Perftoran*® website,[304] mentioned above, provides considerable detail.

19.20 As far back as 1996 a far-sighted Russian registered in London a company aptly named *Perftoran West Limited.* Significantly it held the patent, licensing rights and intellectual property for *Perftoran*®. In December 2014 those rights were then acquired by a newly formed US company named Fluor0^2 Therapeutics Inc. registered in Delaware but based in Boca Raton, Florida.

19.21 This company has rebranded this product as *Vidaphor* which is a derivative from the words meaning 'life-bearing'. In its promotional material seeking capital investment it firstly claims experience of use in 30,000 patients 'with good results and few side effects'. It then estimated having product sales 12 to 14 months after receipt of funding. Its primary perceived market is Mexico which is said to be 'short an estimated 2.4 million units of blood every year and desperately needs a blood substitute'. The company then plans to expand into Latin America focusing on countries that have mutual recognition agreements with Mexico. Future plans also include initiating studies needed to obtain licensing approval in the US.

19.22 There is clearly some way to go with both the necessary patent and licensing applications in the US and with funding but it does seem that the

---

304 *www.perftoran.ru/Eng*

availability of *Vidaphor*, at least in Mexico and Latin America, is closer to becoming a reality.

19.23 *Perftoran*® was formerly licensed for use in Russia, Ukraine, Kazakhstan and, between 2005 and 2010, Mexico. However it would seem likely that it will be sooner rather than later that it is granted approval for use in the West as it appears to be successfully fulfilling its function as an artificial oxygen carrier and a major tool in conservative transfusion strategies and non-blood management. Its major advantage seems to be the reduced diameter of the particles enabling tissue perfusion of oxygen into the narrower tissue spaces.

19.24 A recent online search of www.fluro2therapeutics.com reveals that the application for a US trademark for *Vidaphor* appears to have lapsed in May 2016 and the inference is that the product is no longer being marketed in the US. However the company says that it will now be manufacturing at 'GMP compliant facilities in collaboration with Bioserv Corporation in San Diego and marketed primarily in Mexico'. The website reports that the 'path to FDA approval is expected to be a very brief one'.

19.25 The following chapter looks at the US and the development of the haemoglobin based oxygen carrier HBOC-201.

Chapter Twenty

The US Experience with HBOC-201

20.1 Whilst Russia was concentrating on developing *Perftoran*® as an artificial oxygen carrier, researchers in the US have gone a different route. They have primarily concentrated on a haemoglobin based oxygen carrier derived from bovine haemoglobin. One of the leaders in this line of research has been the Division of Hematology-Oncology at the Massachusetts General Hospital in Boston.

20.2 They clearly take very seriously not only the care of patients but also the emotional impact on caring staff when a patient chooses not to accept a treatment regime that they believe could save life. Such a situation arose in 2002 for a 50-year-old patient who was a qualified nurse and one of Jehovah's Witnesses. She had successfully undergone treatment for node positive breast cancer from which she appeared to have recovered but was then diagnosed with Acute Monocytic Leukaemia (AML). She recognised that this was an aggressive form of leukaemia and she wanted aggressive treatment that did not include whole blood. She signed an explicit Advance Directive excluding blood and the treating team agreed to accept her on that basis. Although she bravely fought her illness, with the treating team trying what they could within the limitation imposed upon them, she finally succumbed.

20.3 The hospital held what could be described as a de-briefing session, the objective of which included firstly lessons to be learned from a clinical perspective. Secondly it was to provide a therapeutic release to those who had cared for her, especially the nurses who had been close to her and were particularly affected by her death. The discussion was led by a facilitator and those who took part included medical professionals such as an oncologist and a palliative care physician with both general and intensive care nursing staff. Others who contributed included the hospital chaplain. The discussion features in an article that includes 32 references, published in *The Oncologist,* entitled 'Faith, Identity and Leukaemia: When blood products are not an option'.[305] The

[305] *The Oncologist* 2002; 7 pp. 371-380

whole article is a recommended read for those interested in exploring this topic further as it examines a range of related medical, legal and ethical issues.

20.4 There is, however, one area of interest in the context of non-blood management. In the section 'Ethical Controversies' under the sub-heading 'Bovine Hemoglobin', the history of the development of its use is reviewed. Initially there were concerns about anaphylactic shock, renal toxicity and hypertension. Yet, ultrafiltration and purification techniques have significantly decreased such side effects leading to human transfusion. One of the leaders in the development of bovine haemoglobin is *Hemopure®* of which it is claimed:

> 'Has increased capacity for both oxygen uptake in the lungs and oxygen delivery in the tissues. While the administration of bovine hemoglobin has been shown to increase the concentration of methemoglobin, hemoglobin's inactive form, in peripheral blood, it does not appear to significantly alter haematocrit levels or platelet counts'.

20.5 Nevertheless, there is one disturbing comment in the article:

> 'However, there is some question as to whether or not animal-derived products derived from bovine haemoglobin are safe from a public health standpoint. Concerns have been raised about whether animal-derived blood products could potentially lead to human infection by prions. While there have been no firm reports of this type of contamination, more research is needed to determine the potential risk of such transmissions'.

This chimes a US warning not dissimilar to that in the UK where, as has already been noted, the risk of prion infection leading potentially to vCJD is such that a formidable sum of £2,000,000 *per annum* has been set aside for research into just such contamination of the UK blood supply.

20.6 Two years later in 2004 the *Journal of Trauma Injury, Infection and Critical Care* published an article[306] in which HBOC-201 was compared with Hetastarch (HEX) in an uncontrolled liver injury haemorrhagic shock swine model with delayed evacuation. The 11 page article is replete with data but the conclusions find that hypotensive resuscitation with HBOC-201 was superior to HEX and no fluid resuscitation. The article concludes, perhaps optimistically, that 'these data are likely to be replicable in human patients with HS...'

---

[306] *Journal of Trauma Injury, Infection and Critical Care*, Vol 57 No. 4 pp. 726—737

20.7 By 2008, research had advanced to the point where an article could be headed 'HBOC-201: A viable alternative to blood transfusion'. Commenting on the results of a randomised, single blind, controlled multinational study, the author concluded:

> 'HBOC-201 does not require cross matching and can be stored at room temperature for as long as 3 years. In this study its use eliminated the need for transfusion of allogeneic PRBC's in 59% of patients. Its safety profile was inferior to that of PRBC transfusion, including a greater incidence of acute coronary syndromes and strokes which the authors partially attributed to age older than 80, volume overload and under treatment…'.

In passing, the article comments that the product is approved in South Africa for clinical use.

20.8 By 2010, research had further advanced as reported in an article entitled 'When blood is not an option: factors affecting survival after the use of a haemoglobin-based oxygen carrier in 54 patients with life threatening anaemia', was published by clinicians at the Department of Anesthesiology at the University of Maryland, Baltimore. The results concluded that no serious event was attributed to HBOC-201.

20.9 In October 2011 there had occurred the incident involving the 33-year-old woman in Melbourne, Australia who had sustained life-threatening injuries in a car accident, previously referred to in chapter 18. With a fine level of co-operation by all involved, manufacturer, border inspection agencies, an ethics committee and the airline carrier; 10 units of HBOC-201 from the US Navy were flown to the patient in Melbourne. She made a remarkable recovery.

20.10 What will be interesting is to see in due course a full, controlled study of the effectiveness of HBOC-201 in comparison with *Perftoran*® and whether the concerns over the prion in bovine haemoglobin and thus the potential for transmission of vCJD materialise. Until the professionals conclude their research and produce a definitive report, the layman has to make his own assessment of the risks and benefits. Given that the risk of bovine-sourced infection in *Perftoran*® is zero and that of HBOC-201 is known to exist but is still unidentified and unquantifiable, the risk/benefit in the meantime seems to come down firmly on the side of *Perftoran*®.

20.11 A PubMed search reveals little in the way of published material since 2009. In October 2014 an article was published in *Anesthesia & Analgesia Journal*[307] the authors having as diverse backgrounds as Belgium, Johannesburg, Massachusetts and Hamburg. It is entitled, 'A safety and efficacy evaluation of hemoglobin-based oxygen carrier HBOC-201 in a randomized, multicenter red blood cell controlled trial in noncardiac surgery patients'. Unfortunately although published in 2014 the article presents the results of a previously unpublished study conducted in 1998-1999 and so adds little to current writings. It does however confirm that as far back as 23 years ago, 'there were no notable differences in mortality and serious adverse events'.

[307] Anesth Analg. 2014 Oct; 119(4) 766-76

Chapter Twenty One

Namibia and South Africa

Historical Background

21.1 The detailed history of Namibia that led to the present legal system is a topic probably more suitable for historians and experts in constitutional law in sub-Saharan Africa. But a brief explanation of the main issues may lead to better understanding of the background to the events and litigation recounted in this chapter.

21.2 After the long, bitter and vicious war between SWAPO/Angola (supported by Cuba) and South Africa finally came to an end, the former province of South Africa at last gained its independence in 1990 to become Namibia. The decision makers in the new regime and the population generally took a conscious decision to break away from many aspects of the past, and rejected some of its less attractive links with apartheid and with many things Afrikaans, Germanic, Dutch, Boer, and the like. Instead they selected English as the national language for its Constitution and, perhaps more importantly in the context of this chapter, as the basis of its legal system. Basically they embraced the English common law but with appropriate additions in legal statutes, procedures and practices adapted for local needs and customs. Strong links were nevertheless maintained with a South Africa that had, by then, rejected apartheid.

21.3 The Presiding Judge of the Supreme Court based in Windhoek read law at Cambridge University for 3 years and returned later to the UK for a post-graduate year at Warwick University, so the court is well anglicised and versed in the traditions and concepts of the common law. In that respect it probably has more in common with, for instance, Australia, Canada, and New Zealand than with the codified systems of law mainly applicable in Central African states or even the Romano-Dutch law that underlies the South African system.

Due to the comparatively limited work load of a nation with a fairly small population and demand that does not justify a Bench full time, the Supreme Court sits when necessary with appropriately experienced judges seconded from other jurisdictions, especially South Africa and, as appropriate, from its

Constitutional Court bench. Such seconded judges bring an added dimension and breadth of experience that rightly supports the undoubted authority that the court commands.

Informed Consent and HIV

21.4 Sadly Namibia is not immune from the HIV virus that has ravaged the population of so many African countries. In a not unreasonable attempt to contain the spread to new-born children, the government instituted a voluntary programme whereby pregnant mothers who were HIV positive were specifically offered birth by caesarean section. This was expressly so that, as an adjunct to and in the course of that procedure under general anaesthetic, effective and irreversible contraceptive measures could be taken surgically by bilateral tubal ligation (BTL) to prevent further infected pregnancies. These mothers were for the most part on highly active retroviral therapy (HAART). The programme was called the Prevention of Mother to Child Transmission and known by its initials as 'PMTCT'. It was an integral part of the process that such mothers were to be offered advance counselling by a community counsellor who works for the PMTCT clinic so that each mother was properly informed and clearly understood the permanence of what was proposed; any alternative methods of contraception; and the health benefits of sterilisation, before even admission for the delivery, and thus gave properly informed consent. The form for consent was specifically tailored to include a statement by the treating doctor 'that he or she has explained the procedure and related aspects of sterilisation to the patient'.

21.5 Almost inevitably in such a government funded programme there arose a resource problem; corners were cut; and the counselling was either non-existent or left to a very late stage in the pregnancy. Some mothers were either just about to go down to the delivery room or had actually progressed in labour to the point where the level of pain was such that medication had been administered and a caesarean section was being considered as a matter of urgency. Only then was the concurrent process of sterilisation discussed and often rather perfunctorily.

In addition to the language barrier, there was also a culture problem, especially with the husbands, with the premature sterilisation of some very young wives manifestly with years of potential (and indeed almost socially required) child bearing ahead of them. Additionally on investigation it emerged that, in many cases, the appropriate certificate of consultation and explanation to the patient had not been completed by the treating doctor and that in itself hung a major question mark over how thoroughly, if at all, the process of counselling had been followed. This raises an echo of the importance of the 'dialogue' to which the Supreme Court in the UK attached such importance in the leading case of *Montgomery* discussed earlier.

21.6 The upshot was that some young mothers had second thoughts after delivery and irreversible sterilisation by BTL in State hospitals. They took legal advice and actions for damages were brought against the State in the High Court[308] alleging non-consensual sterilisation based on a lack of counselling and understanding of the true implications that thereby vitiated any purported consent. Also wrongful discrimination against them, in breach of their human rights, as being HIV positive, although the court later rejected that part of the claim.

21.7 The real issue was whether the court would uphold patient autonomy. The court at first instance had to give careful consideration to (*inter alia*) the right of the patient to choose treatment options and to give genuinely and properly informed consent. A senior expert witness called on behalf of the patients gave evidence that:

> '...the circumstance under which to secure the consent of a patient in respect of a sterilisation procedure is when the patient is rational and not in pain, has time to consider it, time to discuss it with her partner and relatives and thereafter to come to a reasoned conclusion. It is not a decision to be undertaken under the duress of extreme pain'.

21.8 The plaintiffs invoked (*inter alia*) the decision in *Castell v de Greef*[309] wherein the court coined the phrase 'made a paradigm shift from medical paternalism to patient autonomy'. Perhaps more significantly the doctrine of informed consent was placed within the common law context:

> '...It is clearly for the patient to decide whether he or she wishes to undergo the operation, in the exercise of the patient's fundamental right to self-determination...

[308] *LM; MI; NH v The Government of the Republic*—High Court of Namibia 1603/2008 Hoff J, 30 July 2012

[309] *Castell v de Greef*, 1994 (4) SA 408 C

> It is, in principle, wholly irrelevant that her attitude is, in the eyes of the entire medical profession, grossly unreasonable, because her rights of bodily integrity and autonomous moral agency entitle her to refuse medical treatment'.

In the course of its judgment at first instance, the court ruled:

> 'It should be obvious that the required consent must be given freely and voluntarily and should not have been induced by fear, fraud or force. Such consent must also be clear and unequivocal'.

21.9 These matters then went on appeal to the Supreme Court. The appeal was heard in March 2014 and judgment in favour of the affected mothers delivered on 3 November 2014.[310] The court dismissed the State's appeal but in doing so made a number of references to the law of consent and the right of the patient to decide. At §96 *et seq* it cites with approval the *Ethical Guidelines for Health Professionals.* At §97 it states:

> 'The publication recognises the importance of the principles of informed consent and self-determination, stating that a health professional should "apply the principle of informed consent as an ongoing process" and that he or she should "honour patients'" rights to self-determination or to make their own informed choices, living their lives by their own beliefs, values and preferences'.

21.10 Later at §104 the court is critical of the evidence of one of the government's medical witnesses. Perhaps somewhat unwisely he had expressed the view that the doctor knew what was best for the patient. The criticism of the court was 'this attitude smacks of medical paternalism'. It approved the quote in *Castell v de Greef* of an unpublished doctoral thesis by Van Oosten concluding 'I respectfully endorse these observations'.

The Namibia law on informed consent is encapsulated in a single paragraph:

> 'However, by virtue of the application of the doctrine of informed consent, our law and the policies applicable to Namibian health professionals recognise that **the patient has the final say** in deciding whether or not she should undergo an elective medical procedure...There can be **no place in this day and age for medical paternalism** when it comes to the important moment of deciding whether or not to undergo a sterilisation procedure. The principles of individual autonomy and self-determination are the overriding principles towards which our jurisprudence should move in this area of the law'. [Emphasis added]

[310] *Government of Namibia v LM; MI; and NH.* Case No: SA/49/2012

The sequence in which these two cases were heard in the Supreme Court meant that *LM* was heard and argued in March 2014; the case of *ES* cited below was heard and argued on 31 October 2014; and then the judgment in *LM* was delivered in November 2014. Thus self-evidently the *LM* judgment was not available to have been cited at the time *ES* was argued.

The Case of *ES v AC*[311]

21.11 It was against this background that the case arose. *ES* was an intelligent, educated lady in her late thirties who held down a responsible professional job as a senior lecturer in a reputable academic institute. She was married with 2 children and pregnant with her third. She and her husband are of the Christian faith of Jehovah's Witnesses each with a strongly held belief in the Bible and the scriptural command (*inter alia*) to 'keep abstaining from…blood…'. This belief is described in the relevant Protocol[312] of the Royal College of Surgeons of England as a 'core value'. She had for many years carried a written Advance Directive, signed, dated and witnessed, expressing her personal wishes and choice of non-blood management. Also in the event of her being incapable of communicating her wishes personally, she appointed her husband as her Health Care Agent to give consent on her behalf in accordance with her known wishes.

During her uneventful pregnancy she was under the ante-natal care of her family doctor. As the time for delivery approached, she prepared for the expected admission and caesarean section by updating and validating her fresh Advance Directive which was signed and dated a mere few days before her admission. She was thereby relying on the 'paradigm shift…to patient autonomy'.

21.12 Somewhat surprisingly to those in other jurisdictions accustomed to the surgical procedure of a caesarean section being carried out by an obstetrician/gynaecologist fully qualified in surgery, her GP, the holder of a mere diploma, decided that he would perform the procedure himself. The baby was safely delivered and survived but, given that this was not her first caesarean, he ran into difficulties with adhesions of the placenta to the uterine

311 *ES v AC, Supreme Court of Namibia*. Case No: SA 57/2012 (anonymised in the interests of the minor children)

312 *Code of Practice for the Surgical Management of Jehovah's Witnesses*—The Royal College of Surgeons of England 2002

wall. In attempting separation he started a major haemorrhage. Only then did he seek the help of a fully qualified obstetrician who happened to be 'scrubbed' and immediately available for Theatre. With the benefit of hindsight she should have been brought in much earlier to perform the caesarean section with its almost inevitable consequences of haemorrhage.

She took over at a difficult stage with major blood loss having already occurred. By then she had to perform an emergency hysterectomy (conducted with great professional skill by her and the anaesthetist) by which time the patient had bled down to an Hb of a mere 3.4g d/l. The patient was transferred to Intensive Care where she was successfully stabilised, fluid replaced and managed without blood in accordance with her written expressed wishes and then transferred back to a post-natal ward.

21.13 Although there is peer-reviewed professional literature confirming survival at such levels (and lower),[313] other members of the family (who did not share the patient's religious convictions) decided, quite contrary to law, to take over control. An older fleshly brother, who is prominent in another religion bitterly opposed to Jehovah's Witnesses, flew in to Windhoek and ostensibly took charge and started directing things. He appears somehow to have secured the co-operation of the family doctor who had started the surgery but then had been forced to seek more surgically qualified help. Although legally represented, the GP and the patient's brother went secretly and *ex parte* before a High Court judge. The GP, in what seemed to be manifest breach of his professional duties both to comply with the instructions of his patient and to maintain medical confidentiality to his patient, voluntarily made both a witness statement and, without even a witness summons, gave evidence against his own patient.

21.14 Contrary to all legal precedent and procedural requirements, the judge was not informed of the full facts nor of the relevant law supporting the right of an adult patient to decide her treatment options and was thus persuaded to make the order for transfusion of allogeneic blood that the fleshly brother requested. The case is redolent with similarities to the well-established case in the UK of *S v St George's Hospital NHS Trust* referred to in greater detail earlier in this work.

[313] See especially §6.3-6.13 and article by Viele & Weiskopf (*supra)*

The duty on the applicant in an *ex parte* application is well established:

> 'It cannot be emphasised too strongly that at an urgent without notice hearing for ...any [other] form of interim injunction, there is a high duty to make full, fair and accurate disclosure of material information to the court and to draw the court's attention to significant factual, legal and procedural aspects of the case. It is the particular duty of the advocate to see that the correct legal procedures and forms are used; that a written skeleton argument and a properly drafted order are prepared by him personally and lodged with the court before the oral hearing; and that at the hearing the court's attention is drawn by him to unusual features of the evidence adduced, to the applicable law and to the formalities and procedure to be observed'.—*per* Mummery LJ. [314]

These procedural safeguards, designed to protect the interests of the absent Respondent and ensure fairness, appear to have been almost totally ignored.

21.15 When served with the *ex parte* order, the patient immediately instructed lawyers who applied urgently to the court for it to be discharged and an *inter partes* hearing was duly convened before the same judge with both sides represented by experienced counsel. Despite having clear evidence before him including the actual Advance Directive document, the judge, almost unbelievably, confirmed the earlier order for transfusion together with an unprecedented order for the unfortunate, resisting and opposing patient to pay the costs!

21.16 Significantly the private hospital to which the patient had been admitted and undergone the surgery took no part in the litigation, presumably because they, or more probably their lawyers, were satisfied on the law that the competent adult patient had properly exercised her undoubted legal right of choice of non-blood management as expressed in writing in her Advance Directive. But confronted with an order of a High Court judge (supposedly on the authorities of declaratory force only) that it would be lawful to give blood, it seems they felt constrained at least to attempt to do so.

However they had not reckoned on the strength of conviction of the patient. When they advanced on her with the blood bag, she ripped out the cannula through which they were intending to transfuse and then succeeded in locking herself in the bathroom from which she adamantly refused to emerge. Finally recognising the obvious strength of will and determination of the still unwell

[314] *Sidhu v Memory Corporation plc* [2001] 1 WLR 1443 CA

patient to resist the transfusion, the treating team abandoned the attempt and reverted to the non-blood alternatives to which she consented. The patient was thereafter successfully managed within her choice of treatments and, although her hospital stay was prolonged beyond that which she would have liked or chosen, was finally discharged home without having received blood.

21.17 Regrettably the judge's order was not, as it should have been on the relevant legal authorities, time limited nor did it contain any provision for application by the patient to the court to discharge it. The patient was thus left with no alternative in law but to appeal to the Supreme Court and that she duly did.

In granting leave and ruling that the application was not moot, the court ruled:

> 'The facts of this matter concern some of the most essential human rights likely to arise in litigation. They relate to the right to bodily autonomy, the right to freely practise one's religion, and the freedom from discrimination. The facts also relate to relationships within families and the extent to which familial obligations compromise, or should compromise, one's own individual freedom'.

21.18 The application drew together a range of common law authorities and text book citations together with appropriate Namibian-specific law and some relevant South African law. It considered each of the following:

i) the right to bodily integrity;
ii) the assessment of competence and capacity;
iii) the validity and extent of consent to medical treatment;
iv) the validity and enforcement of a clear and specific Advance Directive following the Canadian case of *Malette v Shulman;*
v) the misuse of the *ex parte* procedure to procure an order overriding the expressed choice of treatment;
vi) the need for properly independent expert evidence;
vii) the right of the patient to confidentiality;
viii) the right to choose non-blood management and the relevant risks and benefits thereof; and
ix) the right to due process of law.

21.19 It further considered Constitutional guarantees entrenched in the *Constitution of the Republic of Namibia*, in particular: the rights to Life (Article 6), Liberty (Article 7), Human Dignity (Article 8), Equality and Freedom from Discrimination (Article 10), Privacy (Article 13), and the Fundamental

Freedom to Practice and Manifest any Religion (Article 21(1)(c)). Also the various international treaties and human rights covenants to which Namibia is a signatory and which are thus incorporated into Namibian domestic law.

21.20 It also reviewed some substantive case law. More than 30 years previously in 1983, in the case of *Phillips v. De Klerk*[315] decided in the South African Supreme Court, the right of the patient to choose was upheld. The patient sustained serious injury in a motor vehicle accident. Although severely injured, he was conscious when admitted to the hospital and refused a blood transfusion. He continued to deteriorate and an urgent application to allow the blood transfusion was granted by the court at first instance. As in the case of this appellant, the blood transfusion was never administered as the patient recovered.

Later, the patient brought an application to the Supreme Court to set aside the earlier order. The application succeeded on the basis that the patient was *compos mentis* at the relevant time and that he was entitled to refuse the blood transfusion. The court ruled that the previous order was made erroneously and accordingly was set aside.

21.21 Commenting on this decision, *The Foundational Principles of South African Medical Law* states:

> 'Undoubtedly, the decision in the case of Phillips v. De Klerk is fully in accordance with the present constitutional principles of patient autonomy and the right to bodily integrity [...] In this regard Strauss correctly states, with reference to the proven facts, that in this case the patient, although seriously injured, was fully capable of expressing his will and of assessing the possible consequences of his refusal [...] and that there is no principle in our law whereby a court can overrule a patient's will in these circumstances'.[316]

21.22 In 1994 the principle of patient autonomy was further developed in *Castell v. de Greef*,[317] the principle being stated by the South African Supreme Court:

[315] *Phillips v. De Klerk* (1983), unreported, discussed in Carstens, P. and Pearmain, D. *Foundational Principles of South African Medical Law* (2007), p.921

[316] *Foundational Principles of South African Medical Law*, *ibid*, p.923, par.2

[317] *Castell v. de Greef* (1994) (4) SA 408 (C), 421C

'It is, in principle, wholly irrelevant that her attitude is, in the eyes of the entire medical profession, grossly unreasonable, because her rights of bodily integrity and autonomous moral agency entitle her to refuse medical treatment'.

21.23 The *Foundational Principles of South African Medical Law*[318] further notes:

'The ultimate decision to undergo (informed consent) or refuse (informed refusal) a medical intervention lies with the patient and not with the physician. This applies even if, from the point of view of the medical profession, a refusal may result in his or her death, and even if the medical profession takes the view that the disclosure of the risks and dangers in such circumstances is unnecessary or undesirable. In the absence of other grounds of justification, medical interventions without the patient's consent on the basis of the "patient's best interest" and the doctor-knows-best criteria constitute a violation of the patient's autonomy'.

21.24 Namibian law similarly recognizes the importance of personal autonomy and protects a person's right to self-determination in regard to his or her own body. In the landmark case of *LM and Others v. Government of the Republic of Namibia,*[319] the Namibian High Court refers with approval to *Castell v. De Greef* cited above:[320]

'Castell v. De Greef 1994 (4) SA 408 (C) is regarded as a leading judgment on the issue of informed consent wherein Ackermann J (as he then was) with Friedman JP and Farlam J concurring, **made a paradigm shift from medical paternalism to patient autonomy.** At 420A the doctrine of informed consent was placed within its common law context where the following appears: [Emphasis added]

It is clearly for the patient to decide whether he or she wishes to undergo the operation, in the exercise of the patient's fundamental right to self-determination'.

21.25 The court in *ES* also had to consider the circumstances in which it might be appropriate to consider appointing a third party to take, on behalf of the patient lacking competence, decisions about medical treatment. In *Cloete and Another v. Moeller and Another,*[321] the Namibian High Court held:

'In terms of the applicable authorities it would appear firstly that a curator to a person is not lightly appointed as "applications of this nature involve serious

[318] *Foundational Principles of South African Medical Law, supra,* pp.882, 883
[319] *LM v. Namibia, supra,* pp.6-7, par.10
[320] *Castell v. Greef supra*
[321] *Cloete and Another v. Moeller and Another* (2012) (A75/12) NAHC 140, par.21

encroachments on a person's liberty, and [...] the court should only make appointments when a real need for them has been shown"'.

It was submitted in the pleadings and in argument that a real and genuine need for the appointment of a curator must be shown in these kinds of applications. In the above quoted case, the real need had by contrast been shown by means of a medical report filed with the court by a specialist psychiatrist, whose views were shared by a general practitioner.[322]

21.26 After a day's hearing in October 2014, judgment was reserved and was delivered in June 2015. The court, by a majority, upheld the basic right of the competent patient to choose her management options and the right of bodily integrity. It also upheld the common law principle of the Canadian case of *Malette v Shulman* that a patient has the absolute right to express his or her wishes as to treatment options in writing in an Advance Directive and that such choices are binding on the treating team even if the patient subsequently loses capacity through, for example, supervening anaesthesia.

Despite extensive argument by the dissenting judge to the contrary, the court rejected the concept that the rights of surviving children to the life of the mother override the right of the mother to exercise her choice. In so doing it followed many similar common law jurisdictions in upholding the right of the mother. See the US cases below.[323]

Comparative Law

21.27 The timing coincides with the ruling in the UK Supreme Court in the case of *Montgomery*[324] that seems finally to lay to rest the controversy of whether medical paternalism rules or whether the law of ***informed*** consent applies in the jurisdiction of the UK (See chapter 9).

On the facts it was a sad obstetric case of mismanaged shoulder dystocia with the added element of alleged negligence in failure to perform a caesarean section in response to abnormalities indicated by cardiotocograph traces. The

---

322 *Cloete and Another v. Moeller, supra,* par.11

323 *Bezio v Dorsey, NY Ct of Appeals* 2013/65; *In re Dubreuil,* 629 Se 2d 819 (1993); *Norwood Hospital v Munoz* (1991) 564 NE 2d 1017 (Mass Sup Jud C); *President of Georgetown College Inc.* (1964) 331 F 2d 1000 and on re-hearing 331 F 2d 2010 (USCADCC); *Fosmire v Nicoleau* 75 NY 2d 218 (1990) at pp. 229-230; Wons v Public Health Trust of Dade County, 500 So 2d 679; Affirmed 541 So 2d (Fla)

324 *Montgomery v Lanarkshire Health Board* [2015] UKSC 11

main judgment is available on *www.bailii.org* and therefore not reviewed here in detail. It is given by the majority and, in conducting a fairly extensive (if historical) review of the development of the law on the duty of disclosure leading to valid and informed consent, runs to 34 pages and 106 paragraphs. However for the reader who prefers the short version, Lady Hale, with her usual crisp precision, concurs but in a judgment that occupies a mere 3 pages and 11 paragraphs to arrive at the same conclusion.

The leading judgment cites with approval not only *Birch*[325] in the UK but, at §70 onwards under the sub-heading 'Comparative Law', the well-known cases of *Reibl v Hughes*[326] in Canada and *Rogers v Whittaker*[327] in Australia and is worth a read for that alone.

21.28 It now seems that there is a consensus in the principal common law jurisdictions, including Australia, Canada, Hong Kong, the UK and now Namibia/South Africa that medical paternalism is consigned to the history books and patient autonomy is the governing law. Hopefully this *ES* Judgment will circulate around sub-Saharan Africa and its common law jurisdictions so that no other mother, or indeed patient, will again be subjected to anything similar to what this patient had to endure. It was a very near miss for indefensible assault by non-consensual medical treatment that would, if completed, have triggered a substantial and probably unanswerable claim in damages.

---

325 *Birch v UCH supra*

326 *Reibl v Hughes* (1980) 114 DLR (3d) 1

327 *Rogers v Whittaker* (1992) 175 CLR 479

Chapter Twenty Two

Expectations, Endpoints and Outcomes

22.1 Within the UK there are some hospitals, and some units within hospitals, that are excellent in having developed a Protocol to establish what precisely are their goals, cost effectiveness, and endpoints in treatment; and have in place procedures for monitoring and recording outcomes. But as a generality, the NHS is not good at this. Indeed, in some grossly overworked and often under-funded and under-staffed hospitals the best they can hope to achieve is to send the patient home promptly, still alive and free from MRSA or other hospital acquired infection and without a complaint against the Trust about sub-optimal care or, worse still, a claim for clinical negligence. For these hospital teams it is enough to move the apparently never ending production line of patients; treat and discharge so that endpoints and outcomes are almost an irrelevance.

22.2 So what is the gold standard? There are two basic criteria for measuring successful outcomes. One is science based and involves a series of objective tests where outcome is capable of fairly accurate measurement. The other is an assessment of improved quality of life which is inevitably more subjective and in which there is likely to be greater variation from patient to patient and condition to condition.

22.3 The simplest of the science based criteria is mortality/survival ranging from perioperative death to death in intensive care and then onwards to 30-day survival and thence to 60 days. Into this mix can be added various factors; such as the inability to walk 10 feet across a room without human assistance at, say, 60 days. The scientific criteria include:

- Distance walked in 6 minutes (6MWT);
- Score on the Borg Category Ratio 10 (CR 10);
- Scale for perception of effort;
- Maximal dominant hand strength; and
- Short Form 36 (SF-36) Quality of Life Assessment.

22.4. The Borg CR10 Scale is a Category Ratio Scale with values of 1 to 10 ranging from 0, nothing at all; 0.5 extremely weak (just noticeable) through to 10 extremely strong (almost maximal). By contrast the Rating of Perceived Exertion (RPE) is defined as the degree of heaviness and strain experienced in physical work as estimated according to a specific rating method. These scales are commonly used in exercise testing, training, rehabilitation and ergonomics.

22.5 The SF-36[328] was constructed to survey health status in the Medical Outcomes Study, in particular for use in clinical practice and research, health policy evaluations and general population surveys. It includes one multi-item scale that assesses 8 health concepts:

- limitation in physical activities because of health problems;
- limitations in social activities because of physical or emotional problems;
- limitations in usual role activities because of physical health problems;
- bodily pain;
- general mental health (psychological distress and well-being);
- limitations in usual role activities because of emotional problems;
- vitality (energy and fatigue); and
- general health problems.

The survey was constructed for self-administration by persons 14-years-of-age and older and for administration by a trained interviewer in person or by telephone. These science-based assessments clearly have a significant role in assessing outcomes.

22.6 One of the more complex measurements[329] used in the United States (The American College of Surgeons National Surgical Quality Improvement Project ACS-NSQIP database) that does not appear to be so extensively deployed in the UK includes composite morbidity consisting of the 7 serious individual morbidities. Serious organ morbidities include the following:

- wound complications (deep organ space surgical site infection, deep surgical wound infection and wound dehiscence);

---

[328] The MOS 36-item Short-Form Health Survey (SF-36). *Medical Care,* June 1992 Vol 30 No.6

[329] 'Surgical outcomes and transfusion of minimal amounts of blood in the operating room' Ferraris et al *Arch Surgery* Vol 147 No 1 49-55

- pulmonary complications including pneumonia, unplanned intubation, pulmonary embolism or deep venous thrombosis and mechanical ventilation for longer than 48 hours;
- renal complications including acute kidney injury or dialysis;
- central nervous system complications including new post-operative stroke or coma;
- cardiac complications including postoperative myocardial infarction or cardiac arrest;
- sepsis including postoperative septic shock or blood borne sepsis; and
- unplanned return to the operating room within 30 days of the initial procedure.

22.7 One starting point for the patient-based subjective assessment, although less scientific and simply as an example, is to look at orthopaedics and the frequently conducted procedures for treating hip fractures and hip replacements. The classic patient is probably aged late 60's to 70's and one or both hips have degenerated to the point where there is an undoubted need for surgical intervention, whether or not the condition has been brought to a crisis by a fall and consequent fracture. The symptoms and consequences are not life-threatening but they have a considerable impact on quality of life. The pain of bone grinding on bone is intermittent but when the hip 'goes out' it is excruciating. A walking stick becomes a fixture. The personal indignity of not being able to put on socks, tie shoelaces or even getting in and out of a bath unaided is considerable. The restriction on engaging in routine household tasks such as mowing the lawn is frustrating.

When travelling, it is impracticable to reach the gate at most airports without having to use the electric buggy provided by ground handling for the disabled and those with impaired mobility. The London Underground, designed for a different era, at times can present an obstacle course that is difficult to negotiate. When on holiday, accompanying family in a walk along the beach becomes no longer a pleasure but a burden. On a Saturday afternoon the walk from the rail station to the local football or rugby stadium becomes less of a pleasure and more of a trial. And even activities involving comparatively mild physical exertion such as golf, tennis or even swimming are relegated to mere spectator sports.

22.8 When the patient finally seeks treatment, often expectations are not high. Relief of the pain is a major priority and if the patient can walk and bend more freely that would be a bonus. One concern for an increasing number of patients is that they want the bloodless surgery that is increasingly available. The better surgeons and anaesthetists are content to take on 70-year-olds for a full hip or knee replacement procedure without blood transfusion, largely because each trusts the skills of their colleagues in their respective roles and the deployment of the extensive non-blood armoury now available. Most outcomes are uneventful, with a blood loss, for what is in many surgical units regarded as a high loss procedure, graphically described in lay terms as half a tea cup. The patient is mobilised early and discharged infection free on elbow crutches. But then the patient drops off the radar in the absence of a monitoring process designed to keep track of medium to long term outcomes. The typical experience is a rapid improvement and the elbow crutches soon discarded. The walking stick is no longer needed. The various restrictions on basic activities described above fall away and quality of life improves dramatically.

22.9 It was at the March 2011 NATA Conference in Dublin that this question of endpoints and outcomes was raised and discussed in quite an animated forum. It was conceded with remarkable frankness that most statistical recording concentrates on 30-day mortality. If the patient survived that long and was discharged alive and infection free, then the treatment was a success! In many cases of those whose movement had been seriously impaired, the standard assessment seems to be the '6 minute walking test'. Whilst undoubtedly representing one indicator of outcome, it does seem a somewhat primitive yardstick to assess the effectiveness of a major and costly hospital intervention. Rehabilitation, restoration of function, and improved quality of life should be capable of more precise measurement and provide realistic endpoints that are capable of being monitored.

22.10 One comment related to discharge of patients still manifestly anaemic—with an Hb at around 8g/dl, which is not at the transfusion threshold but is clearly sub-optimal. This is where the costing of hospital treatment as secondary care comes into conflict with costing in Primary Care Trusts. The treatment and welfare of the patient suggests that action needs to be taken to restore the Hb to an appropriate level. Oral iron may not be well tolerated and *Spatone*® although helping may not provide replacement iron in sufficient quantity or adequate timescale. But who is going to initiate and pay for intravenous iron therapy that would undoubtedly benefit such patients? This raises again the issue of *Venofer*® requiring day-patient administration in hospital compared with *Ferinject*® administered as part of the primary care function in the GP's surgery.

22.11 The lack of follow up for children is quite alarming. The references in chapter 15 include 21 case citations of court involvement and authorisation for treatment. Only 3 of these cases made it into the law reports. The rest left court and effectively vanished, with one notable exception where the judge took a personal interest and involvement in the case and followed through. As to the remainder, apart from the parents and the treating team, no one seems to have retained any interest in the child. In the case of *Baby H,* the repair of the heart defect was carried out successfully by an exceptionally skilled cardiac team. But when, 5 years later, the (probably) immune-suppressed boy contracted severe pneumonia that did not respond to top quality care and the best antibiotics, he was technically still a Ward of Court. However, no attempt was made to involve the court or the Official Solicitor and the treating team simply went ahead and did what they could. The death of a Ward in such circumstances seems to have passed unremarked. But the real significance is with the remaining 20 cases, in which, despite all the time and expense of procuring a court authorisation, no blood was in fact administered. All of that medical and legal experience was simply lost to judges, NHS Trust lawyers, and more especially treating teams and fellow professionals who might have benefited from the details. Regrettably the system is not geared to monitoring even medium term outcomes and endpoints.

22.12 In summary, the NHS is a multi-billion pound operation that seems to be sadly lacking in setting expectations, endpoints and outcomes, and there is considerable scope for improvement. The one area of consensus is that outcomes are significantly improved by giving attention to anaemia pre-operatively, intra-operatively and post-operatively. Naturally, in emergency situations there is unlikely to be time for any pre-operative measures to address the anaemic patient and the treating team have to take him as they find him and do the best they can. But in elective procedures, the simple logic is to send every patient down to theatre with as high a level of Hb as can reasonably be obtained. It has been clearly demonstrated that EPO and Iron treatment given a mere 3 weeks before surgery can have a dramatic effect on outcome. At last this issue is being addressed and for orthopaedic surgery at least there is now a firm recommendation for a pre-operative review at 28 days prior to admission precisely to pick up and treat any anaemia.

22.13 Perhaps the most glaring omission is the failure to have in place any mechanism for recording medium and long term outcomes to give a true comparison of the benefits of treatment with and without donor blood or blood products. The *Viele & Weiskopf* study of survival at Hb levels below 5g/dl was some 22 years ago, way back in 1994. Major advances have been made in managing such severe anaemia and there is a serious case for an update. As described in chapter 1.6–7, there was no truly scientific evaluation of blood transfusion before it was categorised as a 'prescription only medicine' and given a Product Licence of Right. There is a serious school of thought that, if the concept of donor to recipient transfer of blood was now being mooted for the first time and the proposed procedure was forced to submit to the same rigorous scientific tests as new pharmaceutical products coming on the market, then donor blood would be unlikely to pass these tests and would not be granted a Product Licence. One day, perhaps, those in authority may address that.

22.14 In the meantime, the technology, treatment modalities and pharmaceutical products exist to avoid donor blood and blood products in the management of a very wide range of cases—it is attitudes that need to change. And a proper assessment of expectations, endpoints and outcomes should be an integral part of that process. As previously mentioned in chapter 1:

> 'To put these changes into effect in the United Kingdom will require a cultural shift among clinicians, managers and policy makers. No longer should clinicians prefer the convenience and immediate benefits of allogeneic transfusion over more troublesome but safer alternatives…' [330]

---

[330] Making Blood Safer—stricter vigilance and fewer transfusions are the way forward, *BMJ* (Editorial) 2002; 325:400-1,

APPENDIX

EXTRACT FROM THE JUDGMENT OF THE EUROPEAN COURT OF HUMAN RIGHTS [331]

'(iii) Encouragement of suicide or the refusal of medical assistance

131. A further ground for banning the applicant community was the charge that it had encouraged its members to commit suicide and/or to refuse medical assistance in life-threatening situations.

132. The Court observes at the outset that the Russian courts did not elaborate on the allegations of encouragement of suicide or give examples of such incitement in the doctrine or practices of the applicant community or name any community member who had terminated his or her life or sought to do so. In so far as the domestic judgments can be understood to consider that the refusal of a blood transfusion is tantamount to suicide, in the Court's view, this analogy does not hold, for the situation of a patient seeking a hastening of death through discontinuation of treatment is different from that of patients who—like Jehovah's Witnesses—just make a choice of medical procedures but still wish to get well and do not exclude treatment altogether. As the charge of encouragement to suicide did not have any basis in fact, the Court's task will be confined to reviewing the second allegation, namely, that, at the instigation of the community, its members declined medical assistance by refusing the transfusion of blood or its components.

133. It is generally known that Jehovah's Witnesses believe that the Bible prohibits ingesting blood, which is sacred to God, and that this prohibition extends to transfusion of any blood or blood components that are not the patient's own. The religious prohibition permits of no exceptions and is applicable even in cases where a blood transfusion is deemed to be necessary in the best clinical judgment to avoid irreparable damage to the patient's health or even to save his or her life. Some Jehovah's Witnesses, including members of the applicant community, carry an advance medical directive—known in Russia as a 'No Blood' card (see paragraph 68 above)—stating that they refuse blood

[331] *Moscow Community of Jehovah's Witnesses v Russia* ECtHR No. 302/02

transfusions under any circumstances as a matter of religious belief. A few members of the applicant community who had been admitted to hospitals had firmly refused a blood transfusion against the advice of medical specialists who strongly recommended it. These elements had been correctly established by the domestic courts and were not contested by the applicants.

134. The Court recognises that the refusal of potentially life-saving medical treatment on religious grounds is a problem of considerable legal complexity, involving as it does a conflict between the State's interest in protecting the lives and health of its citizens and the individual's right to personal autonomy in the sphere of physical integrity and religious beliefs (see, mutatis mutandis, *Pretty v. the United Kingdom*, no. 2346/02, §62 et seq., ECHR 2002-III). The impugned provision of the Russian Religious Act was apparently designed to protect individuals from religious influence which could lead them to make choices that are considered irrational or unwise as a matter of public policy, such as the decision to refuse medical treatment that is generally regarded as beneficial. It was based on the assumption that the State's power to protect people from the harmful consequences of their chosen lifestyle ought to override the rights of believers to respect for their private life and to freedom to manifest their religion in practice and observance. That assumption made it unnecessary for the Russian courts to carry out a balancing exercise which would have allowed them to weigh considerations of public health and safety against the countervailing principle of personal autonomy and religious freedom (compare *Pretty*, cited above, §74). Accordingly, it falls to the Court to verify whether or not the balance has been upset.

135. The very essence of the Convention is respect for human dignity and human freedom and the notions of self-determination and personal autonomy are important principles underlying the interpretation of its guarantees (see *Pretty*, cited above, §§61 and 65). The ability to conduct one's life in a manner of one's own choosing includes the opportunity to pursue activities perceived to be of a physically harmful or dangerous nature for the individual concerned. In the sphere of medical assistance, even where the refusal to accept a particular treatment might lead to a fatal outcome, the imposition of medical treatment without the consent of

a mentally competent adult patient would interfere with his or her right to physical integrity and impinge on the rights protected under Article 8 of the Convention (see *Pretty,* cited above, §§62 and 63, and *Acmanne and Others v. Belgium*, no. 10435/83, Commission decision of 10 December 1984).

136. The freedom to accept or refuse specific medical treatment, or to select an alternative form of treatment, is vital to the principles of self-determination and personal autonomy. A competent adult patient is free to decide, for instance, whether or not to undergo surgery or treatment or, by the same token, to have a blood transfusion. However, for this freedom to be meaningful, patients must have the right to make choices that accord with their own views and values, regardless of how irrational, unwise or imprudent such choices may appear to others. Many established jurisdictions have examined the cases of Jehovah's Witnesses who had refused a blood transfusion and found that, although the public interest in preserving the life or health of a patient was undoubtedly legitimate and very strong, it had to yield to the patient's stronger interest in directing the course of his or her own life (see the judgments cited in paragraphs 85 to 88 above). It was emphasised that free choice and self-determination were themselves fundamental constituents of life and that, absent any indication of the need to protect third parties—for example, mandatory vaccination during an epidemic, the State must abstain from interfering with the individual freedom of choice in the sphere of health care, for such interference can only lessen and not enhance the value of life (see the *Malette v. Shulman* and *Fosmire v. Nicoleau* judgments, cited in paragraphs 85 and 87 above)...

142. In the light of the above considerations, the Court finds that the domestic courts did not convincingly show any 'pressing social need' or the existence of 'relevant and sufficient reasons' capable of justifying a restriction on the applicants' right to personal autonomy in the sphere of religious beliefs and physical integrity.[332]

[332] Cited with approval in the High Court—*W v M* [2011] EWHC 2443 (Fam) Baker J.

INDEX